Sedation and Analgesia in the ICU: Pharmacology, Protocolization, and Clinical Consequences

Guest Editors

PRATIK P. PANDHARIPANDE, MD, MSCI
E. WESLEY ELY, MD, MPH

ANESTHESIOLOGY CLINICS

www.anesthesiology.theclinics.com

Consulting Editor
LEE A. FLEISHER, MD, FACC

December 2011 • Volume 29 • Number 4

SAUNDERS an imprint of ELSEVIER, Inc.

W.B. SAUNDERS COMPANY
A Division of Elsevier Inc.

1600 John F. Kennedy Boulevard, Suite 1800 • Philadelphia, PA 19103-2899

http://www.theclinics.com

ANESTHESIOLOGY CLINICS Volume 29, Number 4
December 2011 ISSN 1932-2275, ISBN-13: 978-1-4557-3360-6

Editor: Rachel Glover

Anesthesiology Clinics (ISSN 1932-2275) is published quarterly by Elsevier Inc., 360 Park Avenue South, New York, NY 10010-1710. Months of issue are March, June, September, and December. Periodicals postage paid at New York, NY and at additional mailing offices. Subscription prices are $154.00 per year (US student/resident), $313.00 per year (US individuals), $383.00 per year (Canadian individuals), $496.00 per year (US institutions), $615.00 per year (Canadian institutions), $216.00 per year (Canadian and foreign student/resident), $434.00 per year (foreign individuals), and $615.00 per year (foreign institutions). To receive student and resident rate, orders must be accompanied by name of affiliated institution, date of term, and the *signature* of program/residency coordinator on institutions letterhead. Orders will be billed at individual rate until proof of status is received. Foreign air speed delivery is included in all *Clinics'* subscription prices. All prices are subject to change without notice. POSTMASTER: Send address changes to *Anesthesiology Clinics,* Elsevier Health Sciences Division, Subscription Customer Service, 3251 Riverport Lane, Maryland Heights, MO 63043. Customer Service (orders, claims, online, change of address): Elsevier Health Sciences Division, Subscription Customer Service, 3251 Riverport Lane, Maryland Heights, MO 63043. Tel:1-800-654-2452 (U.S. and Canada); 314-447-8871 (outside U.S. and Canada). Fax: 314-447-8029. E-mail: journalscustomerservice-usa@elsevier.com (for print support); journalsonlinesupport-usa@elsevier.com (for online support).

Reprints. For copies of 100 or more of articles in this publication, please contact the Commercial Reprints Department, Elsevier Inc., 360 Park Avenue South, New York, NY 10010-1710. Tel.: 212-633-3812; Fax: 212-462-1935; E-mail: reprints@elsevier.com.

Anesthesiology Clinics, is also published in Spanish by McGraw-Hill Inter-americana Editores S. A., P.O. Box 5-237, 06500 Mexico D. F., Mexico.

Anesthesiology Clinics, is covered in *MEDLINE/PubMed (Index Medicus), Current Contents/Clinical Medicine, Excerpta Medica, ISI/BIOMED*, and *Chemical Abstracts*.

Printed and bound by CPI Group (UK) Ltd, Croydon, CR0 4YY

Transferred to Digital Print 2011

Contributors

CONSULTING EDITOR

LEE A. FLEISHER, MD, FACC
Robert D. Dripps Professor and Chair of Anesthesiology and Critical Care, University
of Pennsylvania School of Medicine, Philadelphia, Pennsylvania

GUEST EDITORS

PRATIK P. PANDHARIPANDE, MD, MSCI
Associate Professor of Anesthesiology, Division of Critical Care, Department of
Anesthesiology, Vanderbilt University School of Medicine, Nashville, Tennessee

E. WESLEY ELY, MD, MPH
Associate Director of Research, Veterans Affairs Geriatric Research Education Clinical
Center; Professor of Medicine, Center for Health Services Research and Division of
Allergy/Pulmonary/Critical Care Medicine, Vanderbilt University School of Medicine,
Nashville, Tennessee

AUTHORS

FREDERICK E. BARR, MD, MSCI
Associate Professor of Pediatrics and Anesthesiology, Division Chief, Critical Care,
Department of Pediatrics, Vanderbilt University School of Medicine, Nashville, Tennessee

LISA BURRY, PharmD, FCCP
Clinical Pharmacy Specialist, Department of Pharmacy; Associate Scientist, Department
of Medicine, Mount Sinai Hospital, University of Toronto, Toronto, Ontario, Canada

JOSEPH F. DASTA, MSc, FCCM, FCCP
Professor Emeritus, The Ohio State University, College of Pharmacy, Columbus, Ohio;
Adjunct Professor, College of Pharmacy, University of Texas, Austin, Texas

JOHN W. DEVLIN, PharmD, FCCM, FCCP
Associate Professor, Northeastern University School of Pharmacy; Adjunct Associate
Professor, Tufts University School of Medicine, Boston, Massachusetts

E. WESLEY ELY, MD, MPH
Associate Director of Research, Veterans Affairs Geriatric Research Education Clinical
Center; Professor of Medicine, Center for Health Services Research and Division
of Allergy/Pulmonary/Critical Care Medicine, Vanderbilt University School of Medicine,
Nashville, Tennessee

GILLES L. FRASER, PharmD, FCCM
Professor of Medicine, Director of Critical Care Pharmacology, University of Vermont
College of Medicine, Burlington, Vermont; Departments of Medicine and Pharmacy,
Maine Medical Center, Portland, Maine

D. CATHERINE FUCHS, MD
Associate Professor of Psychiatry, Division Chief, Child Psychiatry, Department of Psychiatry, Vanderbilt University School of Medicine, Nashville, Tennessee

TIMOTHY D. GIRARD, MD, MSc
Instructor in Medicine, Division of Allergy, Pulmonary, and Critical Care Medicine, Department of Medicine, Center for Health Services Research, Vanderbilt University School of Medicine; Tennessee Valley Geriatric Research, Education and Clinical Center (GRECC), Department of Veterans Affairs Medical Center, Tennessee Valley Healthcare System, Nashville, Tennessee

MICHAEL H. HOOPER, MD
Fellow, Division of Allergy, Pulmonary, and Critical Care Medicine, Department of Medicine, Center for Health Services Research, Vanderbilt University School of Medicine, Nashville, Tennessee

RAMONA O. HOPKINS, PhD
Department of Psychology, Neuroscience Center, Brigham Young University, Provo; Division of Pulmonary and Critical Care, Department of Medicine, Intermountain Medical Center, Murray, Utah

TRACY HUSSELL, BSc, PhD
Professor, Department of Inflammatory Disease, National Heart & Lung Institute, Imperial College London, London, United Kingdom

JAMES C. JACKSON, PsyD
Center for Health Services Research, Vanderbilt University Medical Center, Vanderbilt University School of Medicine, Nashville, Tennessee

SANDRA KANE-GILL, PharmD, MSc, FCCM, FCCP
Associate Professor, School of Pharmacy, University of Pittsburgh, Pittsburgh, Pennsylvania

IAIN MCCULLAGH, MBChB, FRCA
International Fellow, Critical Care, Mount Sinai Hospital, University Health Network, Toronto, Ontario, Canada

MERVYN MAZE, MBChB, FRCP, FRCA, FMedSci
Professor and Head, Department of Surgery, Oncology, Reproductive Biology and Anaesthesia, Imperial College London, London, United Kingdom

SANGEETA MEHTA, MD, FRCPC
Research Director and Associate Professor, Medical Surgical Intensive Care Unit, Department of Medicine, Mount Sinai Hospital, University of Toronto, Toronto, Ontario, Canada

NATHANIEL MITCHELL
Center for Health Services Research, Vanderbilt University Medical Center, Vanderbilt University School of Medicine, Nashville, Tennessee

VIVEK MOITRA, MD
Assistant Professor, Department of Anesthesiology; Assistant Medical Director, Surgical Intensive Care Unit, College of Physicians and Surgeons of Columbia University, New York, New York

PRATIK P. PANDHARIPANDE, MD, MSCI
Associate Professor of Anesthesiology, Division of Critical Care, Department of Anesthesiology, Vanderbilt University School of Medicine, Nashville, Tennessee

OLIVER PANZER, MD
Assistant Professor, Department of Anesthesiology, College of Physicians and Surgeons of Columbia University, New York, New York

SAMMY PEDRAM, MD
Assistant Professor, Division of Pulmonary & Critical Care Medicine, Department of Internal Medicine, Virginia Commonwealth University Health System, Richmond, Virginia

RICHARD R. RIKER, MD, FCCM
Currently, Professor of Medicine, Tufts University School of Medicine, Boston, Massachusetts; Department of Medicine and Neurocritical Care, Neuroscience Institute, Maine Medical Center, Portland, Maine; Formerly, Clinical Associate Professor of Medicine, Director of Critical Care Research, University of Vermont College of Medicine, Burlington, Vermont

RUSSEL J. ROBERTS, PharmD
Critical Care Pharmacy Fellow, Northeastern University School of Pharmacy; Tufts Medical Center, Boston, Massachusetts

ROBERT D. SANDERS, BSc, MBBS, FRCA
Academic Clinical Fellow and Specialist Registrar, Magill, Department of Anaesthetics, Intensive Care and Pain Medicine, Imperial College London, Chelsea; Westminster Hospital, London, United Kingdom

CURTIS N. SESSLER, MD
Orhan Muren Professor of Medicine, Division of Pulmonary & Critical Care Medicine, Department of Internal Medicine, Virginia Commonwealth University Health System; Medical Director of Critical Care, Medical College of Virginia Hospitals, Richmond, Virginia

YOANNA SKROBIK, MD, FRCP(C)
Associate Professor, Department of Medicine (Critical Care), Université de Montreal; Staff Intensivist, Intensive Care Unit, Hôpital Maisonneuve Rosemont, Montreal, Quebec, Canada

ROBERT N. SLADEN, MRCP(UK), FRCP(C), FCCM
Chief, Division of Critical Care; Professor and Vice-Chair, Department of Anesthesiology; Medical Director, Cardiothoracic and Surgical Intensive Care Units, College of Physicians and Surgeons of Columbia University, New York, New York

HEIDI A.B. SMITH, MD, MSCI
Assistant Professor of Pediatrics and Anesthesiology, Division of Critical Care, Department of Pediatrics, Vanderbilt University School of Medicine, Nashville, Tennessee

PAULA L. WATSON, MD
Assistant Professor of Medicine, Department of Medicine, Vanderbilt University School of Medicine, Nashville, Tennessee

GERALD L. WEINHOUSE, MD
Assistant Professor of Medicine, Department of Medicine, Harvard Medical School, Boston, Massachusetts

Contents

Opioids, benzodiazepines, and propofol remain the mainstay by which to optimize patient comfort and facilitate mechanical ventilation in patients who are critically ill. Unfortunately none of these agents share all of the characteristics of the ideal sedative or analgesic agent: rapid onset, rapid recovery, a predictable dose response, a lack of drug accumulation, and no toxicity. To optimize care, critical care clinicians should be familiar with the many pharmacokinetic, pharmacodynamic, and pharmacogenetic variables that can affect the safety and efficacy of these sedatives and analgesics.

In this article, the authors discuss the pharmacology of sedative-analgesic agents like dexmedetomidine, remifentanil, ketamine, and volatile anesthetics. Dexmedetomidine is a highly selective alpha-2 agonist that provides anxiolysis and cooperative sedation without respiratory depression. It has organ protective effects against ischemic and hypoxic injury, including cardioprotection, neuroprotection, and renoprotection. Remifentanil is an ultra–short-acting opioid that acts as a mu-receptor agonist. Ketamine is a nonbarbiturate phencyclidine derivative and provides analgesia and apparent anesthesia with relative hemodynamic stability. Volatile anesthetics such as isoflurane, sevoflurane, and desflurane are in daily use in the operating room in the delivery of general anesthesia. A major advantage of these halogenated ethers is their quick onset, quick offset, and ease of titration in rendering the patient unconscious, immobile, and amnestic.

Patient outcomes are significantly influenced by the choice of sedative and analgesic agents, the presence of over- or undersedation, poor pain control, and delirium. Individualized sedation management using sedation assessment tools, sedation protocols, and daily sedative interruption can improve clinical outcomes. Despite the publication of randomized trials and numerous guidelines, the uptake of proven strategies into routine practice can be slow. Surveys of clinicians' self-reported practice and prospective practice audits characterize sedation and analgesia practices and provide directions for education and future research. The objective of this review is to present the findings of surveys and practice audits, evaluating the management of sedation and analgesia in mechanically ventilated adults in the intensive care unit, and to summarize international critical care sedation practices.

Administering sedative and analgesic medications is a cornerstone of optimizing patient comfort and minimizing distress, yet may lead to unintended consequences including delayed recovery from critical illness and slower liberation from mechanical ventilation. The use of structured approaches to sedation management, including guidelines, protocols, and algorithms can promote evidence-based care, reduce variation in clinical practice, and systematically reduce the likelihood of excessive and/or prolonged sedation. Patient-focused sedation algorithms are multidisciplinary, including physician, nurse, and pharmacist development and implementation. Key components of sedation algorithms include identification of goals and specific targets, use of valid and reliable tools to assess analgesia, agitation, and sedation, and incorporation of logical medication selection. Sedation protocols generally focus on a) algorithms that incorporate treating sedation and analgesia based upon escalation, de-escalation, or changing medications according to specific targets, or b) daily interruption of sedative and opioid analgesic infusions. Many published sedation protocols have been tested in controlled clinical trials, often demonstrating benefits such as shorter duration of mechanical ventilation, reduced ICU length of stay, and/or superior sedation management compared to usual care. Implementation of sedation algorithms in ICUs is a challenging process for which sufficient resources must be allocated.

Liberation from mechanical ventilation is a vital treatment goal in the management of critically ill patients. The duration of mechanical ventilation is affected by strategies for ventilator weaning and sedation. The authors review literature on weaning from mechanical ventilation and delivery of sedation in critically ill patients, including current guidelines recommending the use of spontaneous breathing trials and spontaneous awakening trials. Implementation of these strategies in a wake-up-and-breathe protocol has demonstrated benefit over the use of spontaneous breathing trials alone.

Providing sedation and comfort for intensive care patients has evolved in the last few years. New approaches to improving outcomes for intensive care unit (ICU) patients include providing analgesia before adding sedation and recognizing dangerous adverse effects associated with sedative medications, such as prolonged effects of midazolam, propylene glycol toxicity with lorazepam, propofol infusion syndrome, the deliriogenic effects of benzodiazepines and propofol, and bradycardia with dexmedetomidine. There are now reliable and valid ways to monitor pain and delirium in ICU patients. Dexmedetomidine reduces the incidence of delirium, reduces the duration of mechanical ventilation, and appears to be cost effective.

The need for compassionate care of the critically ill often compels clinicians to treat these patients with pharmacologic sedation. Although patients may appear to be asleep under the influence of these sedating medications, the relationship between sleep and sedation is complex and not fully understood. These medications exert their effects at different points along the central nervous system's natural sleep pathway, leading to similarities and differences between the two states. This relationship is important because critically ill patients sleep poorly and this phenomenon has been linked to poor intensive care unit outcomes. Therefore, greater awareness of the effects of these medications on sleep may lead to sedation protocols that further improve outcomes. This article reviews the relationship between sedation and sleep from physiologic and clinical perspectives.

The management of critically ill patients necessitates the use of sedatives and analgesics to provide patient comfort and cooperation. These drugs exert profound effects on all organ systems, not only the central nervous system, and this article describes the immunologic effects of the commonly used critical care sedatives: propofol, the benzodiazepines, opioids, and α2-adrenoceptor agonists. Benzodiazepines, opioids, and possibly even propofol worsen outcomes in animal models of infection, whereas preliminary evidence suggests that the α2-adrenoceptor agonist, dexmedetomidine, may improve outcomes in the setting of infection. Given the burden of sepsis and secondary infections in critical care, choice of sedation may need to be carefully considered to preserve immune responses in critically ill patients.

Despite considerable information on the pharmacotherapy of sedation in the ICU, there is little published on the pharmacoeconomics of sedation in patients who are critically ill. The purpose of this article is to discuss the various components that contribute to the cost of treating the agitated ICU patient and to critically review the articles published since 2000 that evaluated costs and cost-effectiveness in ICU patients receiving drugs for agitation and/or pain. Clinicians should look beyond the acquisition cost of a sedative and include the effect of sedatives on the cost of care when selecting the most appropriate sedative.

VISIT US ONLINE!
Access your subscription at:
www.theclinics.com

Foreword

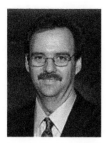

Lee A. Fleisher, MD
Consulting Editor

As perioperative physicians, we are involved with sedation and analgesia in places outside of the operating room. This includes the intensive care unit (ICU), where some of our colleagues actually oversee care. The importance of sedation and analgesia practices in the ICU has increased in recent years as it has become clear that they can influence outcome. It is for this reason that we are publishing this important series of articles, which was also published in *Critical Care Clinics*.

As guest editors for this issue, we are fortunate to have Pratik Pandharipande, MD, MSCI and E. Wesley Ely, MD, MPH. Pratik Pandharipande, MD, MSCI is Associate Professor in the Department of Anesthesiology in the Division of Critical Care and Perioperative Medicine at Vanderbilt University School of Medicine, Nashville, Tennessee. Dr Pandharipande's clinical focus is divided between OR anesthesia and ICU consultancy in the Surgical and Neurological ICU at Vanderbilt University Medical Center. He has published over 45 articles on critical care topics. Dr E. Wesley Ely, MD, MPH is a Professor of Medicine at Vanderbilt University School of Medicine with a subspecialty in Pulmonary and Critical Care Medicine. Dr Ely's research has focused on improving the care and outcomes of critically ill patients with severe sepsis and respiratory failure, with a special emphasis on the problems facing older patients in the ICU. Dr Ely has written or coauthored more than 150 articles, book chapters, and editorials.

Their unique background and experience make them the ideal team to assemble an issue of *Anesthesiology Clinics* on this important topic.

Lee A. Fleisher, MD
University of Pennsylvania School of Medicine
3400 Spruce Street, Dulles 680
Philadelphia, PA 19104, USA

E-mail address:
lee.fleisher@uphs.upenn.edu

Anesthesiology Clin 29 (2011) xiii
doi:10.1016/j.anclin.2011.10.002
1932-2275/11/$ – see front matter © 2011 Elsevier Inc. All rights reserved.

anesthesiology.theclinics.com

Preface

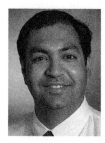 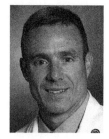

Pratik P. Pandharipande, MD, MSCI   E. Wesley Ely, MD, MPH
Guest Editors

Anyone who has been privileged enough to care for the critically ill over the past 15 years can speak of the rapid evolution of many facets of ICU medicine. Few areas have shifted more than the area of sedation and mechanical ventilation. These inextricably linked components of critical care represent the cornerstones of what we do for patients during their vulnerable course in the ICU. In a nutshell, we have progressed from a culture that embraced nearly universal deep sedation for days on end, with harsh methods of blowing too much air into patients' lungs, to a "kinder and gentler" approach that involves keeping patients much more awake and interactive while delivering much less injurious and smaller puffs of air. Although data from sepsis studies indicate, without a doubt, that early delivery of resuscitation, antibiotics, and other forms of interdisciplinary care are paramount during the first 24 hours to 48 hours of ICU care, a pivotal concept that captures what has changed about sedation and mechanical ventilation is that the timing of their removal (formerly referred to as "weaning," but this term describes a process that is too slow for many patients) turns out to have a very large influence on improving length of stay, cost of care, and complication rates. In short, for sedation and mechanical ventilation, less is more.

Landmark cohort investigations and an emerging body of clinical trials in the last decade have made us acutely aware that patients' brains in the ICU are vulnerable to acute and long-lasting injury that we used to pay very little attention to over the course of diseases such as sepsis and ARDS. Our patients' brains manifest the acute injury as delirium, now thought of as a key feature of the multiple organ dysfunction syndrome. That acute delirium likely represents neuronal injury that, in time, often evolves into a longer-term cognitive impairment, functionally resembling a form of dementia with executive dysfunction and memory deficits. Our role as health care professionals, of course, is to minimize this injury and to reduce any iatrogenic components that are modifiable. These goals have led us to generate this issue of the *Clinics*.

A version of this article appeared in the 25:3 issue of *Critical Care Clinics*.

Anesthesiology Clin 29 (2011) xv–xvi
doi:10.1016/j.anclin.2011.10.001
1932-2275/11/$ – see front matter © 2011 Elsevier Inc. All rights reserved.

anesthesiology.theclinics.com

Routinely administered sedative and analgesic medications, though important for the relief of pain and anxiety, significantly influence patient outcomes independent of comorbidities and severity of illness. The realization that these medications may contribute to both acute and long-term cognitive impairment, and possibly adversely affect quality of life, further attest to the fact that sedation paradigms must continue to evolve through the rigor of science, rather than opinion, in order to optimize recovery for our sickest patients.

This state-of-the-art issue, with contributions from many world-renowned experts in the field of sedation/analgesia and outcomes research, will provide the reader with a comprehensive review of the latest literature that guide quality improvement projects to provide improved safety in all ICUs. This issue of the *Clinics* covers the basic pharmacology of available sedative and analgesic medications, including the role of inhalational anesthetics in critically ill patients, followed by articles identifying the importance of target-based and protocolized sedation, as well as the role of daily spontaneous awakening trials (SATs) and spontaneous breathing trials (SBTs). The articles cover, in detail, conventional agents such as benzodiazepines and propofol, while at the same time detail the use of alternatives such as remifentanil and dexmedetomidine. Because of the importance of the brain as an organ dysfunction and its independent role in survival and long-term functional outcomes, we have included two articles on the assessment and management of this new frontier in critical care. This issue also offers the pediatric ICU specialist a fresh outlook on the evaluation of delirium in children. Other special topics in this issue include the pharmoeconomics of sedation, and the role of sedative and analgesic medications in sleep disturbance, long-term cognitive impairment, and immunomodulation.

We hope that you, as the readers of the *Anesthesiology Clinics*, will find our articles informative and use the information learned to enhance the care of your critically ill patients around the world.

Pratik P. Pandharipande, MD, MSCI
Division of Critical Care
Department of Anesthesiology
Vanderbilt University School of Medicine
Nashville, TN 37232, USA

E. Wesley Ely, MD, MPH
Veterans Affairs Geriatric Research Education Clinical Center (VA-GRECC)
Center for Health Services Research
Division of Allergy/Pulmonary/Critical Care Medicine
Vanderbilt University School of Medicine
Nashville, TN 37232, USA

E-mail addresses:
pratik.pandharipande@vanderbilt.edu (P.P. Pandharipande)
wes.ely@vanderbilt.edu (E.W. Ely)

Pharmacology of Commonly Used Analgesics and Sedatives in the ICU: Benzodiazepines, Propofol, and Opioids

John W. Devlin, PharmD, FCCM, FCCP[a,b,*], Russel J. Roberts, PharmD[a,b]

KEYWORDS

- Sedation • Analgesia • Critical care • Midazolam
- Lorazepam • Propofol • Opioids • Fentanyl

Patients who are critically ill and on mechanical ventilation frequently require sedation and analgesic therapy to optimize patient comfort, facilitate patient-ventilator synchrony, and optimize oxygenation.[1] Despite the 2002 Society of Critical Care Medicine (SCCM) pain and sedation guideline recommendations that sedation and analgesic therapy be titrated to maintain patients in a pain-free and slightly sleepy state, recent data suggests that these endpoints are frequently not obtained.[2–5] For example, one large observational study of sedation practices in 44 French ICUs found that 57% of patients on day 2 and 41% on day 6 were found to be deeply sedated (ie, sedation agitation score $\leq$2).[3] The etiology of oversedation in the ICU is complex and has many drug and nondrug causes.[1] Clinicians in the ICU are often slow to incorporate into practice sedation strategies that have been shown to reduce the duration of mechanical ventilation, such as protocolization and daily interruption of sedative administration.[6–8] Even more important is the failure by clinicians to consider the numerous pharmacokinetic, pharmacodynamic, and pharmacogenetic factors that influence analgesic and sedative response, recovery, and safety in patients who are critically ill.

Although newer sedatives and analgesics such as dexmedetomidine and remifentanil have been the focus of many recent studies and are discussed in other articles

A version of this article appeared in the 25:3 issue of *Critical Care Clinics*.

[a] Northeastern University School of Pharmacy, MU206, 360 Huntington Avenue, Boston, MA 02115, USA

[b] Tufts Medical Center, 800 Washington Street, Boston, MA 02111, USA

* Corresponding author.

E-mail address: j.devlin@neu.edu

Anesthesiology Clin 29 (2011) 567–585

doi:10.1016/j.anclin.2011.09.001
anesthesiology.theclinics.com

in this issue of the *Clinics*, at most centers analgesics and sedatives such as fentanyl, midazolam, lorazepam, and propofol remain the mainstay by which patient comfort is optimized.[9–11] Over the past few years the understanding of the factors that affect the efficacy and safety of these sedatives and analgesics has changed substantially.[1,12] The limited number of methodologically sound clinical trials that have evaluated the use of these agents in the ICU, coupled with the ever-changing dynamics of critical illnesses, requires clinicians to have a thorough knowledge regarding analgesic and sedative pharmacology to optimize patient outcome. The objective of this article is therefore to review the pharmacology of commonly used analgesic and sedative agents including the opioids, benzodiazepines, and propofol. Specifically, this article focuses on the important pharmacokinetic, pharmacodynamic, and pharmacogenetic factors that clinicians should consider when developing an analgesic and sedation regimen that optimizes patient outcomes, reduces oversedation, and prevents medication-related adverse events.

PHARMACOLOGIC PRINCIPLES GUIDING THE USE OF ANALGESICS AND SEDATIVES IN THE CRITICALLY ILL

Several important pharmacologic principles are crucial when formulating an analgesic and sedative regimen in patients who are critically ill. The two pharmacokinetic parameters that will affect the drug response and safety most are volume of distribution (Vd) and clearance. Vd describes the relationship between the amount of drug in the body and the concentration in the plasma after absorption and distribution are completed. Vd is affected by body size, tissue binding, plasma protein binding, regional blood flow, and various physiochemical properties of the drug. Agents that are hydrophilic (ie, do not penetrate the fat well) remain within the plasma (eg, morphine) and have a low Vd (0.5 L/kg), whereas drugs that are lipophilic and sequestered outside the circulation (eg, midazolam) have a much higher Vd.[13,14]

With hepatic dysfunction present in more than half of patients who are critically ill, drug clearance may be reduced because of decreased hepatic drug flow, decreased hepatocellular enzyme activity, and decreased bile flow.[15,16] With shock resulting in a threefold decrease in liver blood flow, the clearance of medications that rely on flow-dependent hepatic clearance (eg, morphine) is reduced. Critical illness may compromise the cytochrome P-450 (CYP450) enzyme system, the primary metabolic pathway for midazolam, fentanyl, and methadone, by decreasing hepatic drug flow, intracellular oxygen tension, and cofactor availability.[16]

Much of the currently available pharmacokinetic data for the benzodiazepines and opioids are derived from single-dose studies completed in healthy volunteers.[16,17] Single-dose studies fail to predict the pharmacokinetic parameters that are seen after long-term infusions of these agents because of the multicompartment behavior of the parent drug and its metabolites.[17] Results of studies completed in healthy volunteers cannot be extrapolated to patients who are critically ill because the alterations in volume status, plasma protein binding, and end-organ function that occur in this population will affect drug bioavailability, volume of distribution, and clearance.[16]

The pharmacodynamic response describes the relationship between drug concentration in both the serum and at the site of action and the observed clinical response. Determining pharmacodynamic response with analgesics and sedatives in patients who are critically ill is challenging given the large Vd of most agents, the difficulty in estimating drug concentrations at the receptor site, and the lack of objective measures of pain and sedation.[13] Many of the genes that encode the proteins dictating drug metabolism, transport, and pharmacodynamic action display genetic polymorphism.[18] This genetic variability may account for up to half of the variability in drug response that is observed in practice and has been shown to affect the metabolism of fentanyl, methadone, and midazolam.[19–22]

ANALGESICS

Opioid analgesic medications remain the mainstay of therapy for alleviating pain in the ICU patient.[1,2] This class of agents is also frequently used because of its sedative properties and to facilitate mechanical ventilation given its potent respiratory depressant effects. Neither acetaminophen nor the nonsteroidal antiinflammatory agents are discussed in this article given their weak analgesic activity and their propensity to cause adverse effects in patients who are critically ill.[2]

Opioids

Pharmacology

Morphine, fentanyl, and hydromorphone are the opioids that are most frequently used in the ICU.[10,11] Opioids elicit their action through stimulation of the μ-, κ-, and δ-opioid receptors, which are widely distributed within the central nervous system and throughout the peripheral tissues.[23] The μ-receptor is the primary site of opioid activity and is subdivided into the μ_1- and μ_2-subreceptors. Stimulation of the μ_1-subreceptor leads to inhibition of neuronal pain, thus altering the perception and response to pain (**Table 1**). Opioids are divided into three primary classes based on chemical structure: (1) Morphine-like agents that include morphine and hydromorphone; (2) Meperidine-like agents that include meperidine, fentanyl, and remifentanil; and (3) Diphenylheptanes that include methadone.[23] Remifentanil is reviewed elsewhere. The use of meperidine should generally be avoided in the ICU given its low potency, its propensity to cause nausea and vomiting, the fact that its use is contraindicated in patients receiving monoamine oxidase inhibitors or serotonin reuptake inhibitors, and the risk for the accumulation of its active metabolite, normeperidine, in patients with renal insufficiency.[2] Normeperidine accumulation is associated with neuroexcitatory effects including tremor, delirium, and seizures.[24] Methadone has N-methyl-D-aspartate (NMDA) receptor antagonistic effects that may be useful in the treatment of neuropathic and opioid-tolerant states.[25,26]

Pharmacokinetics

Most of the currently available pharmacokinetic information regarding opioids is from single-dose studies conducted in either healthy volunteers or patients with chronic diseases.[27] A paucity of data therefore exists surrounding the use of continuously infused opioids in patients who are critically ill—a population with numerous factors that could affect opioid distribution and clearance.[28] The intravenous route of administration is preferred in patients who are critically ill given the fact that it facilitates a faster onset of activity, provides a high bioavailability, and affords better dose titratability. The oral, transdermal, and intramuscular routes of administration are generally not recommended in patients who are hemodynamically unstable given the decreases in drug absorption that will occur in low-perfusion states.[2] Fentanyl patches should be avoided for acute analgesia because the time to reach peak effect is delayed by up to 24 hours after patch application and a prolonged drug effect is seen after patch removal.[2]

The high lipophilicity of fentanyl provides it with a faster onset of activity via the intravenous route (almost immediate) than either morphine or hydromorphone (5–10 minutes for both). However, this high lipophilicity can lead to a prolonged duration of effect after repeated dosing or infusion.[1] The Vd of hydromorphone is similar to

Table 1
Pharmacology of selected analgesics[1,2,23,27,32,97]

Drug	Mechanism of Action	Time to Onset (min)	Half-Life (h)	Lipophilicity	Primary Metabolic Pathway	Presence of Active Metabolites	Pharmacogenetic Implications
Fentanyl	μ-receptor agonist	<1	2–4	+++	N-dealkylation CYP3A4/5 Substrate	Yes	Yes
Hydromorphone	μ-receptor agonist	5–10	2–3	++	Glucuronidation	No	No
Morphine	μ-receptor agonist Weak δ-, κ-receptor agonist	5–10	3–4	+	Glucuronidation	Yes	Yes
Methadone	μ-receptor agonist Weak NMDA receptor antagonist	Oral: 30 IV: 10–20	9–59	+++	N-demethylation CYP3A4/5, 2D6, 2B6, 1A2 Substrate	No	Yes
Meperidine	Weak μ-, κ-receptor agonist	5	3–4	+++	N-demethylation and hydroxylation CYP3A4/2B6 Substrate	Yes	No

that of morphine. Methadone is a unique long-acting synthetic opioid that can be used to treat chronic pain syndromes when patients experience tolerance with other opioids and may help facilitate the down-titration of opioid infusions in the ICU.[22,29] Oral methadone, when administered in the acute care setting, has an onset of action of 30 minutes, reaches a peak effect in 2 to 4 hours, and has a duration of analgesia ranging from 3 to 12 hours—a period far shorter than its half-life.[30]

Following metabolism in the liver, opioid metabolites are excreted via the kidneys.[23] Morphine undergoes glucuronidation producing both a 6-glucuronide and 3-glucuronide metabolite. Morphine-6-glucuronide has significant analgesic activity and may accumulate in patients with decreased renal function.[23] Fentanyl does not have an active metabolite but the parent compound may accumulate in patients with renal insufficiency and thus should be avoided in end-stage renal disease.[31] Hydromorphone has a half-life of 2 to 3 hours and also undergoes glucuronidation similar to morphine. However, the hydromorphone-3-glucuronide metabolite that is produced is inactive, making hydromorphone the opioid of choice for use in patients with end-stage renal disease.[2]

Both fentanyl and morphine are high hepatic extraction ratio drugs; therefore, clearance may be reduced in patients with decreased hepatic blood flow (eg, shock).[27] During the first 3 to 5 days of methadone therapy, a more frequent dosing regimen (eg, every 6–8 hours) may be required secondary to its highly variable elimination half-life, and it may require more aggressive dosing (eg, every 6–8 hours).[32] Drug interactions are possible with both fentanyl and methadone given that each are primarily metabolized by the CYP450 enzyme system. Fentanyl is a substrate CYP3A4 and is affected by CYP3A4 inhibitors (eg, fluconazole) and inducers (eg, phenytoin). Methadone is a substrate of CYP3A4, CYP2D6, and CYP2B6 and therefore is affected by the many inhibitors and inducers associated with these CYP450 isoenzymes.[23]

Pharmacodynamics

A predictable relationship between opioid blood concentrations and analgesic and respiratory depressant effects has not been established.[2,33–35] This is surprising given the increasing evidence that analgesia-based sedation regimens may be as effective as conventional hypnotic-based sedation care.[36,37] Given this lack of pharmacodynamic data, clinicians in the ICU should therefore titrate opioid therapy using a validated pain assessment tool (either verbal or nonverbal) or other physiologic endpoints (eg, heart rate, blood pressure, or respiratory rate).[2]

Dosing and costs for selected opioid analgesics are found in **Table 2**. It is important to note that the maximum dose of an opioid that should be used in the ICU is only limited by the presence of adverse effects.[32] Scheduled intermittent dosing is recommended rather than a continuous infusion to avoid drug accumulation. Patients who may require additional opioid therapy while receiving an opioid infusion should initially receive additional intravenous bolus doses rather than an increase in the infusion rate given the prolonged time it will take to reach a new steady concentration with any increase in the infusion dose. Use of a protocol incorporating daily awakening has been shown to decrease the amount of opioid administered and to shorten both duration of mechanical ventilation and stay in the ICU.[6] When converting from one opioid to another, or switching from the parenteral to oral route of administration, it is important to note that traditional opioid conversion charts are based on studies conducted in healthy volunteers after receiving a single dose of opioid therapy via the intramuscular route and are not reflective of the dosing requirements with continuous intravenous infusions.[38]

Table 2
Dosing and cost of selected analgesics and sedatives[1,2,13,27,32,99]

Drug	Comparative Dose (IV)[a]	Intermittent Dose[e]	Usual Infusion Dose	Cost per Day per 70 kg Patient[f]
Analgesics[b]				
Fentanyl	100–200 mg	0.35–.5 mcg/kg q 0.5–1 h	0.7–10 mcg/kg/h	100 mcg/h: $9.00–23.00
Hydromorphone	1.5 mg	10–30 mcg/kg q 1–2 h	7–15 mcg/kg/h	0.75 mg/h: $9.00–15.50
Morphine	10 mg	0.01–0.15 mg/kg q 1–2 h	0.07–0.5 mg/kg/h	5 mg/h: $5.75–17.75
Methadone	10–20 mg (po)	10–40 mg po q6–12 h	Not recommended	10 mg tid: $0.15–1.00
Meperidine	75–100 mg	Not recommended	Not recommended	—
Sedatives[c,d]				
Diazepam	—	0.03–0.1 mg/kg q 0.5–6 h	—	20 mg q4 h: $4.00–37.00
Lorazepam	0.035 mg/kg/hr	0.02–0.06 mg/kg q 2–6 h	0.01–0.1 mg/kg/h	4 mg/h: $44.00–122.00
Midazolam	0.106 mg/kg/hr	0.02–0.08 mg/kg q 0.5–2 h	0.04–0.2 mg/kg/h	6 mg/h: $51.00–180.00
Propofol	1.66 mg/kg/hr	—	5–80 mcg/kg/min	50 mcg/kg/min: $60.00–262.00

[a] With the exception of methadone, dose equivalents for analgesics and sedatives are based on the intravenous form.
[b] Based on usual accepted opiate conversions derived from single-dose study designs using intramuscular administration.
[c] Comparative doses among sedatives are based on pharmacoeconomic modeling in critically ill patients receiving continuous sedation for 24–72 hours.
[d] Sedative conversions are highly variable and dependent of duration of continuous sedation and numerous pharmacokinetic parameters.
[e] Mechanically ventilated patients may require more frequent dosing to control pain.
[f] Cost based on 2008 average wholesale price from all available manufacturers.

Tolerance, a decrease in a drug's effect over time despite constant plasma concentrations, is a characteristic of all opioid analgesics. Tolerance occurs most frequently when opioids are continuously infused.[39,40] While tolerance likely accounts for substantial dosing increases that are required in the ICU, it is hard to characterize given that opioid dosing requirements may be elevated secondary to increased pain or numerous different pharmacokinetic factors. The changes that occur at the opioid receptor site over time that lead to tolerance may be related in part to genetic adaption that affects receptor transcription.[39] Synthetic opioids (eg, fentanyl) may result in a greater degree of tolerance than nonsynthetic opioids (eg, morphine) given their increased affinity at the opioid receptor.[40,41] Clinicians should consider the use of alternate opioid agents of a different class in those situations where opioid dosing requirements are escalating and adverse effects are observed. Given the role of NMDA receptor system in nociception and the development of tolerance, antagonism of central NMDA receptors through the use of methadone is another strategy that may slow the development of tolerance.[39,40]

Exposure to more than one week of high-dose opioid therapy may lead to the development of neuroadaptation or physiologic dependence in patients who are critically ill.[2] In this situation, rapid discontinuation of opioid therapy, particularly if a short half-life opioid like fentanyl has been used, may lead to withdrawal symptoms that include agitation, hypertension, tachypnea, and sweating. These symptoms may mimic other problems encountered in patients who are critically ill such as delirium. Opioid infusion rates should generally not be decreased by more than 25% each day. Use of methadone may decrease the occurrence of withdrawal effects.[2,29,42]

Pharmacogenetics

Genetic factors have been shown to regulate both opioid pharmacokinetics (ie, metabolizing enzymes and transporters) and pharmacodynamics (ie, target receptor sites and signal transduction elements) and could be a major contributor to the inter-patient variability in response that is observed in clinical practice.[19] More than 100 variants in the μ-opioid receptor gene OPRM1 have been identified of which 20 have a prevalence >1%. The most common single-nucleotide polymorphism of the μ-opioid receptor gene is A118G.[19] It has been associated with greater dose requirements for patients receiving morphine and methadone.[19–21]

The most highly polymorphic CYP450 gene is the CYP2D6 gene, which has been studied extensively and has been found to have large interethnic variations.[21] For example, patients with the CYP2D6 poor metabolizer phenotype are unable to metabolize codeine into its more potent morphine metabolite.[20] Genetic variability in the CYP2D6 gene has been reported to account for some of the interindividual variability associated with methadone.[19] One study found treatment success to be lesser in patients who were ultrarapid metabolizers than in those who were poor metabolizers.[43] Methadone concentrations are increased twofold in patients carrying the CYP2B6*6-variant allele and the risk for corrected QT (QTc) interval prolongation is greater in patients with the CYP2B6 slow metabolizer phenotype.[44,45] Fentanyl clearance may be lower in Caucasians than in non-Caucasians given that CYP3A5, one of its primary metabolic pathways, is highly expressed in only 30% of Caucasians.

Glucuronidation of morphine into its metabolites is catalyzed by the UDP-glucuronosyltransferase (UGT) enzyme, UGT2B7. Allelic variations of this enzyme have been associated with variability in hepatic clearance.[46] P-glycoprotein (P-gp), encoded at the MDR gene, is an efflux pump that is capable of pumping opioids out of the cell and therefore it affects both opioid absorption and elimination. Of the opioids discussed in this article, fentanyl, methadone, and morphine have all been confirmed as P-gp substrates and therefore may have their activity affected by genetic polymorphisms at the MDR1 gene.[19,21]

Safety

Adverse effects related to opioid therapy occur commonly in the ICU.[12,32,47] Opioid-induced respiratory depression is generally dose-related and is most deleterious for the patient in the ICU who is not intubated. Although opioids can cause nausea and vomiting because of their stimulatory effect at the chemoreceptor trigger zone, this is infrequent in the recumbent patient in the ICU. Fentanyl when administered at high doses may cause muscle rigidity. Opioid-induced hypotension occurs most commonly in patients who are hemodynamically unstable, are volume depleted, or have a high sympathetic tone. Compared with fentanyl and hydromorphone, morphine is associated with histamine release and so produces more hypotension, urticaria, pruritus, flushing, and bronchospasm. A synthetic opioid like fentanyl can safely be used in patients with a suspected allergy to morphine.

Excessive sedation from opioids is most often seen with the use of continuous infusions, particularly in patients with end-stage renal disease who are administered fentanyl or morphine. Methadone may cause excessive sedation if the dose is not titrated downwards after the first 5 days of starting therapy or if a CYP3A4 or CYP2D6 inhibitor is concomitantly administered. QTc-interval prolongation can occur with methadone because of its effects on the hERG channel, particularly if the chlorbutanol-containing intravenous formulation is used. Opioids may cause hallucinations, agitation, euphoria, and sleep disturbances and have been associated with the development of delirium.[48] Of the opioids, methadone may be the least deliriogenic because of its antagonistic activity at the NMDA receptor.[49,50] The effects of opioids on intracranial pressure in patients with traumatic brain injury remain unclear.[51]

Gastric retention and ileus are common in patients who are critically ill and receiving opioids, with prokinetic therapy and/or post-pyloric access required in patients prescribed enteral nutrition.[1] Prophylactic use of a stimulant laxative will reduce the incidence of constipation. Methylnaltrexone, an opioid antagonist specific to peripheral receptors, may have a role in treating opioid-induced constipation that fails to respond to laxative therapy.[52] Opioid-induced urinary retention is rarely a problem for patients in the ICU given the widespread use of urinary catheters.

SEDATIVES
Benzodiazepines

Benzodiazepines (eg, diazepam, lorazepam, midazolam) remain the most commonly administered class of sedatives for patients in the ICU given their potent anxiolytic, sedative, and hypnotic effects (**Table 3**). These observed pharmacologic effects depend on the degree to which the benzodiazepine binds to the GABA receptor, with 20% binding associated with anxiolysis, 30%–50% with sedation, and 60% with hypnosis.[53] Although benzodiazepines induce anterograde amnesia, they do not cause retrograde amnesia. They have an opioid-sparing effect by their ability to modulate the anticipatory pain response.[54] Benzodiazepines also have respiratory depressant effects, particularly when administered with an opioid.

Pharmacokinetics
Differences in the clinical response to benzodiazepines are related to both pharmacokinetic and pharmacodynamic factors and are most pronounced when these agents are administered as continuous infusions to patients who are critically ill.[55] Midazolam is a short-acting, water-soluble benzodiazepine that undergoes extensive oxidation in the liver via the CYP450 enzyme system to form water-soluble hydroxylated metabolites, which are excreted in the urine.[17] The primary metabolite of midazolam, 1-hydroxymidazolam glucuronide, has central nervous system (CNS) depressant effects and may accumulate in the patient who is critically ill, especially if kidney failure is present. In one series of patients on prolonged sedation >36 hours after cessation of a midazolam infusion, elevated levels of 1-hydroxymidazolam glucuronide were detected an average of 67 hours after the midazolam infusion was discontinued.[56] Prolonged sedative effects with midazolam have also been observed in patients who are obese or have reduced serum albumin levels.[17] Medications that interfere with CYP3A4 such as erythromycin, intraconazole, and diltiazem inhibit midazolam metabolism. Lorazepam is metabolized by hepatic glucuronidation to inactive metabolites that are cleared by the kidneys. In patients with liver failure, the metabolism of midazolam is more likely to be compromised than the metabolism of lorazepam.[2]

Although the greater lipid solubility of midazolam compared with lorazepam will result in a faster onset of action after a single intravenous bolus dose, it is also associated with a greater likelihood to result in a prolonged sedative effect when it is administered for a prolonged period.[57,58] Patients who are obese are at particularly

Table 3
Pharmacology of selected sedatives[1,2,13,17,27,98]

Drug	Mechanism of Action	Time to Onset (min)	Half-Life (h)	Lipophilicity	Primary Metabolic Pathway	Presence of Active Metabolites	Pharmacogenetic Implications
Diazepam	GABA$_a$/BZ receptor agonist	2–5	20–50	+++	N-desmethylation and hydroxylation (CYP3A4, 2C19 substrate)	Yes	Yes
Lorazepam	GABA$_a$/BZ receptor agonist	5–20	10–20	++	Glucuronidation	No	Yes
Midazolam	GABA$_a$/BZ receptor agonist	2–5	3–12	+++	Hydroxylation (CYP3A4/5 substrate)	Yes	Yes
Propofol	GABA$_a$ receptor agonist	1–2	1.5–12.4	+++	Hydroxylation and glucuronidation (CYP2B6 substrate)	No	Yes

high risk for these effects.[17] These differences lead to recommendations in the 2002 Society of Critical Care Medicine (SCCM) consensus guidelines that midazolam be used only for short-term (<48 hr) therapy and that lorazepam be used for patients in the ICU requiring long-term sedation.[2] Though earlier randomized controlled trials have compared lorazepam with midazolam for long-term sedation and found no difference in the time to awakening between the groups, it should be noted that few of the patients in these comparative studies had renal, hepatic, or neurologic impairment at baseline.[59,60]

Pharmacodynamics
The clinical effects of sedatives are usually measured in terms of time to effect, the ability to maintain sedation within a targeted range, the time to awaken, and the duration of mechanical ventilation. A limited number of studies have compared one or more of these outcomes to benzodiazepine serum drug concentrations.[55,61] A recent study that compared clinical sedation scores with sedative exposure found only a moderate level of agreement to exist between the Richmond agitation sedation score and either the dose of lorazepam administered or the lorazepam plasma drug concentrations achieved.[55] Another study of patients in the ICU that evaluated the pharmacodynamic response of lorazepam and midazolam after long-term continuous infusions concluded that variability in the sedative response to each agent that is observed in practice is an important reason for the oversedation that frequently occurs with the use of this class of agents.[61]

Benzodiazepine dosing requirements are generally lesser in the elderly, given the greater Vd and reduced clearance seen in this population. Older patients require lesser benzodiazepine plasma concentrations to achieve levels of sedation comparable to those in younger patients.[60] Patient-related factors that affect the benzodiazepine pharmacodynamic response are numerous and include age, concurrent pathology, prior alcohol use, and concurrent therapy with other sedative drugs.[2] Benzodiazepine therapy should be initiated using a series of intravenous loading doses. Infusions should only be initiated when scheduled intermittent intravenous dosing does not reach the desired clinical end-point given the association between a prolonged duration of mechanical ventilation and the use of continuous infusions.[62] Interruption of benzodiazepine sedation on a daily basis has been shown to shorten duration of mechanical ventilation without compromising the safety of the patient.[6]

There is emerging evidence that delirium in the ICU is related to the administration of anxiolytic drugs, particularly lorazepam, thus strategies that can avoid this class of agents may help avoid delirium and the numerous negative sequelae associated with it.[63] Delirium may be associated with alterations in level of consciousness, and the agitation that is sometimes present with delirium may lead to the administration of sedative agents, particularly if delirium is not recognized.[64] Although the mechanism by which benzodiazepine drugs predispose patients to delirium remains unclear, the GABA receptor activation that this class of agents induces alters levels of potentially deliriogenic neurotransmitters such as dopamine, serotonin, acetylcholine, norepinephrine, and glutamate.

Posttraumatic stress disorder (PTSD) is frequent in ICU survivors.[65] The amount of benzodiazepine administered during the ICU stay correlates with the severity of PTSD symptoms. In one study, every 10 mg increase in the dose of lorazepam administered was associated with a PTSD 10-Questions Inventory score increase of 0.39 (95% CI 0.17 to 0.61; $P = .04$).[66] Benzodiazepines remain the sedative drug of choice for patients admitted with substance disorders such as alcohol withdrawal. As with opioids, tolerance to benzodiazepines may occur after only a few hours of therapy, and thus dosing requirements may increase.[67] Benzodiazepines must be withdrawn with care, particularly after high-dose, long-term therapy. Administration of enteral lorazepam or diazepam may help prevent benzodiazepine withdrawal and help facilitate the down-titration of benzodiazepine infusions.[68]

Pharmacogenetics

Increasing data suggested that the activity of CYP3A5, the primary isoenzyme that influences midazolam metabolism, is influenced by genetic polymorphism.[69] It has been reported that individuals who are homozygotic for the *CYP3A5*1* allele have increased hepatic levels of the protein CYP3A5 compared with individuals who are homozygotic for the *CYP3A5*3* and *CYP3A5*6* allelic variants. It is also important to note that critical illness itself has been associated with a substantial decrease in CYP450 isoenzyme 3A4 activity, which could also further influence the midazolam-related oversedation.[70] Future research is required to focus the role of CYP3A5 genetic polymorphisms on the predisposition of patients for iatrogenic coma.

Safety

In patients who are not intubated, benzodiazepines must be used with caution because of their respiratory depressant effects. Paradoxic agitation has been described with lorazepam, which may be the result of drug-induced amnesia or disorientation. Lorazepam infusions should be diluted to a concentration of <1 mg/10 mL to prevent precipitation in the intravenous line.

Recent reports have alerted clinicians to the risks for toxicity related to propylene glycol (a diluent used to facilitate drug solubility) accumulation in patients receiving intravenous lorazepam.[71–73] Toxicity from the direct effects of propylene glycol and its metabolites (ie, lactate, pyruvate) may result in hyperosmolar states, cellular toxicity, metabolic acidosis, and acute tubular necrosis. An infusion of 2 mg/h of lorazepam will lead to 19.9 g of propylene glycol per day—an amount that would be more than 11 times the World Health Organization's recommended daily intake for a 70 kg adult. In addition to long-term and high-dose lorazepam therapy, other identified risk factors for propylene glycol toxicity include renal and hepatic derangement, pregnancy, age less than 4 years, and treatment with metronidazole. Monitoring propylene glycol serum concentrations is impractical in most institutions because these assays are rarely available. Instead, clinicians should monitor a daily serum osmol gap in patients who have received a daily lorazepam dose that exceeds 50 mg or 1 mg/kg based on a number of studies showing that an osmol gap greater than 10 to 15 reflects significant propylene glycol accumulation.[71] Hemodialysis effectively removes propylene glycol and corrects hyperosmolar states, but generally discontinuing the parenteral lorazepam is all that is required.[74]

Propofol

Propofol is an intravenous general anesthetic agent that has been widely used as a sedative in the ICU for nearly 20 years.[2,10,11] It exhibits sedative and hypnotic properties at even low doses and has amnestic properties similar to that of the benzodiazepines.[75] Its rapid onset and offset of action provides clinicians with a sedative option that is far more titratable than that of the benzodiazepines, and it is considered the preferred sedative for patients in whom rapid awakening is important.[2] Controversy remains as to whether propofol acts as an effective anticonvulsant or in fact induces seizure activity.[76] Propofol reduces intracranial pressure after traumatic brain injury more effectively than either morphine or fentanyl and also decreases cerebral blood flow and metabolism.[77,78]

Pharmacokinetics

Propofol is hydrophobic and therefore is formulated in an oil-in-water emulsion.[75] It provides 1.1 kcal/mL from fat and should be counted as a caloric source. A water-soluble prodrug of propofol, fospropofol, has recently been approved, although is not well studied in the ICU setting. The lipophilic properties of propofol allow it to cross the blood-brain barrier rapidly. Metabolism of propofol occurs primarily by conjugation in the liver to inactive metabolites, which are eliminated through the kidneys. Clearance does not appear to be significantly altered by hepatic or renal disease, although in critical care populations, clearance is generally slower than in the general population because of decreases in hepatic blood flow.[16] A slightly longer recovery from propofol therapy has been reported with long-term infusions.[79] Elderly patients have decreased clearance and thus maintenance infusions should generally be reduced in an age-related fashion.[75]

Pharmacodynamics

A recent study that evaluated the pharmacokinetics and pharmacodynamics of propofol in patients who are critically ill found that patients who were sicker (based on the sequential organ failure assessment [SOFA] score) were more likely to have a deeper level of sedation that may be related to decreased propofol clearance.[80] In another study, Barr and colleagues[81] showed that the offset of propofol activity can vary considerably and is a function of the depth of sedation, duration of the infusion, and patient size and body composition. For example, the emergence from a deep sedation (to decrease the Ramsey sedation score from 5 to 2) averaged 25 hours for a 24-hour infusion but increased to nearly 3 days for propofol infusions lasting 7 to 14 days.

In response to studies showing that continuous benzodiazepine infusions are associated with a longer duration of mechanical ventilation than propofol therapy, a recent prospective study compared scheduled intermittent lorazepam in conjunction with daily sedation interruption for patients admitted to the medical intensive care unit who required mechanical ventilation for at least 2 days.[2,82] The authors concluded that sedation with propofol resulted in significantly fewer ventilator days than did scheduled intermittent lorazepam (median ventilator days 5.8 vs 8.4; P = .04).

The reasons that patients who receive propofol are on mechanical ventilation for a shorter period compared with patients who receive intermittent benzodiazepine therapy are unclear. One possible explanation may relate to differences in the pharmacokinetic and pharmacodynamic characteristics of each agent. With propofol's shorter half-life, relative to lorazepam, its serum concentrations would be expected to decline more rapidly than lorazepam's, even when lorazepam is administered on a scheduled, intermittent basis.[83] The recent Awakening and Breathing Controlled study found that for those patients randomized to the spontaneous awakening trial arm, the benzodiazepine dose was lower, on average, compared with the dose in the control arm, but the average dose of propofol was not.[84] This suggests that factors other than a reduction in the drug dose were responsible for the benefits observed with the spontaneous awakening trials.

Safety

Hypotension attributable to systemic vasodilation is a well-known adverse effect of propofol, particularly in hypovolemic patients. For this reason, and because of propofol's rapid onset of activity, caution should be exercised when the use of a bolus is needed. Hypertriglyceridemia in ICU receiving propofol infusions occurs rarely and is typically associated with high propofol infusion rates, concurrent administration of parenteral lipids for nutrition or baseline hypertriglyceridemia.[85] Propofol, like any lipid-containing product, has been shown to have immunosuppressant effects, although the clinical importance of these effects remains unclear.[86] Despite the presence of a preservative in all currently marketed formulations of propofol, both the propofol bottle along with the intravenous infusion set should be changed every 12 hours. Whether the preservatives used in commercially available propofol formulations (eg, ethylenediaminetetraacetic acid [EDTA] and sodium metabisulfite) have clinical effects other than their preservative effect remains to be established.

While propofol is generally considered a safe agent when prescribed based on product labeling recommendations, a troublesome syndrome known as the propofol related infusion syndrome (PRIS) has been reported with its use.[87] PRIS was first described in 1992 in a case series of five pediatric patients in the ICU who developed metabolic acidosis with bradyarrhythmia and progressive myocardial failure resulting in death while receiving high dose propofol (>83 mcg/kg/min for >48 hours).[88] Since this report, 38 cases of PRIS have subsequently been published in both adults and children with an associated mortality rate exceeding 80%. PRIS-associated clinical manifestations vary widely and have been reported to include: rhabdomyolysis, myocardial failure, acute renal failure, severe metabolic acidosis, bradyarrhythmias, cardiac arrest, dyslipidemias, and hypotension.[89] Postulated risk factors for PRIS include propofol doses more than 83 mcg/kg/min, a duration of therapy more than 48 hours, concomitant use of catecholamine vasopressors or glucocorticoids, and an age more than 18 years.[89–91] Other potential risk factors include having an inborn error of mitochrondrial fatty acid oxidation or receiving a ketogenic diet.[92,93] Recently, the product labeling of propofol has been changed to increase the prescriber's awareness of PRIS. Current labeling advocates the optimization of hemodynamic and oxygen delivery parameters in all patients in the ICU treated with propofol in addition to the discontinuation of propofol if metabolic acidosis, rhabdomyolysis, hyperkalemia, and/or rapid progressive heart failure occur during therapy.[94]

Although PRIS is associated with a high mortality rate, the disparity between the high use of propofol in the ICU and the small number of published case reports of PRIS leaves the demographic and clinical factors associated with PRIS, particularly those factors associated with death, poorly characterized. One recent analysis of 1139 patients in the FDA MEDWATCH system with suspected PRIS (30% fatal) found that the presence of cardiac failure, rhabdomyolysis, hypotension, metabolic acidosis, and an age more than 18 years were each independently associated with death.[95] Further study is needed to identify the incidence of PRIS and the exact mechanism(s) by which it occurs.

SUMMARY

The ideal sedative or analgesic agent should have a rapid onset of activity, a rapid recovery after drug discontinuation, a predictable dose response, a lack of drug accumulation, and no toxicity.[96] Unfortunately, none of the earlier analgesics, the benzodiazepines, or propofol share all of these characteristics. Patients who are critically ill experience numerous physiologic derangements and commonly require high doses and long durations of analgesic and sedative therapy. There is a paucity of well-designed clinical trials evaluating the safety and efficacy of earlier sedative and analgesic agents in the ICU. In addition, the ever-changing dynamics of patients who are critically ill makes the use of sedation a continual challenge during the course of each patient's admission. To optimize care, clinicians should be familiar with the many pharmacokinetic, pharmacodynamic, and pharmacogenetic variables that can affect the safety and efficacy of sedatives and analgesics.

REFERENCES

1. Sessler CN, Varney K. Patient-focused sedation and analgesia in the ICU. Chest 2008;133(2):552–65.
2. Jacobi J, Fraser GL, Coursin DB, et al. Clinical practice guidelines for the sustained use of sedatives and analgesics in the critically ill adult. Crit Care Med 2002;30(1):119–41.
3. Payen JF, Chanques G, Mantz J, et al. Current practices in sedation and analgesia for mechanically ventilated critically ill patients: a prospective multicenter patient-based study. Anesthesiology 2007;106(4):687–95 [quiz: 891–2].
4. Weinert CR, Calvin AD. Epidemiology of sedation and sedation adequacy for mechanically ventilated patients in a medical and surgical intensive care unit. Crit Care Med 2007;35(2):393–401.
5. Puntillo KA. Pain experiences of intensive care unit patients. Heart Lung 1990; 19(5 Pt 1):526–33.
6. Kress JP, Pohlman AS, O'Connor MF, et al. Daily interruption of sedative infusions in critically ill patients undergoing mechanical ventilation. N Engl J Med 2000; 342(20):1471–7.
7. Devlin JW, Tanios MA, Epstein SK. Intensive care unit sedation: waking up clinicians to the gap between research and practice. Crit Care Med 2006;34(2):556–7.
8. Brook AD, Ahrens TS, Schaiff R, et al. Effect of a nursing-implemented sedation protocol on the duration of mechanical ventilation. Crit Care Med 1999;27(12): 2609–15.
9. Pandharipande PP, Pun BT, Herr DL, et al. Effect of sedation with dexmedetomidine vs lorazepam on acute brain dysfunction in mechanically ventilated patients: the MENDS randomized controlled trial. JAMA 2007;298(22):2644–53.
10. Mehta S, Burry L, Fischer S, et al. Canadian survey of the use of sedatives, analgesics, and neuromuscular blocking agents in critically ill patients. Crit Care Med 2006;34(2):374–80.
11. Martin J, Franck M, Sigel S, et al. Changes in sedation management in German intensive care units between 2002 and 2006: a national follow-up survey. Crit Care 2007;11(6):R124.
12. Riker RR, Fraser GL. Adverse events associated with sedatives, analgesics, and other drugs that provide patient comfort in the intensive care unit. Pharmacotherapy 2005;25(5 Pt 2):8S–18S.
13. Wagner BK, O'Hara DA. Pharmacokinetics and pharmacodynamics of sedatives and analgesics in the treatment of agitated critically ill patients. Clin Pharmacokinet 1997;33(6):426–53.
14. Devlin JW, Barletta JF. Chapter 21: principles of drug dosing in critically ill patients. In: Parrillo JE, Dellinger RP, editors. Critical care medicine: principles of diagnosis and management in the adult. 3rd edition. Philadelphia: Mosby Elsevier; 2008. p. 343–76.
15. Power BM, Forbes AM, van Heerden PV, et al. Pharmacokinetics of drugs used in critically ill adults. Clin Pharmacokinet 1998;34(1):25–56.
16. Bodenham A, Shelly MP, Park GR. The altered pharmacokinetics and pharmacodynamics of drugs commonly used in critically ill patients. Clin Pharmacokinet 1988;14(6):347–73.
17. Spina SP, Ensom MH. Clinical pharmacokinetic monitoring of midazolam in critically ill patients. Pharmacotherapy 2007;27(3):389–98.
18. Weinshilboum R. Inheritance and drug response. N Engl J Med 2003;348(6): 529–37.

19. Somogyi AA, Barratt DT, Coller JK. Pharmacogenetics of opioids. Clin Pharmacol Ther 2007;81(3):429–44.
20. Lotsch J, Skarke C, Liefhold J, et al. Genetic predictors of the clinical response to opioid analgesics: clinical utility and future perspectives. Clin Pharmacokinet 2004;43(14):983–1013.
21. Smith HS. Variations in opioid responsiveness. Pain Physician 2008;11(2): 237–48.
22. Fredheim OM, Moksnes K, Borchgrevink PC, et al. Clinical pharmacology of methadone for pain. Acta Anaesthesiol Scand 2008;52(7):879–89.
23. Trescot AM, Datta S, Lee M, et al. Opioid pharmacology. Pain Physician 2008; 11(2 Suppl):S133–53.
24. Armstrong PJ, Bersten A. Normeperidine toxicity. Anesth Analg 1986;65(5):536–8.
25. Mao J, Price DD, Lu J, et al. Antinociceptive tolerance to the mu-opioid agonist DAMGO is dose-dependently reduced by MK-801 in rats. Neurosci Lett 1998; 250(3):193–6.
26. Pergolizzi J, Boger RH, Budd K, et al. Opioids and the management of chronic severe pain in the elderly: consensus statement of an International Expert Panel with focus on the six clinically most often used World Health Organization step III opioids (buprenorphine, fentanyl, hydromorphone, methadone, morphine, oxyco-done). Pain Pract 2008;8(4):287–313.
27. Hall LG, Oyen LJ, Murray MJ. Analgesic agents. Pharmacology and application in critical care. Crit Care Clin 2001;17(4):899–923, viii.
28. Barr J, Donner A. Optimal intravenous dosing strategies for sedatives and anal-gesics in the intensive care unit. Crit Care Clin 1995;11(4):827–47.
29. Lugo RA, MacLaren R, Cash J, et al. Enteral methadone to expedite fentanyl discontinuation and prevent opioid abstinence syndrome in the PICU. Pharmaco-therapy 2001;21(12):1566–73.
30. Toombs JD, Kral LA. Methadone treatment for pain states. Am Fam Physician 2005;71(7):1353–8.
31. Davies G, Kingswood C, Street M. Pharmacokinetics of opioids in renal dysfunc-tion. Clin Pharmacokinet 1996;31(6):410–22.
32. Gutstein HB, Akil H. Opioid analgesics. In: Brunton LL, Lazo JS, Parker KL, editors. Goodman and Gilman's the pharmacologic basis of therapeutics. 11th edition. New York: McGraw-Hill; 2006. p. 547–90.
33. Walder B, Tramer MR. Analgesia and sedation in critically ill patients. Swiss Med Wkly 2004;134(23-24):333–46.
34. Dahaba AA, Grabner T, Rehak PH, et al. Remifentanil versus morphine analgesia and sedation for mechanically ventilated critically ill patients: a randomized double blind study. Anesthesiology 2004;101(3):640–6.
35. Muellejans B, Lopez A, Cross MH, et al. Remifentanil versus fentanyl for anal-gesia based sedation to provide patient comfort in the intensive care unit: a randomized, double-blind controlled trial [ISRCTN43755713]. Crit Care 2004; 8(1):R1–11.
36. Karabinis A, Mandragos K, Stergiopoulos S, et al. Safety and efficacy of analgesia-based sedation with remifentanil versus standard hypnotic-based regi-mens in intensive care unit patients with brain injuries: a randomised, controlled trial [ISRCTN50308308]. Crit Care 2004;8(4):R268–80.
37. Breen D, Karabinis A, Malbrain M, et al. Decreased duration of mechanical venti-lation when comparing analgesia-based sedation using remifentanil with stan-dard hypnotic-based sedation for up to 10 days in intensive care unit patients: a randomised trial [ISRCTN47583497]. Crit Care 2005;9(3):R200–10.

38. Patanwala AE, Duby J, Waters D, et al. Opioid conversions in acute care. Ann Pharmacother 2007;41(2):255–66.

39. Dumas EO, Pollack GM. Opioid tolerance development: a pharmacokinetic/pharmacodynamic perspective. AAPS J 2008;10:537–51.

40. Tobias JD. Tolerance, withdrawal, and physical dependency after long-term sedation and analgesia of children in the pediatric intensive care unit. Crit Care Med 2000;28(6):2122–32.

41. Hofbauer R, Tesinsky P, Hammerschmidt V, et al. No reduction in the sufentanil requirement of elderly patients undergoing ventilatory support in the medical intensive care unit. Eur J Anaesthesiol 1999;16(10):702–7.

42. Meyer MM, Berens RJ. Efficacy of an enteral 10-day methadone wean to prevent opioid withdrawal in fentanyl-tolerant pediatric intensive care unit patients. Pediatr Crit Care Med 2001;2(4):329–33.

43. Eap CB, Broly F, Mino A, et al. Cytochrome P450 2D6 genotype and methadone steady-state concentrations. J Clin Psychopharmacol 2001;21(2):229–34.

44. Crettol S, Deglon JJ, Besson J, et al. Methadone enantiomer plasma levels, CYP2B6, CYP2C19, and CYP2C9 genotypes, and response to treatment. Clin Pharmacol Ther 2005;78(6):593–604.

45. Eap CB, Crettol S, Rougier JS, et al. Stereoselective block of hERG channel by (S)-methadone and QT interval prolongation in CYP2B6 slow metabolizers. Clin Pharmacol Ther 2007;81(5):719–28.

46. Darbari DS, van Schaik RH, Capparelli EV, et al. UGT2B7 promoter variant -840G>A contributes to the variability in hepatic clearance of morphine in patients with sickle cell disease. Am J Hematol 2008;83(3):200–2.

47. Benyamin R, Trescot AM, Datta S, et al. Opioid complications and side effects. Pain Physician 2008;11(2 Suppl):S105–20.

48. Gaudreau JD, Gagnon P, Roy MA, et al. Opioid medications and longitudinal risk of delirium in hospitalized cancer patients. Cancer 2007;109(11):2365–73.

49. Moryl N, Kogan M, Comfort C, et al. Methadone in the treatment of pain and terminal delirum in advanced cancer patients. Palliat Support Care 2005;3(4):311–7.

50. Benitez-Rosario MA, Feria M, Salinas-Martin A, et al. Opioid switching from transdermal fentanyl to oral methadone in patients with cancer pain. Cancer 2004; 101(12):2866–73.

51. Mirski MA, Hemstreet MK. Critical care sedation for neuroscience patients. J Neurol Sci 2007;261(1-2):16–34.

52. Thomas J, Karver S, Cooney GA, et al. Methylnaltrexone for opioid-induced constipation in advanced illness. N Engl J Med 2008;358(22):2332–43.

53. Amrein R, Hetzel W, Hartmann D, et al. Clinical pharmacology of flumazenil. Eur J Anaesthesiol Suppl 1988;2:65–80.

54. Ghoneim MM, Mewaldt SP. Benzodiazepines and human memory: a review. Anesthesiology 1990;72(5):926–38.

55. Masica AL, Girard TD, Wilkinson GR, et al. Clinical sedation scores as indicators of sedative and analgesic drug exposure in intensive care unit patients. Am J Geriatr Pharmacother 2007;5(3):218–31.

56. McKenzie CA, McKinnon W, Naughton DP, et al. Differentiating midazolam oversedation from neurological damage in the intensive care unit. Crit Care 2005;9(1): R32–6.

57. Shelly MP, Mendel L, Park GR. Failure of critically ill patients to metabolise midazolam. Anaesthesia 1987;42(6):619–26.

58. Bauer TM, Ritz R, Haberthur C, et al. Prolonged sedation due to accumulation of conjugated metabolites of midazolam. Lancet 1995;346(8968):145–7.

59. Swart EL, van Schijndel RJ, van Loenen AC, et al. Continuous infusion of loraze-pam versus medazolam in patients in the intensive care unit: sedation with lora-zepam is easier to manage and is more cost-effective. Crit Care Med 1999;27(8):1461–5.

60. Barr J, Zomorodi K, Bertaccini EJ, et al. A double-blind, randomized comparison of i.v. lorazepam versus midazolam for sedation of ICU patients via a pharmaco-logic model. Anesthesiology 2001;95(2):286–98.

61. Swart EL, Zuideveld KP, de Jongh J, et al. Population pharmacodynamic model-ling of lorazepam- and midazolam-induced sedation upon long-term continuous infusion in critically ill patients. Eur J Clin Pharmacol 2006;62(3):185–94.

62. Kollef MH, Levy NT, Ahrens TS, et al. The use of continuous i.v. sedation is asso-ciated with prolongation of mechanical ventilation. Chest 1998;114(2):541–8.

63. Pandharipande P, Shintani A, Peterson J, et al. Lorazepam is an independent risk factor for transitioning to delirium in intensive care unit patients. Anesthesiology 2006;104(1):21–6.

64. Devlin JW, Fong JJ, Fraser GL, et al. Delirium assessment in the critically ill. Inten-sive Care Med 2007;33(6):929–40.

65. Schelling G, Stoll C, Haller M, et al. Health-related quality of life and posttraumatic stress disorder in survivors of the acute respiratory distress syndrome. Crit Care Med 1998;26(4):651–9.

66. Girard TD, Shintani AK, Jackson JC, et al. Risk factors for post-traumatic stress disorder symptoms following critical illness requiring mechanical ventilation: a prospective cohort study. Crit Care 2007;11(1):R28.

67. Shelly MP, Sultan MA, Bodenham A, et al. Midazolam infusions in critically ill patients. Eur J Anaesthesiol 1991;8(1):21–7.

68. Cigada M, Pezzi A, Di Mauro P, et al. Sedation in the critically ill ventilated patient: possible role of enteral drugs. Intensive Care Med 2005;31(3):482–6.

69. Fukasawa T, Suzuki A, Otani K. Effects of genetic polymorphism of cytochrome P450 enzymes on the pharmacokinetics of benzodiazepines. J Clin Pharm Ther 2007;32(4):333–41.

70. Haas CE, Kaufman DC, Jones CE, et al. Cytochrome P450 3A4 activity after surgical stress. Crit Care Med 2003;31(5):1338–46.

71. Barnes BJ, Gerst C, Smith JR, et al. Osmol gap as a surrogate marker for serum propylene glycol concentrations in patients receiving lorazepam for sedation. Pharmacotherapy 2006;26(1):23–33.

72. Nelsen JL, Haas CE, Habtemariam B, et al. A prospective evaluation of propylene glycol clearance and accumulation during continuous-infusion lorazepam in crit-ically ill patients. J Intensive Care Med 2008;23(3):184–94.

73. Yahwak JA, Riker RR, Fraser GL, et al. Determination of a lorazepam dose threshold for using the osmol gap to monitor for propylene glycol toxicity. Phar-macotherapy 2008;28(8):984–91.

74. Parker MG, Fraser GL, Watson DM, et al. Removal of propylene glycol and correction of increased osmolar gap by hemodialysis in a patient on high dose lorazepam infusion therapy. Intensive Care Med 2002;28(1):81–4.

75. McKeage K, Perry CM. Propofol: a review of its use in intensive care sedation of adults. CNS Drugs 2003;17(4):235–72.

76. Marik PE, Varon J. The management of status epilepticus. Chest 2004;126(2):582–91.

77. Kelly DF, Goodale DB, Williams J, et al. Propofol in the treatment of moderate and severe head injury: a randomized, prospective double-blinded pilot trial. J Neuro-surg 1999;90(6):1042–52.

78. Ravussin P, Guinard JP, Ralley F, et al. Effect of propofol on cerebrospinal fluid pressure and cerebral perfusion pressure in patients undergoing craniotomy. Anaesthesia 1988;43 Suppl:37–41.
79. Bailie GR, Cockshott ID, Douglas EJ, et al. Pharmacokinetics of propofol during and after long-term continuous infusion for maintenance of sedation in ICU patients. Br J Anaesth 1992;68(5):486–91.
80. Peeters MY, Bras LJ, DeJongh J, et al. Disease severity is a major determinant for the pharmacodynamics of propofol in critically ill patients. Clin Pharmacol Ther 2008;83(3):443–51.
81. Barr J, Egan TD, Sandoval NF, et al. Propofol dosing regimens for ICU sedation based upon an integrated pharmacokinetic-pharmacodynamic model. Anesthesiology 2001;95(2):324–33.
82. Carson SS, Kress JP, Rodgers JE, et al. A randomized trial of intermittent lorazepam versus propofol with daily interruption in mechanically ventilated patients. Crit Care Med 2006;34(5):1326–32.
83. de Wit M, Best AM, Epstein SK, et al. Lorazepam concentrations, pharmacokinetics and pharmacodynamics in a cohort of mechanically ventilated ICU patients. Int J Clin Pharmacol Ther 2006;44(10):466–73.
84. Girard TD, Kress JP, Fuchs BD, et al. Efficacy and safety of a paired sedation and ventilator weaning protocol for mechanically ventilated patients in intensive care (Awakening and Breathing Controlled trial): a randomised controlled trial. Lancet 2008;371(9607):126–34.
85. Devlin JW, Lau AK, Tanios MA. Propofol-associated hypertriglyceridemia and pancreatitis in the intensive care unit: an analysis of frequency and risk factors. Pharmacotherapy 2005;25(10):1348–52.
86. Huettemann E, Jung A, Vogelsang H, et al. Effects of propofol vs methohexital on neutrophil function and immune status in critically ill patients. J Anesth 2006; 20(2):86–91.
87. Fodale V, La Monaca E. Propofol infusion syndrome: an overview of a perplexing disease. Drug Saf 2008;31(4):293–303.
88. Bray RJ. Fatal myocardial failure associated with a propofol infusion in a child. Anaesthesia 1995;50(1):94.
89. Bray RJ. Propofol infusion syndrome in children. Paediatr Anaesth 1998;8(6): 491–9.
90. Fudickar A, Bein B, Tonner PH. Propofol infusion syndrome in anaesthesia and intensive care medicine. Curr Opin Anaesthesiol 2006;19(4):404–10.
91. Vasile B, Rasulo F, Candiani A, et al. The pathophysiology of propofol infusion syndrome: a simple name for a complex syndrome. Intensive Care Med 2003; 29(9):1417–25.
92. Baumeister FA, Oberhoffer R, Liebhaber GM, et al. Fatal propofol infusion syndrome in association with ketogenic diet. Neuropediatrics 2004;35(4): 250–2.
93. Wolf A, Weir P, Segar P, et al. Impaired fatty acid oxidation in propofol infusion syndrome. Lancet 2001;357(9256):606–7.
94. Diprivan for I.V. administration vol. 2007.
95. Fong JJ, Sylvia L, Ruthazer R, et al. Predictors of mortality in patients with suspected propofol infusion syndrome. Crit Care Med 2008;36(8):2281–7.
96. Ostermann ME, Keenan SP, Seiferling RA, et al. Sedation in the intensive care unit: a systematic review. JAMA 2000;283(11):1451–9.
97. Ferrari A, Coccia CP, Bertolini A, et al. Methadone–metabolism, pharmacokinetics and interactions. Pharmacol Res 2004;50(6):551–9.

98. Charney DS, Mihic SJ, Harris RA. Hypnotics and sedatives. In: Brunton LL, Lazo JS, Parker KL, editors. Goodman and Gilman's the pharmacological basis of therapeutics. 11th edition. New York: McGraw-Hill; 2006. p. 401–29.
99. MacLaren R, Sullivan PW. Pharmacoeconomic modeling of lorazepam, midazolam, and propofol for continuous sedation in critically ill patients. Pharmacotherapy 2005;25(10):1319–28.

Pharmacology of Sedative-Analgesic Agents: Dexmedetomidine, Remifentanil, Ketamine, Volatile Anesthetics, and the Role of Peripheral Mu Antagonists

Oliver Panzer, MD, Vivek Moitra, MD,
Robert N. Sladen, MRCP(UK), FRCP(C), FCCM*

KEYWORDS

- Sedation • Analgesia • Dexmedetomidine • Remifentanil
- Ketamine • Volatile anesthetics

DEXMEDETOMIDINE
Introduction

Dexmedetomidine is a highly selective alpha-2 agonist that provides anxiolysis and cooperative sedation without respiratory depression. It decreases central nervous system (CNS) sympathetic outflow in a dose-dependent manner and has analgesic effects best described as opioid-sparing. There is increasing evidence that dexmedetomidine has organ protective effects against ischemic and hypoxic injury, including cardioprotection, neuroprotection, and renoprotection. After its approval by the Food and Drug Administration (FDA) in 1999, it has become well established in the United States as a sedative-hypnotic agent.

A version of this article appeared in the 25:3 issue of *Critical Care Clinics*.
Department of Anesthesiology, College of Physicians and Surgeons of Columbia University, 630 West 168th Street, New York, NY 10032, USA
* Corresponding author.
E-mail address: rs543@columbia.edu

Anesthesiology Clin 29 (2011) 587–605
doi:10.1016/j.anclin.2011.09.002
1932-2275/11/$ – see front matter © 2011 Elsevier Inc. All rights reserved.

Receptor Pharmacology

Dexmedetomidine is the *dextro* enantiomer of medetomidine, the methylated derivative of etomidine. Its specificity for the alpha-2 receptor is seven times that of clonidine, with an alpha-2/alpha-1 binding affinity ratio of 1620:1, and its effects are dose-dependently reversed by administration of a selective alpha-2 antagonist such as atipamezole.[1]

Specific alpha-2 receptor subtypes mediate the varied pharmacodynamic effects of dexmedetomidine. For example, agonism at the alpha-2A receptor appears to promote sedation, hypnosis, analgesia, sympatholysis, neuroprotection,[2] and inhibition of insulin secretion.[3] Agonism at the alpha-2B receptor suppresses shivering centrally,[4] promotes analgesia at spinal cord sites, and induces vasoconstriction in peripheral arteries. The alpha-2C receptor is associated with modulation of cognition, sensory processing, mood- and stimulant-induced locomotor activity, and regulation of epinephrine outflow from the adrenal medulla.[5,6] Inhibition of norepinephrine release appears to be equally affected by all three alpha-2 receptor subtypes.[6]

Dexmedetomidine also binds to imidazoline receptors, which recognize the imidazoline or oxaziline structure of alpha-2 agonist agents. This activity may explain some of the non-alpha-2 receptor–related effects of this drug class. Imidazoline receptor subtypes have also been identified. Imidazoline-1 receptors modulate blood pressure regulation and have anti-arrhythmic effects.[7] They are found in the ventrolateral medulla and are linked to G-proteins. Imidazoline-2 receptors have been implicated in neuroprotection in a cerebral ischemia model in animals and in generation of memory.[8] They are typically located on the mitochondrial outer membrane and are not G-protein coupled, but may exert their effects by decreasing tissue norepinephrine levels.[8]

Pharmacokinetics

After intravenous (IV) injection, dexmedetomidine has an onset of action after approximately 15 minutes. Peak concentrations are usually achieved within 1 hour after continuous IV infusion. Analysis by a 2-compartment model demonstrates rapid distribution away from the CNS, with an alpha half-life ($t_{1/2}$ α) of 6 minutes and a terminal elimination half-life ($t_{1/2}$ β) of between 2.0 and 2.5 hours. The drug is highly protein-bound, with a 6% free fraction, and has a relatively large steady state volume of distribution (V_{dss}, 1.33 L/kg). Except for a larger V_{dss}, pharmacokinetics do not appear to be substantially altered in mechanically ventilated patients sedated with dexmedetomidine in an intensive care unit (ICU).[9]

Total plasma clearance of the dexmedetomidine is age independent, thus similar rates of infusion can be used in children and adults to effect a steady state plasma concentration.[10] Plasma protein binding of dexmedetomidine is also similar to adults.[11] In children younger than 2 years of age, the volume of distribution (V_d) at steady state (V_{SS}) is increased, suggesting that higher doses are required to achieve V_{SS}; but $t_{1/2}$ β is prolonged, which may result in increased drug accumulation with time.[10]

Dexmedetomidine is also absorbed systemically through the transdermal,[12] buccal, or intramuscular routes,[13] with a mean bioavailability from the latter 2 routes of 82% and 104% respectively.

Dexmedetomidine is extensively metabolized in the liver through glucuronide conjugation and biotransformation in the cytochrome P450 enzyme system. There are no known active or toxic metabolites. However, hepatic clearance may be decreased by as much as 50% of normal with severe liver disease. Pharmacokinetics are not significantly altered in patients with severe renal impairment,[14] but patients remained sedated for longer than normal controls, suggesting an enhanced pharmacodynamic effect, presumably because of the presence of varying degrees of uremic encephalopathy.[14] Thus, dosages should be decreased in the presence of either hepatic or renal disease. Dexmedetomidine decreases cardiac output in a dose-dependent manner, but the impact of this on clearance does not appear to be clinically relevant.[15]

Dosing and Administration

Phase 1 studies demonstrated that IV doses of dexmedetomidine induced dose-dependent decreases in systolic and diastolic blood pressure and in heart rate and substantial decreases in plasma norepinephrine levels. However, at high-bolus IV doses (50–75 µg), a transient initial hypertensive response may be seen, presumably because of activation of peripheral vascular alpha-2 receptors before the central sympatholytic effect on the vasomotor center.[16] There do not appear to be any reflex or drug-induced alterations in plasma renin activity, atrial natriuretic peptide or arginine vasopressin (AVP).[17] Dexmedetomidine also produces dose-dependent decreases in vigilance and increases in sedation that correlate well with electroencephalogram (EEG)-based spectral entropy monitoring.[18]

Initial studies that targeted plasma dexmedetomidine levels revealed desirable pharmacodynamic effects between 0.5 and 1.2 ng/mL. Subsequent clinical studies designed to achieve these effects used a loading dose of 1 µg/kg during a period of 10 minutes, followed by a continuous IV infusion rate of 0.2 to 0.7 µg/kg/hr, the dosing regimen originally approved by the FDA in 1999.

Studies examining very high dexmedetomidine plasma levels (up to 8.0 ng/mL) demonstrate that the alpha-2C peripheral vasoconstrictor effects become predominant, with increasing systemic vascular resistance and decreasing cardiac index, associated with marked catecholamine suppression and deepening sedation. However, even at these very high plasma levels, there was no clinically significant respiratory depression.[19] Indeed, when administered as the sole agent, dexmedetomidine appears to be remarkably safe. Case reports of large accidental overdoses of dexmedetomidine (192 µg loading dose, 2–30 µg/kg/hr) describe oversedation as the only notable sign, with resolution within an hour of discontinuation.[20] Moreover, dexmedetomidine has been used safely as the sole agent at high rates of infusion (5–15 µg/kg/hr) to anesthetize patients with tracheal stenosis while preserving spontaneous ventilation.[21] In October 2008, the FDA approved an increased dose of dexmedetomidine (up to 1.5 µg/kg/hr) for surgical procedures.

In contrast, there is a risk for excessive bradycardia and even sinus arrest when dexmedetomidine is administered in combination with sympatholytic or cholinergic agents (eg, beta-blockers, fentanyl, neostigmine), especially if there is concomitant vagal stimulation (eg, sternal separation, laparoscopic insufflation, colonoscopy).[22–24]

Based on preliminary studies, the FDA-approved duration of infusion of dexmedetomidine remains 24 hours. However, there are several studies that have demonstrated safe use for a week or longer in mechanically ventilated critically ill patients.[25,26] With prolonged administration, tolerance to dexmedetomidine's hypnotic effects has been demonstrated in animals,[27] but it does not appear to be clinically significant. Unlike clonidine, cessation of administration does not appear to be associated with rebound hypertension or agitation.

Pharmacodynamic Effects

Sedation: anxiolysis, hypnosis, and amnesia
As described earlier, dexmedetomidine provides dose-dependent increases in anxiolysis and sedation. However, the quality of sedation appears to be unique in

comparison with GABAnergic agents such as midazolam or propofol. Arousability is maintained at deep levels of sedation, with good correlation between the level of sedation (Richmond agitation-sedation scale) and the bispectral (BIS) EEG.[28] Once aroused, subjects perform well on tests of vigilance, such as the critical flicker-fusion frequency.[29] To achieve the same result, infusions of midazolam or propofol must be discontinued. This results in so-called "cooperative sedation," in that patients can cooperate with ICU nursing, radiologic, and even airway procedures and undertake sophisticated neurologic testing during craniotomies for tumor dissection or stereotactic implantations.[30,31] In addition, given the demonstrated benefit of daily wake-up trials on outcomes in ICU patients,[32,33] there appears to be particular value in a drug such as dexmedetomidine that facilitates the arousal and rapid orientation of a sedated patient and then allows the patient to return to a sedated state soon afterward.

Sedation induced by dexmedetomidine has the respiratory pattern and EEG changes commensurate with natural sleep.[34] Dexmedetomidine induces sleep by activating endogenous non–rapid eye movement sleep–promoting pathways.[35] Stimulation of alpha-2A receptors in the nucleus ceruleus inhibits noradrenergic neurons and disinhibits gamma-aminobutyric acid (GABAnergic) neurons in the ventrolateral preoptic nucleus (VLPO). In contrast, GABAnergic agents, such as propofol or benzodiazepines, directly enhance the inhibitory effects of the GABAnergic system at the VLPO. Norepinephrine release from the locus ceruleus remains unaffected, thus leading to less restful sleep. Functional MRI studies show that unlike GABAnergic agents, dexmedetomidine preserves a cerebral blood flow pattern akin to natural sleep.[36]

The amnestic effects of dexmedetomidine are far less than the benzodiazepines, which provide profound anterograde amnesia that may contribute to confused states on emergence. In contrast, amnesia is achieved with dexmedetomidine only at high plasma levels ($\geq$1.9 ng/mL), without retrograde amnesia.[19]

Analgesia

Dexmedetomidine appears to exert analgesic effects at the spinal cord level and at supraspinal sites. However, there has been considerable debate as to whether its analgesic effects are primary or simply opioid-sparing. Early studies suggested that part of its analgesic benefit might be mediated by attenuation of the affective-motivational component of pain.[37] Nonetheless, in comparison with hypnotic agents such as propofol, or postoperative opioids used alone, dexmedetomidine significantly decreases opioid requirement.[38,39]

Dexmedetomidine may also provide antinociception through nonspinal mechanisms—intra-articular administration during knee surgery improves postoperative analgesia, with less sedation than the IV route.[40] Suggested mechanisms are activation of alpha-2A receptors,[41] inhibition of the conduction of nerve signals through C and Aδ fibers, and the local release of encephalin.

Cardiovascular effects

Dexmedetomidine causes dose-dependent decreases in heart rate and blood pressure, concomitant with decreasing plasma catecholamines. This is of considerable benefit in tachycardiac, hypertensive patients, and dexmedetomidine typically improves hemodynamic stability in the perioperative period. However, these effects may be unwanted in patients with congestive heart failure, whose cardiac output is rate dependent, or with conduction system disease. As mentioned, high-dose boluses may result in a biphasic response, with bradycardia and hypertension consequent to initial stimulation of peripheral alpha-2B vascular receptors, followed by central sympatholysis and a decline in blood pressure.[19]

Respiratory effects
Unlike opioids, dexmedetomidine is able to achieve its sedative, hypnotic, and analgesic effects without causing any clinically relevant respiratory depression, even when dosed to plasma levels up to 15 times those normally achieved during therapy.[19] Compared with remifentanil, hypercapnic arousal is preserved, and the apnea threshold is actually decreased.[34] Administration of dexmedetomidine during sevoflurane or desflurane anesthesia with spontaneous ventilation has no effect on end-tidal carbon dioxide.[42] Arterial saturation is better preserved with dexmedetomidine than propofol in children undergoing MRI procedures.[43] A similar improvement in oxygenation was observed in extubated patients in an ICU.[44]

In contrast to infusions of opioids, benzodiazepines, or propofol, dexmedetomidine can safely be infused through tracheal extubation and beyond. It has been used successfully to facilitate tracheal extubation in patients who had previously failed extubation because of excessive agitation[45,46] and with similar benefit in agitated patients requiring noninvasive ventilation.[47] Dexmedetomidine is effective in achieving excellent sedation without respiratory depression during fiberoptic intubation or other difficult airway procedures.[21,48–50] Intubating conditions are further enhanced because dexmedetomidine decreases saliva production and airway secretions.[1]

Despite the lack of respiratory depression, dexmedetomidine was originally approved by the FDA for use in "initially intubated, mechanically ventilated patients," that is, it had to be started on ventilated patients but could be continued through and beyond tracheal extubation. In October 2008, dexmedetomidine was FDA-approved for procedural sedation in nonintubated patients.

Metabolic effects
Dexmedetomidine and other alpha-2 agonists suppress shivering, possibly by their activity at alpha-2B receptors in the hypothalamic thermoregulatory center of the brain.[4] Low-dose dexmedetomidine has an additive effect with meperidine on lowering the shivering threshold, when these drugs are combined.[51] Dexmedetomidine may be beneficial in decreasing patient discomfort from postoperative shivering[52] and controlling shivering that may delay therapeutic hypothermia for acute stroke or CNS injury. However, bradycardia has been noted when dexmedetomidine was added to remifentanil during therapeutic hypothermia in children.[53]

Organ protective effects
The ability of alpha-2 agonists to decrease tachycardia and hypertension suggests that they may play a role in cardioprotection by enhancing myocardial oxygen balance. There is as yet little evidence that dexmedetomidine enhances myocardial ischemic preconditioning or attenuates reperfusion injury. Most of the evidence is inferred; for example, when used after cardiac surgery, dexmedetomidine decreased the incidence of ventricular arrhythmias from 5% to zero, compared with propofol.[54]

A large European study demonstrated that perioperative infusion of mivazerol, another alpha-2 agonist, significantly decreased cardiac death after vascular surgery in patients with known coronary artery disease.[55] A meta-analysis of noncardiac vascular surgery patients receiving any alpha-2 agonist agent demonstrated decreased risk of myocardial infarction and death,[56] but a more recent meta-analysis of dexmedetomidine alone on cardiovascular outcomes after noncardiac surgery did not show statistical significance.[57] Larger studies are required to clearly establish the cardioprotective effect of dexmedetomidine; they should include patients at sufficiently high cardiac risk, and the dexmedetomidine infusion should be continued for at least 48 to 72 hours postoperatively.[57]

There is considerably more experimental evidence that dexmedetomidine has neuroprotective effects by several mechanisms. These include sympatholysis, preconditioning, and attenuation of ischemia-reperfusion injury.[58] There is also evidence that dexmedetomidine decreases cerebral blood flow,[59,60] but its ratio with cerebral metabolic rate (ie, flow-metabolism coupling) appears to be preserved.[61]

Alpha-2 adrenergic agonists, such as clonidine, have an established role in the treatment of central hyperadrenergic states induced by withdrawal of drugs, including cocaine, alcohol, or opioids. Numerous case reports of successful treatment of withdrawal using dexmedetomidine have been published,[62–69] but to date, no randomized trials have been performed.

The effects of dexmedetomidine on renal function are complex. Alpha-2 agonists exert a diuretic effect by inhibiting the antidiuretic action of AVP at the collecting duct, most likely through alpha-2A receptors, resulting in decreased expression of aquaporin-2 receptors and decreased salt and water reabsorption.[70,71] They also enhance osmolal clearance through non–AVP-dependent pathways, possibly mediated by the alpha-2B receptor.[72]

There is experimental evidence that dexmedetomidine attenuates murine radiocontrast nephropathy by preserving cortical blood flow.[73] This mechanism is supported by the observation that dexmedetomidine decreases the renal cortical release of norepinephrine.[74] There is also evidence that dexmedetomidine attenuates murine ischemia-reperfusion injury.[75] However, prospective human studies establishing a benefit are not yet available.

REMIFENTANIL

Remifentanil is an ultra–short-acting opioid that acts as a mu-receptor agonist; it is 250 times more potent than morphine. In 1996, the FDA approved remifentanil as an analgesic agent for the induction and maintenance of anesthesia. In 2002, the European Medicines Agency approved its use for analgesia in mechanically ventilated adult patients in intensive care for up to 3 days.[76] Although remifentanil is used and studied extensively in the operating room, its popularity in the critical care arena is growing.[77]

The pharmacokinetic profile of remifentanil is unique in its class. Described as a "forgiving opioid," remifentanil is characterized by a rapid onset and offset.[78,79] Infusion of remifentanil has an onset of action of 1 minute[78] and rapidly achieves steady-state plasma levels. Its action dissipates within 3 to 10 minutes after discontinuation of an infusion. Remifentanil has a $t_{1/2}$ β of approximately 10 to 20 minutes and a context sensitive half-time of 3 to 4 minutes, regardless of the duration of infusion.[78,80,81]

Remifentanil is metabolized directly in the plasma by nonspecific esterases. Its primary metabolite is remifentanil acid, which has negligible pharmacologic activity. Thus, although remifentanil acid is eliminated by the kidneys, remifentanil's action is not prolonged to a significant extent by renal injury or prolonged infusion in patients in intensive care.[82] Dose adjustments are not required in patients with hepatic dysfunction, but patients with liver disease can be more sensitive to the ventilatory depressant effects of remifentanil.[76,83,84] In contrast to other opioids such as morphine and fentanyl, which can accumulate in organ dysfunction, continuous infusions of remifentanil are not associated with a prolongation of effect. Several publications report the successful use of a remifentanil infusion for up to 33 days with signs of recovery within 10 minutes of discontinuation of the infusion.[76,82,85,86] On the other hand, inadvertent or sudden discontinuation of remifentanil may result in rapid return of the underlying pain. Thus, a longer-acting opioid should be administered before stopping the remifentanil infusion if it is anticipated that analgesic requirements are ongoing.

Similar to other opioids, remifentanil can cause bradycardia, hypotension, respiratory depression, nausea, and skeletal muscle rigidity. Bolus injections of remifentanil are not recommended because they may cause thoracic muscle rigidity with difficult mask or pressure-controlled ventilation.[76]

Several cases of acute withdrawal syndrome have been reported after cessation of remifentanil infusions in the ICU. Tachycardia, hypertension, sweating, mydriasis, and myoclonus have occurred within 10 minutes of discontinuation of remifentanil-based sedation. Symptoms persisted after administration of morphine and clonidine and were resolved only after remifentanil was reinitiated.[87] Gradual tapering of the infusion from 24 to 48 hours may decrease the incidence of a withdrawal syndrome.[87,88]

The rapid offset of the analgesic effect of remifentanil has generated considerable interest in its use to shorten mechanical ventilator times in the ICU. A regimen using remifentanil infusion (0.1–0.15 µg/kg/min) with midazolam, added as needed, shortened the duration of prolonged mechanical ventilation by more than 2 days compared with a midazolam infusion with the addition of fentanyl or morphine.[85] In a randomized controlled trial, the duration of mechanical ventilation, extubation times, and the interval after extubation to ICU discharge were significantly shorter with remifentanil infusion (0.15 µg/kg/min) compared with morphine infusion.[89] When remifentanil-midazolam was compared with sufentanil-midazolam for a median duration of 6 days of mechanical ventilation, mean weaning time was 22 hours compared with 96 hours, even though the sufentanil dose was down-titrated before extubation.[90]

In contrast, there was no difference in time to tracheal extubation when combined infusions of remifentanil (0.15 µg/kg/min) and propofol were compared with fentanyl and propofol after short-term ventilation (12–72 hours). Moreover, patients who received remifentanil complained of more pain during and after tracheal extubation.[91] In a subsequent study by the same group, mechanical ventilation time after cardiac surgery was decreased, and ICU discharge was earlier with a remifentanil-propofol regimen than with a fentanyl-midazolam regimen.[92] These two studies suggest that the duration of ventilation was more influenced by the duration of action of the hypnotic agent (midazolam vs propofol) than the opioid (fentanyl vs remifentanil).

Remifentanil has been evaluated in the neurointensive care setting. Because of its short half-life, remifentanil may facilitate frequent awakening to evaluate neurologic and respiratory parameters.[76,93] In a study of patients with traumatic brain injury who were mechanically ventilated, intracranial pressure (ICP) and cerebral perfusion pressure were maintained with remifentanil.[94] However, in patients with severe traumatic brain injury, even high doses of remifentanil (up to 1.0 µg/kg/min) were insufficient to suppress coughing and elevation of ICP, and increased doses of vasopressor drugs were required to maintain cerebral perfusion pressure.[95]

KETAMINE

Clinical reports of the use of ketamine, a nonbarbiturate phencyclidine derivative, first appeared more than four decades ago.[96] Because it provides analgesia and apparent anesthesia with relative hemodynamic stability, ketamine was considered an ideal "battlefield anesthetic" and was popularized during the Vietnam war.[97]

Ketamine binds with N-methyl-D-aspartate (NMDA) and sigma opioid receptors to produce intense analgesia and a state termed dissociative anesthesia; patients become unresponsive to nociceptive stimuli, but may keep their eyes open and maintain their reflexes. Blood pressure is maintained, and spontaneous breathing and laryngeal reflexes are preserved. Ketamine crosses the blood-brain barrier rapidly and reaches maximal effect in 1 minute. The duration of a single dose of ketamine (2 mg/kg IV) is 10 to 15 minutes. Effective plasma levels of ketamine can be achieved by IV, intramuscular, sublingual, or rectal routes, making it a useful agent in pediatric patients.

In comparison to etomidate, propofol, and midazolam, ketamine appears to act as a cardiac stimulant through sympathetic-mediated mechanisms.[98] At clinical concentrations, ketamine has a positive inotropic action and induces vasoconstriction,[99,100] probably by inhibiting endothelial nitric oxide production,[101] which preserves hemodynamic stability even in septic shock.[102] In animal studies, ketamine acts as a myocardial depressant at very high plasma concentrations, particularly in a catecholamine-depleted state, but this manifestation appears extremely rare in clinical medicine. Although vasoconstriction and inotropy are preferable in certain situations, ketamine increases myocardial oxygen demand, limiting its use in patients with active coronary ischemia. Its sympathomimetic activity is attenuated by concomitant administration of benzodiazepines.[103] Ketamine has bronchodilator activity and may be helpful in the setting of status asthmaticus and bronchospasm,[104,105] although this benefit may be counteracted by its propensity to increase oral secretions.

Ketamine has antiinflammatory properties. It decreases the formation of the cytokine precursor, nuclear factor kappa-light-chain-enhancer of activated B cells (NF-κB), and thereby decreases interleukin-, cytokine-, and endotoxin-induced tumor necrosis factor alpha production.[101,106–109]

Ketamine is still used in clinical anesthesia, but its popularity is limited because of its undesirable side-effect profile of hallucinations (during dissociative anesthesia), emergence delirium and unpleasant recall, increased oral secretions, lacrimation, tachycardia, and the potential for exacerbating myocardial ischemia. Clinicians have avoided ketamine in patients at risk for elevated ICP, which may occur in patients who are spontaneously ventilating. This observation contrasts with studies that show that ketamine does not increase cerebral blood flow or ICP if normal carbon dioxide levels are maintained.[110,111] In combination with benzodiazepines, ketamine prevents increases and decreases in ICP.[112–114] Hemodynamic variables appear to be preserved in brain or spinal cord injured ICU patients.[115] These results suggest that the depth of sedation is more important than the choice of sedative in the management of elevated ICP.

Concerns for the psychotropic effects of ketamine have restricted its use as a sedative-analgesic in the ICU. However, there is evidence that low-dose (60–120 μg/kg/h) ketamine infusions in combination with opioids may not be associated with untoward effects and may improve outcomes in the critically ill. There are several explanations for this benefit. The analgesic effects of ketamine occur at plasma concentrations lower than those associated with its psychotropic activity,[116–119] which are in any event attenuated by simultaneous administration of hypnotics such as propofol or midazolam.[116,120–122] When patients received ketamine infusions as an adjunct to opioid therapy in the ICU, morphine consumption decreased without adverse side effects.[123] Similar findings were noted in a randomized controlled trial of patients who had cardiac surgery, with improvement in patient satisfaction.[124] Prolonged infusion of opioids, such as fentanyl and morphine, inhibits bowel function and promotes constipation or even prolonged ileus. Ketamine does not inhibit bowel mobility and may reduce the feeding complications associated with opioids.[125]

There are other benefits of concomitant administration of ketamine. Major surgery, burns, trauma, and painful procedures in the ICU induce prolonged noxious stimuli, which can cause central sensitization and lead to allodynia (a painful response to an innocuous stimulus), hyperalgesia (an exaggerated response to a painful stimulus), and eventually chronic pain syndromes.[126–128] Opioids themselves can induce hyperalgesia. Ketamine antagonizes the NMDA receptor to block these responses, reducing windup pain and central hyperexcitability. Several studies report that ketamine decreases opioid-induced hyperalgesia.[129,130] Potentially, ketamine can decrease opioid requirements, tolerance, and prevent chronic pain.[97] In summary, ketamine prevents opioid-induced hyperalgesia, decreases inflammation, and ameliorates bronchoconstriction.[130–133] For these reasons, ketamine has regained its popularity as a "battlefield anesthetic" in the Iraq war for the treatment of acute and chronic pain and burns.[97,134]

There are few reports of adverse long-term psychological sequelae after ketamine. Its administration has actually been associated with a decreased incidence of post-traumatic stress disorder (PTSD) in soldiers in the Iraq war.[134,135] There is also evidence that a single dose of IV ketamine rapidly improves symptoms in patients with treatment-resistant depression.[136] Because PTSD and depression can occur in patients who are critically ill, randomized controlled trials to investigate ketamine as a novel therapeutic agent would appear to be warranted.

VOLATILE ANESTHETIC AGENTS

Volatile anesthetics such as isoflurane, sevoflurane, and desflurane are in daily use in the operating room in the delivery of general anesthesia. A major advantage of these halogenated ethers is their quick onset, quick offset, and ease of titration in rendering the patient unconscious, immobile, and amnestic. Although volatile anesthetics are generally associated with stable hemodynamics with little variation, dose-dependent vasodilatation, cardiac depression, and arrhythmias can occur.[137–139] Isoflurane, sevoflurane, and desflurane provide cardioprotection through pharmacologic preconditioning; troponin levels and length of ICU stay are decreased.[140–142] Volatile anesthetics are also bronchodilators and can be prescribed as therapeutic agents for the treatment of bronchospasm and status asthmaticus.[143–146]

Administering sedation through the lung is a dependable route for delivery and elimination. Characterized by a steep dose-response curve, inhalation anesthesia offers a more consistent onset time with less variability compared with traditional IV sedation.[147] Because newer volatile anesthetics (eg, isoflurane, sevoflurane, desflurane) are primarily eliminated by the lungs, there is very little accumulation in patients with renal and hepatic dysfunction, and shorter and more predictable emergence times are observed.[138,148–150] Potential concerns for the accumulation of inorganic fluorides and possible renal dysfunction have not been realized.[151,152]

Intensivists use sedation scales to titrate sedatives in the ICU. In contrast, volatile anesthetics can be monitored by their end-tidal concentration or fraction. This allows excellent control of the drug's actions and can provide a guide to the expected concentration at target organs. In an ICU study, isoflurane end-tidal concentrations correlated with the clinical assessment of sedation depth better than with the BIS index.[153] Adverse effects can be reversed by immediately decreasing the inspired concentration. The term median alveolar concentration (MAC) is defined as the specific vapor end-tidal concentration needed to prevent motor response to a painful stimulus in 50% of subjects; the exact value depends on the potency of the volatile anesthetic.[139] In general, it is recommended that, in the ICU, volatile anesthetics be delivered at an end-tidal concentration of 0.5 MAC.[138,151]

Several clinical trials have compared volatile anesthetics to IV sedation in critical care. Preliminary studies evaluating isoflurane in the ICU found that it was safe, effective, and associated with shorter emergence times than midazolam or propofol.[148–150,154] Compared with propofol, sevoflurane sedation was associated with shorter extubation times and length of hospital stay in patients after cardiac surgery.[151] Similar observations have been made when desflurane was compared with propofol after surgery, and patients appeared to have better cognitive function after emergence.[138] Long-term (6-month) follow-up of patients found a trend toward fewer hallucinations and delusions if they had received isoflurane versus midazolam sedation in the ICU.[155]

Given these benefits, a number of major restrictions remain that govern the routine delivery of volatile anesthesia in the ICU—cost, environmental pollution, and the anesthesiologist's expertise.[156] The need for a cumbersome circuit to deliver the volatile anesthetic and the uneconomical anesthetic consumption in an open ICU ventilator circuit have limited their effectiveness. Non-rebreathing ICU ventilators require a scavenging system to avoid environmental pollution. Several published studies have used a new and fairly simple device, the "Anesthetic Conserving Device" (AnaConDa, Hudson RCI, Uppslands Väsby, Sweden) that allows infusion of liquid volatile anesthetic through the breathing circuit of a standard ICU ventilator. By incorporating a vaporizer chamber with a charcoal reflection filter it creates a semi-closed rebreathing circuit that retains 90% of the inhaled anesthetic. Modifications are still required to enhance safety. Changes in ventilator settings affect the delivery of the anesthetic, and it is possible that the volatile anesthetic syringe could inadvertently be connected to an IV infusion line, but there is little escape of the anesthetic into the atmosphere.[157]

PERIPHERAL OPIOID RECEPTOR ANTAGONISTS

Opioids remain the primary class of analgesic drugs in the ICU and may be infused for many days in critically ill patients. Undesired side effects are legion, and in addition to nausea, vomiting, pruritus, and urinary retention, they include delayed gastric emptying, suppression of bowel motility, constipation, and ileus. Methylnaltrexone and alvimopan are members of a new class of drugs—peripherally acting mu opioid receptor antagonists (PAMORAs). In contrast to naloxone, these medications do not cross the blood-brain barrier to antagonize the central effects of opioids. Instead, they antagonize the peripheral side effects of opioids—notably constipation and ileus—while preserving analgesia. The FDA has approved subcutaneous methylnaltrexone for the relief of opioid-induced constipation and oral alvimopan to facilitate the return of gut dysfunction after anastomotic bowel surgery.

The PAMORAs have the potential to markedly benefit the management of ICU patients, and further trials are warranted. Enteral feeding promotes gut function and the immune system; by delaying gastric emptying, opioids predispose patients to vomiting and pulmonary aspiration. Methylnaltrexone reverses opioid-induced delayed gastric emptying time[158,159] and thereby may not only decrease aspiration risk but also improve absorption of orally administered medications in the critically ill.[160]

Opioids enhance the ability of the human immunodeficiency virus (HIV) to enter macrophages by modulating coreceptors such as beta-chemokines and chemokine (C-C motif) receptor 5 (CCR5). This activity is completely reversed by methylnaltrexone, which may be of benefit to HIV patients receiving or abusing opioids.[161]*Pseudomonas aeruginosa*, a common pathogen in ICU patients, is endowed with mu opioid receptors, which when activated produce factors that enhance gut wall permeability and allow the bacteria to spread systemically. Methylnaltrexone blocks the production of these factors and may help curtail systemic invasion in patients receiving opioids.[160]

REFERENCES

1. Scheinin H, Aantaa R, Anttila M, et al. Reversal of the sedative and sympatholytic effects of dexmedetomidine with a specific alpha2-adrenoceptor antagonist atipamezole: a pharmacodynamic and kinetic study in healthy volunteers. Anesthesiology 1998;89:574–84.
2. Ma D, Hossain M, Rajakumaraswamy N, et al. Dexmedetomidine produces its neuroprotective effect via the alpha 2A-adrenoceptor subtype. Eur J Pharmacol 2004;502:87–97.
3. Fagerholm V, Scheinin M, Haaparanta M. Alpha2A-adrenoceptor antagonism increases insulin secretion and synergistically augments the insulinotropic effect of glibenclamide in mice. Br J Pharmacol 2008;154:1287–96.
4. Takada K, Clark DJ, Davies MF, et al. Meperidine exerts agonist activity at the alpha(2B)-adrenoceptor subtype. Anesthesiology 2002;96:1420–6.
5. Fagerholm V, Rokka J, Nyman L, et al. Autoradiographic characterization of alpha(2C)-adrenoceptors in the human striatum. Synapse 2008;62:508–15.
6. Moura E, Afonso J, Hein L, et al. Alpha2-adrenoceptor subtypes involved in the regulation of catecholamine release from the adrenal medulla of mice. Br J Pharmacol 2006;149:1049–58.
7. Khan ZP, Ferguson CN, Jones RM. Alpha-2 and imidazoline receptor agonists. Their pharmacology and therapeutic role. Anaesthesia 1999;54:146–65.
8. Takamatsu I, Iwase A, Ozaki M, et al. Dexmedetomidine reduces long-term potentiation in mouse hippocampus. Anesthesiology 2008;108:94–102.
9. Venn RM, Karol MD, Grounds RM. Pharmacokinetics of dexmedetomidine infusions for sedation of postoperative patients requiring intensive caret. Br J Anaesth 2002;88:669–75.
10. Vilo S, Rautiainen P, Kaisti K, et al. Pharmacokinetics of intravenous dexmedetomidine in children under 11 yr of age. Br J Anaesth 2008;100:697–700.
11. Petroz GC, Sikich N, James M, et al. A phase I, two-center study of the pharmacokinetics and pharmacodynamics of dexmedetomidine in children. Anesthesiology 2006;105:1098–110.
12. Kivisto KT, Kallio A, Neuvonen PJ. Pharmacokinetics and pharmacodynamics of transdermal dexmedetomidine. Eur J Clin Pharmacol 1994;46:345–9.
13. Anttila M, Penttila J, Helminen A, et al. Bioavailability of dexmedetomidine after extravascular doses in healthy subjects. Br J Clin Pharmacol 2003;56:691–3.
14. De Wolf AM, Fragen RJ, Avram MJ, et al. The pharmacokinetics of dexmedetomidine in volunteers with severe renal impairment. Anesth Analg 2001;93:1205–9.
15. Dutta S, Lal R, Karol MD, et al. Influence of cardiac output on dexmedetomidine pharmacokinetics. J Pharm Sci 2000;89:519–27.
16. Talke P, Richardson CA, Scheinin M, et al. Postoperative pharmacokinetics and sympatholytic effects of dexmedetomidine. Anesth Analg 1997;85:1136–42.
17. Kallio A, Scheinin M, Koulu M, et al. Effects of dexmedetomidine, a selective alpha 2-adrenoceptor agonist, on hemodynamic control mechanisms. Clin Pharmacol Ther 1989;46:33–42.
18. Bulow NM, Barbosa NV, Rocha JB. Opioid consumption in total intravenous anesthesia is reduced with dexmedetomidine: a comparative study with remifentanil in gynecologic videolaparoscopic surgery. J Clin Anesth 2007;19:280–5.

19. Ebert TJ, Hall JE, Barney JA, et al. The effects of increasing plasma concentrations of dexmedetomidine in humans. Anesthesiology 2000;93:382–94.

20. Jorden VS, Pousman RM, Sanford MM, et al. Dexmedetomidine overdose in the perioperative setting. Ann Pharmacother 2004;38:803–7.

21. Ramsay MA, Luterman DL. Dexmedetomidine as a total intravenous anesthetic agent. Anesthesiology 2004;101:787–90.

22. Jalowiecki P, Rudner R, Gonciarz M, et al. Sole use of dexmedetomidine has limited utility for conscious sedation during outpatient colonoscopy. Anesthesiology 2005;103:269–73.

23. Muntazar M, Kumar FC. Cardiac arrest, a preventable yet a possible risk of dexmedetomidine: fact or fiction? Anesthesiology 2004;101:1478–9 [author reply: 9–80].

24. Shah AN, Koneru J, Nicoara A, et al. Dexmedetomidine related cardiac arrest in a patient with permanent pacemaker; a cautionary tale. Pacing Clin Electrophysiol 2007;30:1158–60.

25. Riker RR, Shehabi Y, Bokesch PM, et al. Dexmedetomidine vs midazolam for sedation of critically ill patients: a randomized trial. JAMA 2009;301:489–99.

26. Venn M, Newman J, Grounds M. A phase II study to evaluate the efficacy of dexmedetomidine for sedation in the medical intensive care unit. Intensive Care Med 2003;29:201–7.

27. Reid K, Hayashi Y, Guo TZ, et al. Chronic administration of an alpha 2 adrenergic agonist desensitizes rats to the anesthetic effects of dexmedetomidine. Pharmacol Biochem Behav 1994;47:171–5.

28. Turkmen A, Altan A, Turgut N, et al. The correlation between the Richmond agitation-sedation scale and bispectral index during dexmedetomidine sedation. Eur J Anaesthesiol 2006;23:300–4.

29. Aantaa R. Assessment of the sedative effects of dexmedetomidine, an alpha 2-adrenoceptor agonist, with analysis of saccadic eye movements. Pharmacol Toxicol 1991;68:394–8.

30. Bekker A, Sturaitis MK. Dexmedetomidine for neurological surgery. Neurosurgery 2005;57(1 Suppl):1–10 [discussion: 1–10].

31. Elias WJ, Durieux ME, Huss D, et al. Dexmedetomidine and arousal affect subthalamic neurons. Mov Disord 2008;23:1317–20.

32. Girard TD, Kress JP, Fuchs BD, et al. Efficacy and safety of a paired sedation and ventilator weaning protocol for mechanically ventilated patients in intensive care (Awakening and Breathing Controlled trial): a randomised controlled trial. Lancet 2008;371:126–34.

33. Kress JP, O'Connor MF, Pohlman AS, et al. Sedation of critically ill patients during mechanical ventilation. A comparison of propofol and midazolam. Am J Respir Crit Care Med 1996;153:1012–8.

34. Hsu YW, Cortinez LI, Robertson KM, et al. Dexmedetomidine pharmacodynamics: part I: crossover comparison of the respiratory effects of dexmedetomidine and remifentanil in healthy volunteers. Anesthesiology 2004;101:1066–76.

35. Nelson LE, Lu J, Guo T, et al. The alpha2-adrenoceptor agonist dexmedetomidine converges on an endogenous sleep-promoting pathway to exert its sedative effects. Anesthesiology 2003;98:428–36.

36. Coull JT, Jones ME, Egan TD, et al. Attentional effects of noradrenaline vary with arousal level: selective activation of thalamic pulvinar in humans. Neuroimage 2004;22:315–22.

37. Kauppila T, Kemppainen P, Tanila H, et al. Effect of systemic medetomidine, an alpha 2 adrenoceptor agonist, on experimental pain in humans. Anesthesiology 1991;74:3–8.

38. Arain SR, Ebert TJ. The efficacy, side effects, and recovery characteristics of dexmedetomidine versus propofol when used for intraoperative sedation. Anesth Analg 2002;95:461–6.
39. Arain SR, Ruehlow RM, Uhrich TD, et al. The efficacy of dexmedetomidine versus morphine for postoperative analgesia after major inpatient surgery. Anesth Analg 2004;98:153–8.
40. Al-Metwalli RR, Mowafi HA, Ismail SA, et al. Effect of intra-articular dexmedetomidine on postoperative analgesia after arthroscopic knee surgery. Br J Anaesth 2008;101:395–9.
41. Yoshitomi T, Kohjitani A, Maeda S, et al. Dexmedetomidine enhances the local anesthetic action of lidocaine via an alpha-2A adrenoceptor. Anesth Analg 2008;107:96–101.
42. Deutsch E, Tobias JD. Hemodynamic and respiratory changes following dexmedetomidine administration during general anesthesia: sevoflurane vs desflurane. Paediatr Anaesth 2007;17:438–44.
43. Koroglu A, Teksan H, Sagir O, et al. A comparison of the sedative, hemodynamic, and respiratory effects of dexmedetomidine and propofol in children undergoing magnetic resonance imaging. Anesth Analg 2006;103:63–7.
44. Venn RM, Hell J, Grounds RM. Respiratory effects of dexmedetomidine in the surgical patient requiring intensive care. Crit Care 2000;4:302–8.
45. Arpino PA, Kalafatas K, Thompson BT. Feasibility of dexmedetomidine in facilitating extubation in the intensive care unit. J Clin Pharm Ther 2008;33:25–30.
46. Siobal MS, Kallet RH, Kivett VA, et al. Use of dexmedetomidine to facilitate extubation in surgical intensive-care-unit patients who failed previous weaning attempts following prolonged mechanical ventilation: a pilot study. Respir Care 2006;51:492–6.
47. Akada S, Takeda S, Yoshida Y, et al. The efficacy of dexmedetomidine in patients with noninvasive ventilation: a preliminary study. Anesth Analg 2008; 107:167–70.
48. Bergese SD, Khabiri B, Roberts WD, et al. Dexmedetomidine for conscious sedation in difficult awake fiberoptic intubation cases. J Clin Anesth 2007;19:141–4.
49. Grant SA, Breslin DS, MacLeod DB, et al. Dexmedetomidine infusion for sedation during fiberoptic intubation: a report of three cases. J Clin Anesth 2004;16: 124–6.
50. Stamenkovic DM, Hassid M. Dexmedetomidine for fiberoptic intubation of a patient with severe mental retardation and atlantoaxial instability. Acta Anaesthesiol Scand 2006;50:1314–5.
51. Doufas AG, Lin CM, Suleman MI, et al. Dexmedetomidine and meperidine additively reduce the shivering threshold in humans. Stroke 2003;34:1218–23.
52. Elvan EG, Oc B, Uzun S, et al. Dexmedetomidine and postoperative shivering in patients undergoing elective abdominal hysterectomy. European journal of anaesthesiology 2008;25:357–64.
53. Tobias JD. Bradycardia during dexmedetomidine and therapeutic hypothermia. J Intensive Care Med 2008;23:403–8.
54. Herr DL, Sum-Ping ST, England M. ICU sedation after coronary artery bypass graft surgery: dexmedetomidine-based versus propofol-based sedation regimens. J Cardiothorac Vasc Anesth 2003;17:576–84.
55. Oliver MF, Goldman L, Julian DG, et al. Effect of mivazerol on perioperative cardiac complications during non-cardiac surgery in patients with coronary heart disease: the European Mivazerol Trial (EMIT). Anesthesiology 1999;91: 951–61.

56. Wijeysundera DN, Naik JS, Beattie WS. Alpha-2 adrenergic agonists to prevent perioperative cardiovascular complications: a meta-analysis. Am J Med 2003; 114:742–52.
57. Biccard BM, Goga S, de Beurs J. Dexmedetomidine and cardiac protection for non-cardiac surgery: a meta-analysis of randomised controlled trials. Anaesthesia 2008;63:4–14.
58. Dahmani S, Rouelle D, Gressens P, et al. Effects of dexmedetomidine on hippocampal focal adhesion kinase tyrosine phosphorylation in physiologic and ischemic conditions. Anesthesiology 2005;103:969–77.
59. Prielipp RC, Wall MH, Tobin JR, et al. Dexmedetomidine-induced sedation in volunteers decreases regional and global cerebral blood flow. Anesth Analg 2002;95:1052–9 table of contents.
60. Zornow MH, Maze M, Dyck JB, et al. Dexmedetomidine decreases cerebral blood flow velocity in humans. J Cereb Blood Flow Metab 1993;13:350–3.
61. Drummond JC, Dao AV, Roth DM, et al. Effect of dexmedetomidine on cerebral blood flow velocity, cerebral metabolic rate, and carbon dioxide response in normal humans. Anesthesiology 2008;108:225–32.
62. Maccioli GA. Dexmedetomidine to facilitate drug withdrawal. Anesthesiology 2003;98:575–7.
63. Multz AS. Prolonged dexmedetomidine infusion as an adjunct in treating sedation-induced withdrawal. Anesth Analg 2003;96:1054–5 table of contents.
64. Baddigam K, Russo P, Russo J, et al. Dexmedetomidine in the treatment of withdrawal syndromes in cardiothoracic surgery patients. J Intensive Care Med 2005;20:118–23.
65. Kent CD, Kaufman BS, Lowy J. Dexmedetomidine facilitates the withdrawal of ventilatory support in palliative care. Anesthesiology 2005;103:439–41.
66. Farag E, Chahlavi A, Argalious M, et al. Using dexmedetomidine to manage patients with cocaine and opioid withdrawal, who are undergoing cerebral angioplasty for cerebral vasospasm. Anesth Analg 2006;103:1618–20.
67. Rovasalo A, Tohmo H, Aantaa R, et al. Dexmedetomidine as an adjuvant in the treatment of alcohol withdrawal delirium: a case report. Gen Hosp Psychiatry 2006;28:362–3.
68. Stemp LI, Karras GE Jr. Dexmedetomidine facilitates withdrawal of ventilatory support. Anesthesiology 2006;104:890 [author reply: 890].
69. Darrouj J, Puri N, Prince E, et al. Dexmedetomidine infusion as adjunctive therapy to benzodiazepines for acute alcohol withdrawal. Ann Pharmacother 2008;42:1703–5.
70. Junaid A, Cui L, Penner SB, et al. Regulation of aquaporin-2 expression by the alpha(2)-adrenoceptor agonist clonidine in the rat. J Pharmacol Exp Ther 1999; 291:920–3.
71. Rouch AJ, Kudo LH, Hebert C. Dexmedetomidine inhibits osmotic water permeability in the rat cortical collecting duct. J Pharmacol Exp Ther 1997;281:62–9.
72. Intengan HD, Smyth DD. Clonidine-induced increase in osmolar clearance and free water clearance via activation of two distinct alpha 2-adrenoceptor sites. Br J Pharmacol 1996;119:663–70.
73. Billings FT 4th, Chen SW, Kim M, et al. Alpha2-Adrenergic agonists protect against radiocontrast-induced nephropathy in mice. Am J Physiol Renal Physiol 2008;295:F741–8.
74. Taoda M, Adachi YU, Uchihashi Y, et al. Effect of dexmedetomidine on the release of [3H]-noradrenaline from rat kidney cortex slices: characterization of alpha2-adrenoceptor. Neurochem Int 2001;38:317–22.

75. Kocoglu H, Ozturk H, Yilmaz F, et al. Effect of dexmedetomidine on ischemia-reperfusion injury in rat kidney: a histopathologic study. Ren Fail 2009;31:70–4.
76. Wilhelm W, Kreuer S. The place for short-acting opioids: special emphasis on remifentanil. Crit Care 2008;12(Suppl 3):S5 [abstract].
77. Martin J, Franck M, Sigel S, et al. Changes in sedation management in German intensive care units between 2002 and 2006: a national follow-up survey. Crit Care 2007;11:R124. Available at: http://ccforum.com/content/11/6/R124. Accessed June 15, 2009.
78. Egan TD, Lemmens HJ, Fiset P, et al. The pharmacokinetics of the new short-acting opioid remifentanil (GI87084B) in healthy adult male volunteers. Anesthesiology 1993;79:881–92.
79. Rosow C. Remifentanil: a unique opioid analgesic. Anesthesiology 1993;79: 875–6.
80. Kapila A, Glass PS, Jacobs JR, et al. Measured context-sensitive half-times of remifentanil and alfentanil. Anesthesiology 1995;83:968–75.
81. Westmoreland CL, Hoke JF, Sebel PS, et al. Pharmacokinetics of remifentanil (GI87084B) and its major metabolite (GI90291) in patients undergoing elective inpatient surgery. Anesthesiology 1993;79:893–903.
82. Pitsiu M, Wilmer A, Bodenham A, et al. Pharmacokinetics of remifentanil and its major metabolite, remifentanil acid, in ICU patients with renal impairment. Br J Anaesth 2004;92:493–503.
83. Dershwitz M, Rosow CE. The pharmacokinetics and pharmacodynamics of remifentanil in volunteers with severe hepatic or renal dysfunction. J Clin Anesth 1996;8:88S–90S.
84. Dumont L, Picard V, Marti RA, et al. Use of remifentanil in a patient with chronic hepatic failure. Br J Anaesth 1998;81:265–7.
85. Breen D, Karabinis A, Malbrain M, et al. Decreased duration of mechanical ventilation when comparing analgesia-based sedation using remifentanil with standard hypnotic-based sedation for up to 10 days in intensive care unit patients: a randomised trial [ISRCTN47583497]. Crit Care 2005;9:R200–10.
86. Evane TN, Park GR. Remifentanil in the critically ill. Anaesthesia 1997;52:800–1.
87. Delvaux B, Ryckwaert Y, Van Boven M, et al. Remifentanil in the intensive care unit: tolerance and acute withdrawal syndrome after prolonged sedation. Anesthesiology 2005;102:1281–2.
88. Jacobi J, Fraser GL, Coursin DB, et al. Clinical practice guidelines for the sustained use of sedatives and analgesics in the critically ill adult. Crit Care Med 2002;30:119–41.
89. Dahaba AA, Grabner T, Rehak PH, et al. Remifentanil versus morphine analgesia and sedation for mechanically ventilated critically ill patients: a randomized double blind study. Anesthesiology 2004;101:640–6.
90. Baillard C, Cohen Y, Le Toumelin P, et al. Remifentanil-midazolam compared to sufentanil-midazolam for ICU long-term sedation. Ann Fr Anesth Reanim 2005; 24:480–6 [in French].
91. Muellejans B, Lopez A, Cross MH, et al. Remifentanil versus fentanyl for analgesia-based sedation to provide patient comfort in the intensive care unit: a randomized, double-blind controlled trial [ISRCTN43755713]. Crit Care 2004;8:R1–11.
92. Muellejans B, Matthey T, Scholpp J, et al. Sedation in the intensive care unit with remifentanil/propofol versus midazolam/fentanyl: a randomised, open-label, pharmacoeconomic trial. Crit Care 2006;10:R91. Available at: http://ccforum. com/content/10/3/R91. Accessed June 15, 2009.

93. Karabinis A, Mandragos K, Stergiopoulos S, et al. Safety and efficacy of analgesia-based sedation with remifentanil versus standard hypnotic-based regimens in intensive care unit patients with brain injuries: a randomised, controlled trial [ISRCTN50308308]. Crit Care 2004;8:R268–80.
94. Engelhard K, Reeker W, Kochs E, et al. Effect of remifentanil on intracranial pressure and cerebral blood flow velocity in patients with head trauma. Acta Anaesthesiol Scand 2004;48:396–9.
95. Leone M, Albanese J, Viviand X, et al. The effects of remifentanil on endotracheal suctioning-induced increases in intracranial pressure in head-injured patients. Anesth Analg 2004;99:1193–8 table of contents.
96. Domino EF, Chodoff P, Corssen G. Pharmacologic effects of Ci-581, a new dissociative anesthetic, in man. Clin Pharmacol Ther 1965;6:279–91.
97. Malchow RJ, Black IH. The evolution of pain management in the critically ill trauma patient: emerging concepts from the global war on terrorism. Crit Care Med 2008;36:S346–57.
98. Gelissen HP, Epema AH, Henning RH, et al. Inotropic effects of propofol, thiopental, midazolam, etomidate, and ketamine on isolated human atrial muscle. Anesthesiology 1996;84:397–403.
99. Saegusa K, Furukawa Y, Ogiwara Y, et al. Pharmacologic analysis of ketamine-induced cardiac actions in isolated, blood-perfused canine atria. J Cardiovasc Pharmacol 1986;8:414–9.
100. Reich DL, Silvay G. Ketamine: an update on the first twenty-five years of clinical experience. Can J Anaesth 1989;36:186–97.
101. Chen RM, Chen TL, Lin YL, et al. Ketamine reduces nitric oxide biosynthesis in human umbilical vein endothelial cells by down-regulating endothelial nitric oxide synthase expression and intracellular calcium levels. Crit Care Med 2005;33:1044–9.
102. Yli-Hankala A, Kirvela M, Randell T, et al. Ketamine anaesthesia in a patient with septic shock. Acta Anaesthesiol Scand 1992;36:483–5.
103. Doenicke A, Angster R, Mayer M, et al. The action of S-(+)-ketamine on serum catecholamine and cortisol. A comparison with ketamine racemate. Anaesthesist 1992;41:597–603 [in German].
104. Park GR, Manara AR, Mendel L, et al. Ketamine infusion. Its use as a sedative, inotrope and bronchodilator in a critically ill patient. Anaesthesia 1987;42:980–3.
105. Sarma VJ. Use of ketamine in acute severe asthma. Acta Anaesthesiol Scand 1992;36:106–7.
106. Mazar J, Rogachev B, Shaked G, et al. Involvement of adenosine in the antiinflammatory action of ketamine. Anesthesiology 2005;102:1174–81.
107. Gurfinkel R, Czeiger D, Douvdevani A, et al. Ketamine improves survival in burn injury followed by sepsis in rats. Anesth Analg 2006;103:396–402, table of contents.
108. Kawasaki T, Ogata M, Kawasaki C, et al. Ketamine suppresses proinflammatory cytokine production in human whole blood in vitro. Anesth Analg 1999;89:665–9.
109. Takenaka I, Ogata M, Koga K, et al. Ketamine suppresses endotoxin-induced tumor necrosis factor-alpha production in mice. Anesthesiology 1994;80:402–8.
110. Pfenninger E, Grunert A, Bowdler I, et al. The effect of ketamine on intracranial pressure during haemorrhagic shock under the conditions of both spontaneous breathing and controlled ventilation. Acta Neurochir (Wien) 1985;78:113–8.
111. Schwedler M, Miletich DJ, Albrecht RF. Cerebral blood flow and metabolism following ketamine administration. Can Anaesth Soc J 1982;29:222–6.
112. Himmelseher S, Durieux ME. Revising a dogma: ketamine for patients with neurological injury? Anesth Analg 2005;101:524–34, table of contents.

113. Strebel S, Kaufmann M, Maitre L, et al. Effects of ketamine on cerebral blood flow velocity in humans. Influence of pretreatment with midazolam or esmolol. Anaesthesia 1995;50:223–8.
114. Albanese J, Arnaud S, Rey M, et al. Ketamine decreases intracranial pressure and electroencephalographic activity in traumatic brain injury patients during propofol sedation. Anesthesiology 1997;87:1328–34.
115. Hijazi Y, Bodonian C, Bolon M, et al. Pharmacokinetics and haemodynamics of ketamine in intensive care patients with brain or spinal cord injury. Br J Anaesth 2003;90:155–60.
116. Himmelseher S, Durieux ME. Ketamine for perioperative pain management. Anesthesiology 2005;102:211–20.
117. Bowdle TA, Radant AD, Cowley DS, et al. Psychedelic effects of ketamine in healthy volunteers: relationship to steady-state plasma concentrations. Anesthesiology 1998;88:82–8.
118. Hartvig P, Valtysson J, Lindner KJ, et al. Central nervous system effects of subdissociative doses of (S)-ketamine are related to plasma and brain concentrations measured with positron emission tomography in healthy volunteers. Clin Pharmacol Ther 1995;58:165–73.
119. Tucker AP, Kim YI, Nadeson R, et al. Investigation of the potentiation of the analgesic effects of fentanyl by ketamine in humans: a double-blinded, randomised, placebo controlled, crossover study of experimental pain[ISRCTN83088383]. BMC Anesthesiol 2005;5:2. Available at: http://www.biomedcentral.com/1471-2253/5/2. Accessed June 15, 2009.
120. Badrinath S, Avramov MN, Shadrick M, et al. The use of a ketamine-propofol combination during monitored anesthesia care. Anesth Analg 2000;90:858–62.
121. Friedberg BL. Propofol-ketamine technique: dissociative anesthesia for office surgery (a 5-year review of 1264 cases). Aesthetic Plast Surg 1999;23:70–5.
122. Morse Z, Sano K, Kanri T. Effects of a midazolam-ketamine admixture in human volunteers. Anesth Prog 2004;51:76–9.
123. Guillou N, Tanguy M, Seguin P, et al. The effects of small-dose ketamine on morphine consumption in surgical intensive care unit patients after major abdominal surgery. Anesth Analg 2003;97:843–7.
124. Lahtinen P, Kokki H, Hakala T, et al. S(+)-ketamine as an analgesic adjunct reduces opioid consumption after cardiac surgery. Anesth Analg 2004;99:1295–301 table of contents.
125. Zielmann S, Grote R. The effects of long-term sedation on intestinal function. Anaesthesist 1995;44(Suppl 3):S549–58 [in German].
126. Li J, Simone DA, Larson AA. Windup leads to characteristics of central sensitization. Pain 1999;79:75–82.
127. Oye I. Ketamine analgesia, NMDA receptors and the gates of perception. Acta Anaesthesiol Scand 1998;42:747–9.
128. Mao J, Price DD, Mayer DJ. Mechanisms of hyperalgesia and morphine tolerance: a current view of their possible interactions. Pain 1995;62:259–74.
129. Stubhaug A, Breivik H, Eide PK, et al. Mapping of punctuate hyperalgesia around a surgical incision demonstrates that ketamine is a powerful suppressor of central sensitization to pain following surgery. Acta Anaesthesiol Scand 1997;41:1124–32.
130. Joly V, Richebe P, Guignard B, et al. Remifentanil-induced postoperative hyperalgesia and its prevention with small-dose ketamine. Anesthesiology 2005;103:147–55.
131. Angst MS, Clark JD. Opioid-induced hyperalgesia: a qualitative systematic review. Anesthesiology 2006;104:570–87.

132. De Kock M, Lavand'homme P, Waterloos H. 'Balanced analgesia' in the perioperative period: is there a place for ketamine? Pain 2001;92:373–80.
133. Lois F, De Kock M. Something new about ketamine for pediatric anesthesia? Curr Opin Anaesthesiol 2008;21:340–4.
134. McGhee LL, Maani CV, Garza TH, et al. The correlation between ketamine and posttraumatic stress disorder in burned service members. J Trauma 2008;64: S195–8 [discussion: S7–8].
135. Hersack RA. Ketamine's psychological effects do not contraindicate its use based on a patient's occupation. Aviat Space Environ Med 1994;65:1041–6.
136. Zarate CA Jr, Singh JB, Carlson PJ, et al. A randomized trial of an N-methyl-D-aspartate antagonist in treatment-resistant major depression. Arch Gen Psychiatry 2006;63:856–64.
137. De Hert SG. Volatile anesthetics and cardiac function. Semin Cardiothorac Vasc Anesth 2006;10:33–42.
138. Meiser A, Sirtl C, Bellgardt M, et al. Desflurane compared with propofol for postoperative sedation in the intensive care unit. Br J Anaesth 2003;90:273–80.
139. Campagna JA, Miller KW, Forman SA. Mechanisms of actions of inhaled anesthetics. N Engl J Med 2003;348:2110–24.
140. De Hert SG, Cromheecke S, ten Broecke PW, et al. Effects of propofol, desflurane, and sevoflurane on recovery of myocardial function after coronary surgery in elderly high-risk patients. Anesthesiology 2003;99:314–23.
141. De Hert SG, ten Broecke PW, Mertens E, et al. Sevoflurane but not propofol preserves myocardial function in coronary surgery patients. Anesthesiology 2002;97:42–9.
142. Belhomme D, Peynet J, Louzy M, et al. Evidence for preconditioning by isoflurane in coronary artery bypass graft surgery. Circulation 1999;100:II340–4.
143. Bierman MI, Brown M, Muren O, et al. Prolonged isoflurane anesthesia in status asthmaticus. Crit Care Med 1986;14:832–3.
144. Johnston RG, Noseworthy TW, Friesen EG, et al. Isoflurane therapy for status asthmaticus in children and adults. Chest 1990;97:698–701.
145. Maltais F, Sovilj M, Goldberg P, et al. Respiratory mechanics in status asthmaticus. Effects of inhalational anesthesia. Chest 1994;106:1401–6.
146. Revell S, Greenhalgh D, Absalom SR, et al. Isoflurane in the treatment of asthma. Anaesthesia 1988;43:477–9.
147. Kong KL, Bion JF. Sedating patients undergoing mechanical ventilation in the intensive care unit–winds of change? Br J Anaesth 2003;90:267–9.
148. Millane TA, Bennett ED, Grounds RM. Isoflurane and propofol for long-term sedation in the intensive care unit. A crossover study. Anaesthesia 1992;47:768–74.
149. Kong KL, Willatts SM, Prys-Roberts C. Isoflurane compared with midazolam for sedation in the intensive care unit. BMJ 1989;298:1277–80.
150. Spencer EM, Willatts SM. Isoflurane for prolonged sedation in the intensive care unit; efficacy and safety. Intensive Care Med 1992;18:415–21.
151. Rohm KD, Wolf MW, Schollhorn T, et al. Short-term sevoflurane sedation using the Anaesthetic Conserving Device after cardiothoracic surgery. Intensive Care Med 2008;34:1683–9.
152. Bito H, Atsumi K, Katoh T, et al. Effects of sevoflurane anesthesia on plasma inorganic fluoride concentrations during and after cardiac surgery. J Anesth 1999;13:156–60.
153. Sackey PV, Radell PJ, Granath F, et al. Bispectral index as a predictor of sedation depth during isoflurane or midazolam sedation in ICU patients. Anaesth Intensive Care 2007;35:348–56.

154. Sackey PV, Martling CR, Granath F, et al. Prolonged isoflurane sedation of intensive care unit patients with the anesthetic conserving device. Crit Care Med 2004;32:2241–6.
155. Sackey PV, Martling CR, Carlsward C, et al. Short- and long-term follow-up of intensive care unit patients after sedation with isoflurane and midazolam–a pilot study. Crit Care Med 2008;36:801–6.
156. Maccioli GA, Cohen NH. General anesthesia in the intensive care unit? Is it ready for "prime time"? Crit Care Med 2005;33:687–8.
157. Berton J, Sargentini C, Nguyen JL, et al. AnaConDa reflection filter: bench and patient evaluation of safety and volatile anesthetic conservation. Anesth Analg 2007;104:130–4.
158. Murphy DB, Sutton JA, Prescott LF, et al. Opioid-induced delay in gastric emptying: a peripheral mechanism in humans. Anesthesiology 1997;87:765–70.
159. Yuan CS, Foss JF, O'Connor M, et al. Effects of low-dose morphine on gastric emptying in healthy volunteers. J Clin Pharmacol 1998;38:1017–20.
160. Moss J, Rosow CE. Development of peripheral opioid antagonists' new insights into opioid effects. Mayo Clin Proc 2008;83:1116–30.
161. Ho WZ, Guo CJ, Yuan CS, et al. Methylnaltrexone antagonizes opioid-mediated enhancement of HIV infection of human blood mononuclear phagocytes. J Pharmacol Exp Ther 2003;307:1158–62.

Current Sedation Practices: Lessons Learned from International Surveys

Sangeeta Mehta, MD, FRCPC[a,d],*, Iain McCullagh, MBChB, FRCA[b], Lisa Burry, PharmD, FCCP[c,d]

KEYWORDS

- Critical care • Survey • Sedation • Analgesia • Delirium
- Protocol • Daily interruption

Most critically ill patients experience pain, stress, fear, and anxiety. Sedative, anxiolytic, and analgesic pharmacotherapies are fundamental to the care of critically ill patients, to facilitate the use of life-supporting therapies (ie, mechanical ventilation [MV] or extracorporeal life support) and to ensure patients safety, comfort, and amnesia as needed.[1–3] The last 3 decades have witnessed the development of new therapeutic agents and a gradual evolution in the methods of administering and monitoring these agents.[4–7] The extent of sedative-analgesic use during MV was recently emphasized in an international cohort of more than 5000 adult intensive care unit (ICU) patients, in which these agents were administered to approximately 70% of all patients at some point during the course of ventilation.[8] Despite the ubiquitous use of sedatives and analgesics in the critical care setting, administration of these agents to achieve balanced sedation can be complex, as the medications have numerous limitations, including unpredictable pharmacokinetics/dynamics and significant side effects, particularly in patients with multiorgan failure.

What constitutes the ideal level of sedation in the ICU is still controversial. In the past, the practice of ICU sedation has focused on the extensive use of sedatives to achieve deep sedation or "detachment" from the environment.[4–7] Recent evidence suggests that

A version of this article appeared in the 25:3 issue of *Critical Care Clinics*.

[a] Medical Surgical Intensive Care Unit, Mount Sinai Hospital, 600 University Avenue Room 18-216, Toronto, Ontario M5G 1X5, Canada

[b] Critical Care, Mount Sinai Hospital, University Health Network, 600 University Avenue Room 18-216, Toronto, Ontario M5G 1X5, Canada

[c] Department of Pharmacy, Mount Sinai Hospital, University of Toronto, 600 University Avenue Room 18-216, Toronto, Ontario M5G 1X5, Canada

[d] Department of Medicine, Mount Sinai Hospital, University of Toronto, 600 University Avenue Room 18-216, Toronto, Ontario M5G 1X5, Canada

* Corresponding author.

E-mail address: geeta.mehta@utoronto.ca

Anesthesiology Clin 29 (2011) 607–624

doi:10.1016/j.anclin.2011.09.003

1932-2275/11/$ – see front matter © 2011 Elsevier Inc. All rights reserved.

patient outcomes are significantly influenced by the choice of agent, the presence of over- or undersedation, poor pain control, and delirium.[8–12] Thus, there is a trend toward lighter sedation guided by sedation assessment tools. Two pivotal trials form the scientific foundation of this new era of lighter sedation: a trial evaluating a nurse-driven sedation protocol and a trial evaluating daily sedative interruption.[9,10] These trials demonstrated reductions in the durations of MV and ICU stay in patients managed with the intervention compared with usual care. To optimize the use of these high-risk medications, several guidelines have been published detailing the selection of the agents and the administration and monitoring techniques that have been shown to improve clinical outcomes.[1,13,14] Knowledge gained from surveys about the uptake of these guidelines can identify areas for education and further research. The objective of this review is to discuss the findings of surveys and practice audits evaluating the management of sedation and analgesia and to summarize international critical care sedation practices.

SURVEYS PUBLISHED IN THE LAST DECADE

Surveys can be a powerful tool for collecting data on human characteristics, attitudes, thoughts, and behaviors, and they are sometimes the only available methodological option for acquiring the data necessary to answer an important research question. The results of surveys present important insights into the practice of sedation for critically ill patients. They offer a reflection of actual practice, highlighting the gaps between clinical practice and current recommendations and potentially serving as a basis for the elaboration of guidelines and educational programs.

To identify all relevant articles published between 1999 and 2009, a computerized search of Medline was performed, using the following terms: *sedation*, *analgesia*, *intensive care*, *critical care*, *critical illness*, and *survey*. Relevant articles were retrieved and their bibliographies were reviewed for surveys not identified through the computerized search. Included surveys could have used a postal or electronic questionnaire, to seek the opinions of ICU directors, physicians, nurses, or other allied health care providers, or they could have been conducted as an audit of practice.

Table 1 summarizes the demographics and methodologies of the identified surveys evaluating the use of sedation and analgesia in a critical care setting. Although the vast majority of surveys reflect self-reported practice (ie, perceived practice), a few identified reports provide a snapshot of actual sedative-analgesic drug selection and administration to critically ill, mechanically ventilated patients.

SELECTION OF SEDATIVES AND ANALGESICS

The ideal sedative regimen in ICU patients should (1) provide adequate coverage for pain, sedation, and anxiety; (2) have evidence to support routine or extended use in various critical care populations; (3) have favorable kinetics and clinical effect (eg, rapid onset of action, short half-life, minimal bioaccumulation or drug interactions); (4) be easily titrated and monitored; (5) have tolerable adverse effects; and (6) have a reasonable cost. Unfortunately, none of the commonly available agents satisfy all of these criteria. There are significant limitations associated with each drug, many fitting the definition of "high-risk medications"—those that have the highest risk of causing injury when misused.[34,35] Propofol is associated with hypotension, respiratory depression, hypertriglyceridemia, immune modulation, and propofol infusion syndrome.[36–38] Midazolam and morphine, both associated with hypotension, have active metabolites and unpredictable kinetics in the critically ill or those with significant organ dysfunction,[39] potentially resulting in delayed awakening and liberation from MV compared with short-acting agents. High-dose lorazepam infusions may result in propylene glycol toxicity because of accumulation of the diluent.[40] Furthermore, benzodiazepine use seems to increase the risk of delirium,[41,42] which is an independent predictor of ICU mortality.[42,43] Dexmedetomidine, a centrally acting α_2-adrenergic agonist, provides both sedation and analgesia with minimal respiratory depression. Although dexmedetomidine has recently shown promise for longer-term sedation in the ICU,[11,44] it is not yet commonly available. For a detailed review of sedative and analgesic medications available for clinical use, see the articles by Drs Devlin and Sladen in this edition of the *Clinics.*

The 2002 Society of Critical Care Medicine (SCCM) guidelines for sustained use of sedatives and analgesics recommend propofol or midazolam for short-term sedation, lorazepam for longer-term sedation (>24 hours), and morphine or fentanyl for analgesia.[1] There is a paucity of data available on the choice of sedative, and only a few agents used in the critical care setting have been evaluated by more than one randomized trial. Furthermore, randomized trials have yielded mixed results regarding the "best" regimen to use in critically ill, ventilated patients. Trials comparing propofol with midazolam have found no difference in the quality of sedation overall.[45,46] Despite the higher acquisition cost of propofol, the more rapid awakening associated with this drug leads to similar ICU costs when compared with midazolam and lower costs compared with lorazepam.[47,48]

Table 2 summarizes the survey findings regarding the primary sedative and analgesic choices for both short- and long-term sedation and analgesia and illustrates the wide variation in clinical practice. Most surveys, regardless of country, identified midazolam or propofol as the top two choices for both short-term (<24 hours) and prolonged sedation. The choice of analgesic drugs varies more with geography, with no consistent trend identified across surveys. In the largest European survey, Soliman and colleagues[17] surveyed 674 ICU physicians in 17 western European countries using a short electronic questionnaire. This group found substantial variations in drug choice, particularly for analgesic agents. For patients requiring continuous intravenous analgesia, 33% used morphine often or always, 33% used fentanyl, and 24% sufentanil, with significant differences among countries. For example, morphine was used more commonly than the other agents in the UK, Sweden, Norway, Switzerland, the Netherlands, Spain, and Portugal, whereas fentanyl was preferred in France, Germany, and Italy. Midazolam was used as a sedative most often or always by 63% of respondents and propofol by 35%, but the primary sedative choice varied tremendously internationally, and the use of propofol was more frequent in surgical than medical units. Lorazepam was used extremely rarely (<0.5%). In contrast, the North American surveys document high use of lorazepam and midazolam, with only a small proportion of respondents citing propofol as their primary choice—13% in the study by Mehta and colleagues and 26% in the study by Tanios and colleagues.[22,24] In both the surveys, morphine was the most commonly administered analgesic, with fentanyl a second choice.

Most recently, OConnor and Bucknall[31] reported the results of their Internet-based survey of 348 Australian-New Zealand critical care clinicians, 75% of whom were nurses. For sedation, midazolam and propofol were equally used (approximately 50% each). For analgesia, 67% of respondents used morphine primarily, with only 13% using fentanyl primarily. The data show that newer agents, such as dexmedetomidine and remifentanil, which more closely resemble the definition of the "ideal sedative," are still used much less commonly than the traditional agents.

Several groups have conducted sequential surveys to evaluate change in practice over time. The Danish group noted a significant reduction in the use of benzodiazepines and opioids, as well as an increase in the use of propofol.[15,25] Between 2002 and 2006,

Table 1
Surveys published between 1999 and 2009 evaluating the use of sedation and analgesia

Author, Year	Country/Region	Sampling Period	n, Population	Response Rate (%)	Methodology
Christensen & Thunedberg, 1999[15]	Denmark	1996	49 Physicians	92	Postal questionnaire
Murdoch & Cohen, 2000[16]	UK	1998	255 ICUs	79	Postal questionnaire
Soliman et al, 2001[17]	Europe	NR	647 Physicians	20	E-mail questionnaire
Samuelson et al, 2003[18]	Sweden	2000	89 ICUs—head nurses	98	Postal questionnaire
Rhoney & Murry, 2003[19]	US	1998	457 Physicians 393 Institutions	50	Postal questionnaire
Guldbrand et al, 2004[20]	Nordic	2002	Part I: 88 ICUs Part II: 202 patients	36	Part I: self-administered survey Part II: 5 days of patient data. Internet-based
Kamel et al, 2005[21]	Maghreb	N/A	50 Physicians	36	Postal questionnaire
Tanios et al, 2005[22]	USA	2004	904 Physicians, nurses, pharmacists	<1[a]	Web-based questionnaire
Martin et al, 2005[23]	Germany	2002	220 ICU directors—all anesthesiologists	84	Postal questionnaire
Arroliga et al, 2005[8]	International	NR	5183 Adult patients >12 h MV	N/A	Prospective practice audit
Mehta et al, 2006[24]	Canada	2002	273 Physicians	60	Postal questionnaire
Egerod et al, 2006[25]	Denmark	2003	39 Physician leaders	81	Postal questionnaire

Study	Country	Year	Sample	Response rate (%)	Method
Martin et al, 2006[26]	Germany	2002	305 Patients	84	Postal questionnaire: audit of 1–3 patients, arbitrarily selected
Martin et al, 2007[27]	Germany	2006	214 ICU directors	82	Postal questionnaire, same questionnaire as 2002
Ahmad et al, 2007[28]	Malaysia	N/A	37 ICU directors—all anesthesiologists	92	Postal questionnaire
Payen et al, 2007[29]	France	2004	1382 Patients	N/A	Prospective audit on days 2, 4, and 6 of ICU stay
Reschreiter et al, 2008[30]	UK	2006–2007	192 ICUs	64	Postal questionnaire
OConnor & Bucknall, 2009[31]	Australia	2006–2007	348 ICU staff, 75% nurses	16	Web-based questionnaire
Burry et al, 2009[32,b]	Canada	2008–2009	52 ICUs—clinical pharmacists	N/A	Prospective practice audit
Patel et al, 2009[33]	International	2006–2007	1384 Physicians, nurses, respiratory therapists, pharmacists	N/A	Paper and Web-based questionnaire

Abbreviations: NR, not reported; N/A, not applicable.
[a] <1% of 12,994 SCCM members.
[b] Published as an abstract.

Table 2
Most commonly used pharmacotherapeutic agents

Author, Year	Sedation	Analgesia	Comments
Christensen & Thunedberg, 1999[15]	Midazolam > propofol > diazepam	Morphine > fentanyl > sufentanil	NMBAs <20% patients Haloperidol rarely used
Murdoch & Cohen, 2000[16]	<72 h: Propofol > midazolam Midazolam > propofol	<72 h: Alfentanil >72 h: Morphine	NMBAs administered to 10% of patients
Soliman et al, 2001[17]	Midazolam > propofol	Morphine = fentanyl > sufentanil	Haloperidol used in 9% Clonidine 1.8%
Samuelson et al, 2003[18]	Propofol or midazolam	Opioid	
Rhoney & Murry, 2003[19]	<48 h: Midazolam & propofol >72 h: Lorazepam	<24 h: Fentanyl & meperidine >72 h: Morphine	Reversal agents naloxone & flumazenil commonly used
Guldbrand et al, 2004[20]	Propofol = midazolam	Fentanyl or ketobemidon	Morphine <25%
Kamel et al, 2005[21]	Midazolam	Fentanyl	<14% use propofol
Tanios et al, 2005[22]	Benzodiazepine > propofol	NR	
Martin et al, 2005[23]	<24 h: Propofol >24 h: Midazolam	<24 h: Sufentanil or fentanyl >24 h: Fentanyl	Clonidine used in 66% of patients during weaning
Arroliga et al, 2005[8]	Propofol > diazepam	Fentanyl > morphine	NMBAs used ≥1 day in 13% of patients
Mehta et al, 2006[24]	Midazolam > propofol = lorazepam	Morphine >> fentanyl	

Study			
Egerod et al, 2006[25]	Propofol > midazolam	Fentanyl > sufentanil	Phenobarbital & clonidine used for sedative withdrawal
Martin et al, 2006[26]	<72 h or Weaning: propofol >72 h: Midazolam	<72 h: Piritramide >72 h: Sufentanil	Clonidine as adjuvant in 39% patients during weaning
Martin et al, 2007[27]	<24 h: Propofol > midazolam	<24 h: Sufentanil >24 h: Remifentanil	Ketamine for sedation >72 h and for weaning
Ahmad et al, 2007[28]	Midazolam	Morphine	
Payen et al, 2007[29]	Midazolam > propofol	Sufentanil = fentanyl	Nonopioid analgesia in 35% of patients
Reschreiter et al, 2008[30]	<24 h: Propofol >24 h: Propofol = midazolam	Alfentanil > fentanyl or morphine	Clonidine commonly used for weaning
OConnor & Bucknall, 2009[31]	Midazolam = propofol	Morphine > fentanyl	
Burry et al, 2009[32]	Midazolam > propofol	Fentanyl > morphine	40% received antipsychotics

Abbreviations: NR, not reported; NMBAs, neuromuscular blocking agents.

67% of German ICUs made changes in sedation management as a result of published literature, national guidelines, and scientific lectures.[23,26,27] Propofol was reportedly used more frequently for short-term sedation (83%) and midazolam was used significantly less frequently in 2006 compared with the earlier survey. Clonidine, used as an adjuvant for sedation, was used in a high percentage of both short- and longer-term sedation. Fentanyl was used less frequently in all stages of sedation as sufentanil and remifentanil use increased, and the use of morphine remained stable. Patient-controlled analgesia techniques and neuraxial regional analgesia were more frequently used in all stages of sedation compared with the preliminary survey findings. All three German studies found sedative and analgesic usage to be consistent with their national guidelines.[12] Two surveys from the UK show few major changes in practice over 8 years, and practices were comparable with the rest of Europe.[16,30] The later study noted that choice of agent was largely determined by the duration of drug action rather than cost, and the most frequently used agents were propofol and alfentanil for short-term sedation, and propofol, midazolam, and morphine for longer-term sedation.[30]

Because there may be a substantial gap between physicians statements and clinical practice, there is a need to document what is done daily in ICUs. Payen and colleagues performed a prospective audit of sedation practices, collecting data on 1381 adults admitted to 44 ICUs in France.[29] In contrast to the other European surveys, midazolam was the most commonly used sedative (70%), with propofol used only 20% of the time. Sufentanil (40%) and fentanyl (35%) were the most frequently used opioids, with morphine (15%–20%) and remifentanil (10%) used less often. An extremely important finding of this study was the low incidence of providing specific analgesia during procedural pain (<25%), specifically during suctioning and mobilization. Burry and colleagues, in a prospective audit of 52 ICUs across Canada, found that the most commonly used agents were midazolam (24%) and propofol (19%) for sedation, and fentanyl (22%) and morphine (16%) for analgesia.[32]

Surveys published to date generally show fairly similar preferences for sedative agents, with differences mainly in the proportion of midazolam and propofol used. There is a growing trend toward the use of propofol for short-term sedation, with an overall increase in propofol use in some regions, such as Australia. Lorazepam use is largely confined to North America, possibly demonstrating the influence that national guidelines have on practice, and there seems to be more variation in the selection of analgesic agents. Morphine is still a favored analgesic for most clinicians, but the use of fentanyl and newer, short-acting fentanyl derivatives is increasing. Overall, the variation in practice likely relates to the heterogeneity in the published data supporting the use of these agents, the clinical limitations associated with each drug, familiarity with the products, the severity of patients illness, the anticipated duration of ventilation, and the habits and resources of each site.

INTERMITTENT DOSES, CONTINUOUS INFUSIONS, AND DAILY INFUSION INTERRUPTIONS

Administration of sedatives and analgesics by way of intermittent dosing can result in fluctuation in plasma concentrations, and peaks and troughs can be associated with periods of oversedation and pain or anxiety, respectively. Continuous infusion produces more predictable pharmacokinetics, maximizing the therapeutic benefit and minimizing side effects by avoiding major fluctuations in plasma concentration.[49] However, time to awakening after discontinuation of continuous infusions may be prolonged, presumably due to drug bioaccumulation.[50] One nonrandomized study found a longer duration of MV in patients managed with sedative infusions compared with intermittent dosing.[50] In contrast, Carson and colleagues found that patients managed with propofol infusions had a shorter duration of MV than those treated with intermittent lorazepam.[11] However, because there is no trial comparing continuous with intermittent benzodiazepines, it is not yet clear which strategy results in superior patient outcomes.

Several surveys have explored the proportion of mechanically ventilated patients who receive sedatives and analgesics as continuous infusions versus intermittent dosing. Rhoney and colleagues[19] found that intermittent dosing was most commonly used for morphine (56%), lorazepam (61%), midazolam (56%), and haloperidol (81%), whereas propofol and fentanyl were more likely to be administered as continuous infusions, 87% and 96%, respectively. Recent surveys describe more frequent use of continuous infusions, particularly in France (>90%),[29] Sweden (99%),[18] and Australia (>70%).[31] In the survey of Canadian physicians, 26% use infusions in few patients (<25%), 38% in some patients (25%–75%), and 26% in most or all patients.[24] This group also found that lorazepam was primarily administered as intermittent bolus (64%), midazolam by either intermittent bolus (53%) or infusion (45%), and propofol as a continuous infusion (79%). Tanios and colleagues[22] found that 64% of respondents administer sedatives by continuous infusion, with only 10% using bolus doses. Among commonly cited reasons for the use of infusions are (1) ICU patients barriers to communicating their sedative requirements; (2) randomized trials demonstrating that the maintenance of adequate continuous opioid blood concentration improves patients analgesia[51]; and (3) increasing evidence from randomized trials that the continuous administration of opioids decreases morbidity, and may decrease mortality, compared with intermittent administration.[52]

To minimize the potential of oversedation with the use of continuous infusions, the concept of daily drug interruption with reintroduction of the infusions at a reduced rate, if necessary, has been explored.[6,10,43] Daily interruption of sedative and analgesic infusions allows better assessment of a patients sedative needs, reduces drug bioaccumulation, and has been shown to significantly reduce the duration of MV and ICU and hospital lengths of stay compared with usual care.[10] Other notable benefits of daily sedation interruption include a reduced incidence of posttraumatic stress disorder,[53] reduced complications of critical illness,[53,54] and no increase in risk of myocardial ischemia.[55] In a more recent randomized controlled trial, Girard and colleagues randomized patients to daily sedative interruption or routine sedative management, with both groups receiving daily spontaneous breathing trials. The daily interruption group had more ventilator-free days and earlier ICU and hospital discharge, at the expense of a higher incidence of self-extubation (16 vs 6 patients, $P = .03$), although reintubation rates were similar.[43] Another study has also raised concern that daily interruption may not be ideal for all ICU patients. In a single-center trial that was terminated prematurely by the Data Monitoring Committee, patients randomized to daily interruption had more days of MV and longer ICU and hospital lengths of stay compared with patients managed with a sedation protocol.[56] These investigators proposed the high proportion of patients with alcohol and drug use disorders as an explanation for their findings, suggesting that daily sedative interruption may not be appropriate for these patients. However, given the early trial termination, no firm conclusions can be made. Daily interruption is now officially endorsed by the UK Department of Health[57] (www.clean-safe-care.nhs.uk), the Institute for Healthcare Improvement (www.IHI.org), Safer Health Care Now! (www.saferhealthcarenow.ca), and the Surviving Sepsis Campaigns[58] (www.survivingsepsis.org).

Table 3 presents the proportion of ICUs/physicians who report the use of daily interruption. Since the first description of daily sedative interruption was published in

Table 3
Reported use of sedation strategies in published surveys

Author, Year	Assessment Tools	Protocol-Directed Sedation	Daily Sedative/Analgesic Interruption
Christensen & Thunedberg, 1999[15]	16% (all Ramsay)	33%	NR
Murdoch & Cohen, 2000[16]	67% (28% Ramsay)	NR	NR
Soliman et al, 2001[17]	43% (74% Ramsay)	NR	NR
Samuelson et al, 2003[18]	16% (Ramsay, Addenbrooke, Newcastle, SAS)	27%	1%
Rhoney & Murry, 2003[19]	78% (43% GCS, 42% Ramsay)	33%	NR
Guldbrand et al, 2004[20]	53% (34% MAAS, 9% Ramsay)	41%	15%
Martin et al, 2005[23]	31% (8% Ramsay)	21%	NR
Arroliga et al, 2005[8]	NR	NR	NR
Kamel et al, 2005[21]	14% (all Ramsay)	20%	NR
Tanios et al, 2005[22]	NR	64%	40%
Mehta et al, 2006[24]	49% (67% Ramsay, 10% SAS, 9% GCS, 8% MAAS)	29%	40%
Egerod et al, 2006[25]	44% (mostly Ramsay)	23%	31%
Martin et al, 2006[26]	46% (mostly Ramsay)	52%	34%
Martin et al, 2007[27]	35% (mostly Ramsay)	38%	14%
Ahmad et al, 2007[28]	28% (48% Ramsay, 16% RASS, 15% SAS)	36%	0%
Payen et al, 2007[29]	88% (66% Ramsay)	80%	78%
Reschreiter et al, 2008[30]	75% (GCS 56%, SAS 25%, 8% RASS)	54% sedation 51% analgesia	62%
OConnor & Bucknall, 2009[31]	8%	43%	Sedative 20% of days Analgesic 9% of days
Patel et al, 2009[33]	88% (38% Ramsay, 26% RASS)	71%	22% practice drug interruption on 75%–100% of days

Abbreviations: SAS, sedation agitation scale; GCS, Glasgow Coma Scale; MAAS, motor activity assessment scale; RASS, Richmond agitation sedation scale; NR, not reported.

2000,[10] the use of this strategy seems to be increasing. Compared with a rate of 15% in the Nordic countries, reported by Guldbrand and colleagues in 2004,[20] the reported proportion of ICUs practicing daily interruption in 2006 was 40% in Canada, 31% in Denmark, and 34% in Germany.[24,25,27] However, the Canadian group reported that 63% of physicians interrupt infusions in only some patients, often avoiding this approach in patients who are extremely ill.[24] A more recent survey reported a higher overall rate of 62% in Australia and New Zealand, with 58% using it in more than 25% of patients, and 25% in more than 75% of patients.[31] In 2008, Reschreiter and colleagues reported a rate of 78% in the UK; however, only 56% of ICUs audit the performance of daily interruption, and find variable compliance.[30] Surprisingly, none of the 44 French ICUs participating in the prospective audit of sedation practice reported the use of daily sedative interruption.[29] In their 2008 prospective audit of sedation practices in 52 Canadian ICUs, Burry and colleagues observed that sedative and analgesic interruptions were done on 20% and 9% of days, respectively, in contrast to 40% self-reported use in 2006.[24,32] These data suggest that the actual number of ICUs or clinicians practicing daily sedative interruption is lower than the percent identified from self-report.

There are many reasons why ICU clinicians are not practicing daily sedative interruption. In a US study, the three most common barriers to the use of daily interruption, reported by physicians, nurses, or pharmacists, were fear of respiratory compromise (26%), lack of nursing acceptance (22%), and concern about patient-initiated device removal (20%).[22] Other surveys have identified clinical reasons why individual patients may not be suitable, such as cardiovascular, respiratory, or neurologic instability. More clinical trials are needed to better identify "ideal" patients and to further demonstrate the safety of this strategy. OConnor and Bucknall[31] found that nurses were more likely than physicians to believe that daily sedative interruption could make their jobs more difficult.

USE OF SEDATION PROTOCOLS AND ASSESSMENT TOOLS

Sedation protocols are algorithms by which nurses adjust sedatives based on written guidelines and patient assessment. These protocols decrease variability in sedation practices, promote a consistent approach to sedation, and reduce treatment delays by eliminating the need for physician orders. The strongest data to support the use of a protocol are from Brook and colleagues,[9] who randomized 322 ventilated adults to usual sedation care or to a nurse-driven protocol, whereby nurses titrated sedatives according to the patients level of sedation, as measured by the Ramsay scale. In this study, the use of a sedation protocol reduced the duration of MV by 1.5 days, as well as ICU and hospital stays (1 and 6 days, respectively). Quality assurance studies have shown that incorporation of a sedation protocol and scale into routine practice can reduce the incidence of oversedation, the duration of MV, and ICU length of stay.[59,60] **Table 3** shows the reported use of sedation protocols since the publication of the trial by Brook and colleagues. Although earlier surveys report rates of 20% to 30%, there seems to be a trend toward an increasing use of sedation protocols, with the highest rates reported in Australia (54%),[31] Germany (52%),[27] United States (64%),[22] and United Kingdom (80%).[30] In Canada, the use of protocols increased from 29% in 2002 to 43% in 2008[24,32]; most of the protocols in use were developed locally.[17] Besides improving communication and standardizing therapy, Payen and colleagues[29] found increased dedicated education aimed at pain and sedation in sites where protocols were in use.

Regardless of the sedative-analgesic regimen selected, clinicians face the challenge of avoiding over- and undersedation. The key to providing patients with balanced therapy is combining knowledge of the desired clinical effects and possible adverse effects, with dose adjustment based on frequent individualized patient assessment. Assessing sedative-analgesic requirements can be challenging in ventilated patients, with whom communication is invariably limited. The use of a sedation scale may improve clinical assessment. A sedation assessment tool should be developed by a multidisciplinary team and have discrete criteria that are easy to recall, use, and interpret.[61] There are many validated scales with good inter-rater reliability, including the Ramsay scale,[62] the sedation agitation scale,[63] and the motor activity assessment scale.[64] Several newer scales, such as the Richmond agitation and sedation scale,[65] have also been shown to accurately reflect changes in sedation status over time (responsiveness). For the assessment of pain, two tools are available besides the visual analog scale: the behavior pain scale and critical-care pain observation tool, both with acceptable validity and reliability.[66–69] A newer generation of scales, such as the Vancouver interactive and calmness scale,[70] the Minnesota sedation assessment tool,[71] and the adaptation to the intensive care environment instruments[72] evaluate multiple domains, such as consciousness, agitation, motor activity, sleep, and patient-ventilator synchrony. Although the choice of scales may be overwhelming, no single tool has been identified, at this point, as offering complete assessment of the various essential domains of pain, sedation, anxiety, delirium, and patient-ventilator synchrony. Further study is needed to extend the use of these tools to various ICU patient populations and to address limitations, such as assessment of pain in the presence of delirium or deep sedation.

Table 3 describes the reported frequency of use of a sedation scale, and the particular scale used. The Ramsay scale, published in 1974, seems to be the most commonly adopted scale, even in recent surveys, despite not being designed for use in ICU patients.[62] Despite the publication of guidelines recommending routine incorporation of a pain scale,[1,73] the surveys reveal infrequent use. In Germany, the use of a pain scale increased from 9 to 33 of 214 units between 2002 and 2006.[23,27] Although a protocol was used to assess and manage pain in 56% of Australian and New Zealand ICUs, there was no comment about the use of a pain scale.[31] In Canada, 49% of physicians reported using a sedation scale in 2002,[24] but a subsequent audit in 2008 revealed that only 8% of patients had their sedation adjusted using a scale.[32] Several surveys have found a difference between target and actual levels of sedation,[26,29,74] meaning that many patients are more deeply sedated than desired. Another disturbing finding is the discrepancy between the percentage of patients receiving sedation and analgesia, and the percentage who have formal assessment using a sedation scale.[29]

DELIRIUM

Delirium has been strongly associated with poor outcomes, including longer ICU and hospital lengths of stay and higher mortality.[41,42] Although the incidence of delirium in the ICU may be as high as 60% to 80%, it is often overlooked or misdiagnosed because of the difficulty in assessing the mental status of intubated patients. The confusion assessment method for the ICU (CAM-ICU) and intensive care delirium-screening checklist are valid and reliable tools for the diagnosis of delirium in ICU patients, and can be applied by physicians, nurses, or pharmacists.[75,76] Either of these tools can be used to detect hypo- or hyperactive delirium, as they assess clarity of thought rather than focusing on the level of consciousness.

Very few surveys have queried the use of delirium assessment tools or antipsychotics in the ICU. Several surveys have reported haloperidol use, but there are no data regarding the newer atypical agents, such as risperidone and quetiapine. Mehta and colleagues found that haloperidol was used often in 50% of patients, and routinely in 11%, yet a delirium scale was rarely used.[24] In their follow-up prospective audit of sedation practices in 52 Canadian ICUs, 40% of patients received antipsychotics, most commonly haloperidol (33%), but a delirium scale was used in fewer than 1% of patients.[32] In Europe, Soliman and colleagues found that 58% of respondents used haloperidol.[17] Rhoney and colleagues reported that 37% of respondents used haloperidol frequently, 49% occasionally, and 11% routinely.[19] In the survey by Patel and colleagues, delirium was considered a serious problem by most health care providers. They found that 59% of respondents screened for delirium, with 33% using a specific screening tool, most commonly the CAM-ICU, and haloperidol was the antipsychotic of choice for more than 80% of respondents.[33]

DETERMINANTS OF PRACTICE

Several studies have explored the determinants of sedation practices. For Canadian and US physicians, frequently cited reasons for choice of agent are clinician familiarity, rapid onset of action, and adverse drug effects.[19,24] In Canada, intensivists working in university-affiliated hospitals and larger ICUs ($\geq$15 beds) were more likely to use sedation protocols and scales, and younger physicians ($\leq$40 years) were more likely to use daily sedative interruption.[24]

In the UK, Reschreiter and colleagues[30] noted that the choice of agent was largely determined by the duration of drug action rather than cost. Samuelson reported that local ICU tradition and personal attitudes play a major role in sedation practice in Swedish ICUs.[18] In Australia and New Zealand, the most important determinants of sedation management decisions were level of experience, level of education, support from medical staff, and directions from medical staff.[31] In Malaysia, the reported determinants of sedative choice were familiarity, pharmacology, the expected duration of sedation, the patients diagnosis, and cost.[28] In the UK, 52% of ICUs quoted cost as "important" when considering sedation choices,[30] and 64% of Maghrebian intensivists stated that cost was important.[21] To illustrate the difference in cost with some of the newer agents, in Australia, remifentanil is 70 times more expensive than morphine per day.[31] Notwithstanding the potential advantages of remifentanil over morphine, it is clear why its use is not more widespread.

SUMMARY

Limitations are inherent to surveys. Most surveys have low response rates, which raises the issue of responder bias. Another limitation of self-report surveys stems from the possible differences between stated and actual practice. That is, what physicians report that they do in surveys often contrasts significantly with what they do in observational studies, as highlighted by the Canadian surveys conducted in 2002 and 2008.[24,32] Some surveys report estimates provided by ICU nurse managers[18] or physician directors,[30] potentially resulting in inaccurate estimates or data reflecting the individuals practice rather than the entire ICU. Surveys may not reflect how different specialists practice; for example, the German surveys collected data only in ICUs run by anesthesiologists.[23,26,27]

Notwithstanding these limitations, surveys provide a wealth of information on current practice and determinants of practice, and serve as a useful tool to guide future research and educational interventions. The authors identified substantial international variation in the use of sedative and analgesic drugs, and marked changes over the last 10 years. Overall, there is a trend toward lighter sedation, along with a shift from benzodiazepines toward propofol, and from morphine toward fentanyl and remifentanil. Despite the publication of numerous studies and guidelines for sedation and analgesia, actual practice differs from recommended practice, suggesting that the impact of clinical trials and guidelines on physician practice is quite low. It is clear that there remain substantial barriers to the incorporation of sedation scales, protocols, and daily interruption into routine ICU care.

REFERENCES

1. Jacobi J, Fraser GL, Coursin DB, et al. Clinical practice guidelines for the sustained use of sedatives and analgesics in the critically ill adult: sedation and analgesia task force of the American College of Critical Care Medicine (ACCM) of the Society of Critical Care Medicine. Crit Care Med 2002;30:119–41.
2. Ostermann ME, Keenan SP, Seiferling RA, et al. Sedation in the intensive care unit: a systematic review. JAMA 2000;283:1451–9.
3. Aitkenhead AR. Analgesia and sedation in intensive care. Br J Anaesth 1989; 63(2):196–206.
4. Dasta J, Fuhrman TM, McCandles C. Patterns of prescribing and administering drugs for agitation and pain in patients in a surgical intensive care unit. Crit Care Med 1994;22:974–80.
5. Merriman H. The techniques used to sedate ventilated patients. Intensive Care Med 1981;7:217–24.
6. Hansen-Flaschen J, Brazinsky S, Basile C, et al. Use of sedating drugs and neuromuscular blocking agents in patients requiring mechanical ventilation for respiratory failure: a national survey. JAMA 1991;266:2870–5.
7. Bion JF, Ledingham IM. Sedation in intensive care: a postal survey. Intensive Care Med 1987;13:215–6.
8. Arroliga A, Frutos-Vivar F, Hall J, et al. International Mechanical Ventilation Study Group. Use of sedatives and neuromuscular blockers in a cohort of patients receiving mechanical ventilation. Chest 2005;128(2):496–506.
9. Brook AD, Ahrens TS, Schaiff R, et al. Effect of a nursing implemented sedation protocol on the duration of mechanical ventilation. Crit Care Med 1999;27:2609–15.
10. Kress JP, Pohlman AS, OConnor MF, et al. Daily interruption of sedative infusions in critically ill patients undergoing mechanical ventilation. N Engl J Med 2000; 342(20):1471–7.
11. Carson SS, Kress JP, Rodgers JE, et al. A randomized trial comparing intermittent bolus lorazepam and continuous infusions of propofol with daily interruption in mechanically ventilated patients. Crit Care Med 2006;34(5):1326–32.
12. Pandharipande P, Pun BT, Herr DL, et al. Effect of sedation with dexmedetomidine vs lorazepam on acute brain dysfunction in mechanically ventilated patients: the MENDS randomised controlled trial. JAMA 2007;298(22):2644–53.
13. Martin J, Basell K, Burkle H, et al. Analgesie und sedierung in der intensivmedizin-S2-leitlinien der Deutschen gesellschaft fur anaesthesiologie und intensivmedizin. Anasth Intensivmed 2005;46:1–20 [German].
14. Lui LL, Gropper MA. Postoperative analgesia and sedation in the adult intensive care unit: a guide to drug selection. Drugs 2003;63:755–67.
15. Christensen BV, Thunedberg IP. Use of sedatives, analgesics and neuromuscular blocking agents in Danish ICUs 1996/97. A national survey. Intensive Care Med 1999;25:186–91.

16. Murdoch S, Cohen A. Intensive care sedation: a review of current British practice. Intensive Care Med 2000;26:922–8.
17. Soliman HM, Melot C, Vincent JL. Sedative and analgesic practice in the intensive care unit: the results of a European survey. Br J Anaesth 2001;87:186–92.
18. Samuelson KA, Larsson S, Lundberg D, et al. Intensive care sedation of mechanically ventilated patients: a national Swedish survey. Intensive Crit Care Nurs 2003;19:350–62.
19. Rhoney DH, Murry KR. National survey of the use of sedating drugs, neuromuscular blocking agents, and reversal agents in the intensive care unit. J Intensive Care Med 2003;18:139–45.
20. Guldbrand P, Berggren L, Brattebo G, et al. Survey of routines for sedation of patients on controlled ventilation in Nordic intensive care units. Acta Anaesthesiol Scand 2004;48:944–50.
21. Kamel S, Tahar M, Nabil F, et al. Sedative practice in intensive care units; results of a Maghrebian survey. Tunis Med 2005;83(11):657–63.
22. Tanios MA, Devlin JW, Epstein SK, et al. Perceived barriers to implementing strategy of daily interruption of sedative in the intensive care unit for critically ill patients. Journal of Critical Care 2009;24:66–73.
23. Martin J, Parsch A, Franck M, et al. Practice of sedation and analgesia in German intensive care units: results of a national survey. Crit Care 2005;9:R117–23.
24. Mehta S, Burry L, Fischer S, et al. Canadian survey of the use of sedatives, analgesics, and neuromuscular blocking agents in critically ill patients. Crit Care Med 2006;34(2):374–80.
25. Egerod I, Christensen BV, Johansen L. Trends in sedation practices in Danish intensive care units in 2003: a national survey. Intensive Care Med 2006;32:60–6.
26. Martin J, Franck M, Fischer M, et al. Sedation and analgesia in German intensive care units: how is it done in reality? Results of a patient based survey of analgesia and sedation. Intensive Care Med 2006;32:1137–42.
27. Martin J, Franck M, Sigel S, et al. Changes in sedation management in German intensive care units between 2002 and 2006: a national follow up survey. Crit Care 2007;11:R124.
28. Ahmad N, Tan CC, Balan S. The current practice of sedation and analgesia in intensive care units in Malaysian public hospitals. Med J Malaysia 2007;62(2):122–6.
29. Payen JF, Chanques G, Mantz J. Current practices in sedation and analgesia for mechanically ventilated critically ill patients: a prospective multicenter patient-based study. Anesthesiology 2007;107:687–95.
30. Reschreiter H, Maiden M, Kapila A. Sedation practice in the intensive care unit: a UK national survey. Crit Care 2008;12:R152.
31. OConnor M, Bucknall T. Sedation management in Australian and New Zealand ICUs: doctors and nurses practice and opinions. Am J Crit Care 2010;19(3):285–95.
32. Burry L, Perreault M, Williamson D, et al. A prospective evaluation of sedative, analgesic, anti-psychotic and paralytic practices in Canadian mechanically ventilated adults. Proc Am Thorac Soc 2009;179:A5492.
33. Patel RP, Gambrell M, Speroff T, et al. Delirium and sedation in the intensive care unit: survey of behaviours and attitudes of 1384 healthcare professionals. Crit Care Med 2009;37(3):825–32.
34. Institute for Safe Medication Practices (ISMP) Canada Bulletins. Lowering the risk of medication errors: independent double checks. 2005. Available at: http://www.ismp-canada.org. Accessed March 1, 2009.

35. Riker RR, Fraser GL. Adverse events associated with sedatives, analgesics and other drugs that provide patient comfort in the intensive care unit. Pharmacotherapy 2005;25(5 Pt 2):8S–18S.
36. Kam PC, Cardone D. Propofol infusion syndrome. Anaesthesia 2007;62:690–701.
37. Fong JJ, Sylvia L, Ruthazer R, et al. Predictors of mortality in patients with suspected propofol infusion syndrome. Crit Care Med 2008;36(8):2281–7.
38. Marik PE. Propofol: an immunomodulating agent. Pharmacotherapy 2005;25 (5 Pt 2):28S–33S.
39. Spina SP, Ensom MHH. Clinical pharmacokinetic monitoring of midazolam in critically ill patients. Pharmacotherapy 2007;27(3):389–98.
40. Arroliga AC, Shehab N, McCarthy K, et al. Relationship of continuous infusion lorazepam to serum propylene glycol concentration in critically ill adults. Crit Care Med 2004;32(8):1709–14.
41. Pandharipande P, Ely EW. Sedative and analgesic medications: risk factors for delirium and sleep disturbances in the critically ill. Crit Care Clin 2006;22:313–27.
42. Ely EW, Shintani A, Truman B, et al. Delirium as a predictor of mortality in mechanically ventilated patients in the intensive care unit. JAMA 2004;291(14):1753–62.
43. Girard TD, Kress JP, Fuchs BD, et al. Efficacy and safety of a paired sedation and ventilator weaning protocol for mechanically ventilated patients in intensive care (awakening and breathing controlled trial): a randomised controlled trial. Lancet 2008;371:126–34.
44. Riker RR, Shehabi Y, Wisemandle W, et al. Dexmedetomidine improves outcomes for long term ICU sedation when compared to midazolam: the SEDCOM study. JAMA 2009;301(5):489–99.
45. Chamorro C, De Latorre FJ, Montero A, et al. Comparative study of propofol versus midazolam in the sedation of critically ill patients: results of a prospective randomised controlled trial. Crit Care Med 1996;24(6):932–40.
46. Ronan KP, Gallagher TJ, George B, et al. Comparison of propofol and midazolam for sedation in intensive care unit patients. Crit Care Med 1995;23(2):286–93.
47. Barrientos-Vega R, Sanchez-Soria MM, Morales-Garcia C, et al. Prolonged sedation of critically ill patients with midazolam or propofol: impact on weaning and costs. Crit Care Med 1997;25(1):33–41.
48. Cox CE, Reed SD, Govert JA, et al. Economic evaluation of propofol and lorazepam for critically ill patients undergoing mechanical ventilation. Crit Care Med 2008;36(3):706–10.
49. Pohlman A, Simpson K, Hall J. Continuous intravenous infusions of lorazepam versus midazolam for sedation during mechanical ventilatory support: a prospective, randomized study. Crit Care Med 1994;22:1241–7.
50. Kollef MH, Levy NT, Ahrens TS, et al. The use of continuous IV sedation is associated with prolongation of mechanical ventilation. Chest 1998;114(2):541–8.
51. Richman PS, Baram D, Varela M, et al. Sedation during mechanical ventilation: a trial of benzodiazepine and opiate in combination. Crit Care Med 2006;34(5):1395–401.
52. Elliot R, McKinley S, Aitken LM, et al. The effect of an algorithm-based sedation guideline on the duration of mechanical ventilation in an Australian intensive care unit. Intensive Care Med 2006;32:1506–14.
53. Kress JP, Gehlbach B, Lacy M, et al. The long term psychological effects of daily sedative interruption on critically ill patients. Am J Respir Crit Care Med 2003;168: 1457–61.
54. Schweickert WD, Gehlbach BK, Pohlman AS, et al. Daily interruption of sedative infusions and complications of critical illness in mechanically ventilated patients. Crit Care Med 2004;32:1272–6.

55. Kress JP, Vinayak AG, Levitt J, et al. Daily sedative interruption in mechanically ventilated patients at risk for coronary artery disease. Crit Care Med 2007; 35(2):365–71.
56. De Wit M, Gennings C, Jenvey WI, et al. Randomized trial comparing daily interruption of sedation and nursing-implemented sedation algorithm in medical intensive care unit patients. Crit Care 2008;12(3):R70.
57. Department of Health. The Health Act 2006—code of practice for the prevention and control of healthcare associated infections. London: Department of Health; 2006. Available at: http://www.dh.gov.uk/assetRoot/04/13/93/37/04139337.pdf. Accessed March 1, 2009.
58. Dellinger RP, Levy MM, Carlet JM, et al. Surviving sepsis campaign: international guidelines for management of severe sepsis and septic shock 2008. Intensive Care Med 2008;36(1):296–327.
59. Brattebo G, Hofoss D, Flaaten H, et al. Effect of a scoring system and protocol for sedation on duration of patients need for ventilator support in a surgical intensive care unit. BMJ 2002;324:1386–9.
60. De Jonghe B, Bastuji-Garin S, Fangio P, et al. Sedation algorithm in critically ill patients without acute brain injury. Crit Care Med 2005;33:120–7.
61. Weinert CR, Chlan L, Gross C. Sedating critically ill patients: factors affecting nurses delivery of sedative therapy. Am J Crit Care 2001;10:156–67.
62. Ramsay MA, Savage TM, Simpson BR, et al. Controlled sedation with alphaxalone-alphadolone. BMJ 1974;2:81–4.
63. Riker R, Picard JT, Fraser GL. Prospective evaluation of the sedation-agitation scale for adult critically ill patients. Crit Care Med 1999;27:1325–9.
64. Devlin JW, Boleski G, Mlynarek M, et al. Motor activity assessment scale: a valid and reliable sedation scale for use with mechanically ventilated patients in an adult surgical intensive care unit. Crit Care Med 1999;27:1271–5.
65. Sessler CN, Gosnell MS, Grap MJ, et al. The Richmond agitation-sedation scale: validity and reliability in adult intensive care patients. Am J Respir Crit Care Med 2002;166:1338–44.
66. Payen JF, Bru O, Bosson J, et al. Assessing pain in critically ill sedated patients by using a behavioural pain scale. Crit Care Med 2001;29(12):2258–63.
67. Gelinas C, Fillion L, Puntillo KA, et al. Validation of the critical-care pain observation tool in adult patients. Am J Crit Care 2006;15(4):420–7.
68. Young J, Siffleet J, Nikoletti S, et al. Use of a behavioural pain scale to assess pain in ventilated, unconscious and/or sedated patients. Intensive Crit Care Nurs 2006;22(1):32–9.
69. Li D, Puntillo K, Miakowski C, et al. A review of objective pain measures for use with critical care adult patients unable to self-report. J Pain 2008;9(1): 2–10.
70. de Lemos J, Tweeddale M, Chittock D. Measuring quality of sedation in adult mechanically ventilated critically ill patients. The Vancouver interaction and calmness scale. Sedation Focus Group. J Clin Epidemiol 2000;53(9):908–19.
71. Weinert C, McFarland L. The state of intubated ICU patients: development of a two-dimensional sedation rating scale for critically ill adults. Chest 2004; 126(6):1883–90.
72. De Jonghe B, Cook D, Griffith L, et al. Adaptation to the Intensive Care Environment (ATICE): development and validation of a new sedation assessment instrument. Crit Care Med 2003;31(9):2344–54.
73. Mattia C, Savoia G, Paoletti F, et al. SIAARTI recommendations for analgosedation in intensive care unit. Minerva Anestesiol 2006;72(10):769–805.

74. Weinert CR, Calvin AD. Epidemiology of sedation and sedation adequacy for mechanically ventilated patients in a medical and surgical intensive care unit. Crit Care Med 2007;35(2):393–401.
75. Ely EW, Inouye SK, Bernard GR, et al. Delirium in mechanically ventilated patients: validity and reliability of the confusion assessment method for the intensive care unit (CAM-ICU). JAMA 2001;286(21):2703–10.
76. Bergeron N, Dubois MJ, Dumont M, et al. Intensive care delirium screening checklist: evaluation of a new screening tool. Intensive Care Med 2001;27(5): 859–64.

Protocolized and Target-based Sedation and Analgesia in the ICU

Curtis N. Sessler, MD[a,b,*], Sammy Pedram, MD[a]

KEYWORDS

- Sedation • Analgesia • Protocol • Guidelines
- Patient-focused • Outcomes

Important goals in the management of patients who are critically ill include prevention and relief of suffering and distress and the provision of safe and effective care that leads to optimal outcomes. Administration of sedatives and analgesics is a cornerstone for optimizing patient comfort and minimizing distress, particularly for patients on mechanical ventilation, yet it may lead to unintended consequences including adverse drug effects and delayed recovery from critical illness.[1–5] As with all aspects of medical management, thoughtful patient-focused care should be based on sound principles and evidence from relevant research. Although individual care for patients, led by experienced clinicians, is central to effective sedation and analgesia management, this aspect of care is particularly well-suited to a structured approach because of the ever-changing patient status that requires repeated evaluation and medication titration at the bedside and the multidisciplinary nature of the care.[6]

Within the context of a comprehensive review of the many aspects of sedation and analgesia in patients who are critically ill in this issue of *the Clinics*, this article will focus on structured approaches to sedation management with emphasis on protocolized, target-based care. The use of protocolized care, with structured approaches that prioritize avoiding the accumulation of drugs and metabolites that could lead to a slower recovery, is supported by a rapidly expanding body of evidence.[1,7] Such strategies embrace the notion of administering the right drug(s) in the right dose to the right patient at the right time for the right reasons. Decision making by clinicians at the bedside—primarily nurses—regarding sedation and analgesia is complex,

A version of this article appeared in the 25:3 issue of *Critical Care Clinics*.

[a] Division of Pulmonary & Critical Care Medicine, Department of Internal Medicine, Virginia Commonwealth University Health System, Box 980050, Richmond, VA 23298-0050, USA

[b] Medical College of Virginia Hospitals, Richmond, VA, USA

* Corresponding author. Division of Pulmonary and Critical Care, Virginia Commonwealth University Health System, Box 980050, Richmond, VA 23298-0050.

E-mail address: csessler@vcu.edu

Anesthesiology Clin 29 (2011) 625–650

doi:10.1016/j.anclin.2011.09.004

1932-2275/11/$ – see front matter © 2011 Elsevier Inc. All rights reserved.

anesthesiology.theclinics.com

reflecting assessment, physiology, and treatment aspects of care.[8] The consequences of off-target sedation include inadequate treatment resulting in excessive pain and anxiety, agitation, self-removal of tubes and catheters, violence toward caregivers, myocardial ischemia, patient-ventilator asynchrony, hypoxemia, and pain-related immune suppression. In contrast, excessive and/or prolonged sedation can lead to skin breakdown, nerve compression, delirium, unnecessary testing for altered mental status, prolonged mechanical ventilation and associated problems such as ventilator-associated pneumonia (VAP), and perhaps posttraumatic stress disorder (PTSD).

It is widely recognized that many patients in the ICU are deeply sedated—a suspicion confirmed by epidemiologic studies that show deep sedation in one-third to half of the patients assessed.[9,10] Deep sedation may be accepted as an expected state, as indicated by the low rates (2.6% in one study) at which bedside nurses judge patients to be oversedated, particularly during nighttime hours.[10] An important impetus for taking a more structured approach to sedation management is the observation that while continuous infusion sedation promotes a smooth course of comfort, it is an independent risk factor for longer duration of mechanical ventilation and longer ICU and hospital length of stay (LOS).[11] A variety of pharmacologic factors conspire to increase the likelihood of excessive and/or prolonged sedative effect in the patient who is critically ill, which include altered pharmacokinetic and pharmacodynamic characteristics with prolonged administration, altered protein binding and volume status, and end-organ dysfunction.[12] Other evidence links sedative management with pace of recovery from respiratory failure. In many modern ventilator weaning protocols assessment of mental status has become a component of the screening phase.[13–19] Depressed level of consciousness is independently associated with lower maximal inspiratory pressure, an effort-dependent measure of inspiratory muscle strength,[20] and recently a strategy that couples interruption of continuous sedation ("spontaneous awakening trial [SAT]") with a spontaneous breathing trial (SBT) was associated with beneficial effects.[21] Accordingly, clinicians have developed strategies with a primary goal of avoiding excessive and/or prolonged sedation.

STRUCTURED APPROACHES TO SEDATION AND ANALGESIA IN THE ICU

Several ideas underlie successful design, implementation, and sustainability of a structured approach to care (**Box 1**). It is important to recognize that such a tool will be implemented primarily by nurses at the bedside and involves the manipulation of

---

Box 1
Principles for developing and implementing protocolized sedation management

1. Perform multidisciplinary development and implementation

2. Establish treatment goals and specific targets that should be frequently re-evaluated

3. Measure key components (pain, agitation, and sedation) using validated scales

4. Select medications based on important characteristics and evidence

5. Incorporate key patient-considerations in selection of medication and management, including safety screening for at-risk populations

6. Design the protocol to prevent over-sedation, yet control pain and agitation.

7. Promote multidisciplinary acceptance and integration into routine care

medications—underscoring the importance of taking a multidisciplinary approach to design and implementation by involving physicians, nurses, and pharmacists. In most algorithms, the nurse at the bedside is responsible for actual application of the algorithm-based interventions such as escalating or de-escalating medications. Marshall and colleagues,[22] however, showed that adding a daily intervention consisting primarily of enforcing the sedation algorithm by a clinical pharmacist improved quality of management and led to better outcomes. The structure should be sufficiently robust to incorporate major differences in patient characteristics, yet simple enough to promote ease of use. The targets for intervention should be clear, and key parameters such as pain, agitation, and sedation should be measured with valid reliable instruments. Selection of medication should reflect current evidence for safety and efficacy. Given that oversedation is a key driver for delayed recovery, the protocol should be specifically designed to minimize this likelihood, and yet relieve pain and anxiety. Finally, ease of use and incorporation into standard practice is crucial for sustainability. Using a structured approach is likely to promote management that has been developed considering viewpoints from different professionals, is logical, is evidence-based, and is consistently applied to all patients who are eligible. In its 2002 guidelines, the expert panel from the Society of Critical Care Medicine (SCCM) recommends (a) titration of a sedative dose to defined endpoints with systematic tapering of the dose or daily interruption with re-titration to minimize prolonged sedative effects, and (b) use of sedation guidelines, an algorithm, or a protocol.[2] Major components for further discussion include sedatives and analgesics, tools to measure pain, agitation, and sedation, and protocol design. Detailed review of the medications commonly used as analgesics and sedatives is beyond the scope of this paper. The reader is referred to other publications[1–3,12,23] and other articles in this issue of the *Clinics*.

Assessment of Pain, Sedation, and Agitation for Patients in the ICU

Careful assessment of key behaviors using valid and reliable tools is a cornerstone of effective management. Existing guidelines and expert opinion support frequent objective assessment of pain, sedation, agitation, and perhaps delirium. Such assessments should be consistently documented, the results communicated among caregivers, and management based on the results of assessment made, noting the response to therapy.[1,2,6,24] The 2002 SCCM guidelines for management of sedation and analgesia recommend (a) establishing and regularly redefining a sedation goal or endpoint, (b) documenting sedation and pain assessment and response to therapy regularly, and (c) using validated assessment scales.

Pain is common and the majority of algorithms incorporate testing for pain. Patient self-report is the most accurate means of assessment if the patient is able to understand and communicate.[2,24,25] Self-report is facilitated using a numerical rating scale (NRS) or visual aid. Pain assessment in patients who are noncommunicative is more challenging. A number of tools for pain observation, such as the behavior pain scale (BPS)[26] and the critical care pain observation tool (CPOT),[27] which are based on observation of behaviors (facial expression, body movement, muscle tension, and ventilator synchrony), have been validated with acceptable results from patients in the ICU.[28–30] The validity declines with increasing depth of sedation and additional work is needed for pain assessment in this population.

The use of a scale to assess level of consciousness dates to the introduction of a 6-point scale by Ramsay and colleagues 25 years ago.[31] Sedation scales are used to assess the depth of sedation, awakeness, and arousal to stimuli, as in the Ramsay sedation scale (RSS),[31] and testing of cognition as in Richmond agitation sedation scale (RASS) developed by Sessler and colleagues[32] and adaptation to the intensive care environment (ATICE) developed by De Jonghe and colleagues.[33] Recently developed scales often combine the sedation/arousal domain with an assessment of agitation, including the sedation agitation scale (SAS) developed by Riker and colleagues,[34] the motor activity assessment scale (MAAS) by Devlin and colleagues,[35] RASS, and ATICE. Desirable features of a good sedation instrument for use in the ICU include rigorous multidisciplinary development; ease of administration, recall, and interpretation; well designed discreet criteria for each level; sufficient sedation levels for effective drug titration; assessment of agitation; and demonstration of inter-rater reliability and validity in relevant patient populations.[36] Among existing sedation-agitation scales, SAS and RASS have been extensively validated in multiple populations and by different groups of investigators.[24] RSS has also been extensively tested but does not grade agitation.[31] Use of a sedation-agitation scale is a key component of sedation algorithms, and it can be used to direct the management of agitation and to establish a target level of sedation for medication titration and to detect oversedation when the target level is exceeded. Virtually all sedation algorithms reviewed by the authors used a sedation scale, with RSS, RASS, and SAS being most common.

Although delirium in patients in the ICU is achieving greater recognition as an important component of brain failure[37] and the SCCM guidelines recommend the routine assessment for the presence of delirium,[2] formal testing for delirium was rarely a component of published sedation algorithms that were reviewed by the authors. This echoes the low rate of implementation of delirium testing using formal assessment tools such as confusion assessment method for the intensive care unit (CAM-ICU)[38] or the intensive care delirium checklist[39] noted in surveys.[40–42]

The introduction of a sedation scale into clinical practice has been shown to result in fewer hours of oversedation and reduced sedation costs.[43] Botha and Mudhalker also showed decreased use of sedatives and analgesics, and also a reduction in the amount of vasopressor therapy for hypotension after introducing a sedation scale.[44] Detection and quantification of pain and agitation can be used to target specific therapy, whereas assessment of the level of sedation is often used to avoid oversedation. Chanques and colleagues[45] showed that by using an explicit protocol to detect and manage pain and agitation, they were able to reduce the incidence of pain and agitation and decrease the duration of mechanical ventilation and the incidence of nosocomial infections. **Table 1** contains details regarding the protocols used in various prospective studies, including scales to measure pain, agitation, and sedation.

Protocol Design

Prospective clinical trials that tested various sedation protocols are listed by year of publication with randomized controlled trials (RCT)s listed first and 2-phase observational studies second in **Table 1**. The authors specifically omitted published studies in which the comparison is primarily between two or more medications and instead focused on the process of delivery of care. In **Table 1** information regarding the protocol construction and the study design is given. Published protocols range in complexity from simple guidelines for selection of medication and introduction of a sedation scale to comprehensive algorithms that evaluate and treat multiple domains (ie, sedation, agitation, pain, and patient-ventilator synchrony). The authors categorize these approaches generally as (a) implementation of a guideline, algorithm, or protocol for sedation management, including those that emphasize intermittent therapy or analgesia as a priority, and (b) protocols that emphasize daily interruption of sedation (DIS).

PROSPECTIVE TRIALS OF SEDATION PROTOCOLS

Most of the validation studies are comparisons between a new structured approach and "baseline," "standard," or "conventional" management in a before-after 2-phase design. This before-after design is subject to concerns regarding historical controls and other unreported concomitant changes in practice. Numerous studies reviewed by the authors were RCTs, denoting a higher level of evidence.

Sedation Protocols, Algorithms, and Guidelines

One of the earliest studies introduced a sedation scale that showed improved quality of sedation with a significant reduction in hours of oversedation.[43] However, the modern era of protocolized sedation management was introduced a decade ago in two published reports. Brook and colleagues[46] tested a nursing-directed algorithm that emphasized the reduction of continuous infusion sedation in favor of intermittent sedation, and Kress and co-investigators[47] examined the impact of a strategy for DIS.

In their RCT, Brook and colleagues[46] compared a complicated algorithm that emphasized intermittent therapy, primarily with fentanyl for analgesia and lorazepam for sedation, to nonprotocolized sedation. A significant reduction in the duration of mechanical ventilation, shorter ICU and hospital LOS, and fewer tracheostomies with the protocol were shown.[46] Since 2000, other sedation algorithms, protocols, and guidelines have focused on the use of a sedation scale, rational and/or cost-effective selection of medication, and other components of sedative and analgesic management.[48–55] In some studies, use of a sedation algorithm was linked to shorter duration of mechanical ventilation and/or shorter ICU LOS.[50,51,53,54] In many studies, however, no difference was seen in the duration of mechanical ventilation or ICU LOS in comparison to baseline practice, although some studies may have been underpowered to detect a difference.[48,49,52,55] Other beneficial outcomes linked to the use of a sedation algorithm or protocol in controlled studies included more "on-target" sedation,[56] less pain,[49] reduced direct drug costs or medication use,[50,54] less patient-ventilator asynchrony,[56] and decreased incidence of VAP.[53] Negative effects of the sedation algorithm were not commonly reported, although longer ICU LOS following introduction of an algorithm was reported by Elliot and colleagues.[52] It is possible that publication bias, in which negative studies are not submitted for publication, or may be more readily rejected, confounds the results.

A number of investigators have designed protocols that are "analgesia-based" or so-called "co-sedation."[56–58] Richman and colleagues[56] showed that the combination of fentanyl plus midazolam (co-sedation) resulted in "better" sedation with less "off-target" sedation and less patient-ventilator asynchrony than midazolam without an opioid, although no difference in duration of mechanical ventilation or ICU LOS was reported. Many sedation protocols and algorithms incorporate evaluation and management of pain and agitation and management of over-sedation within a single algorithm. A typical starting place with patient assessment is to ask if "the patient is comfortable." The first decision point for the patient who is not on target addresses the question, "is the patient in pain?" with management directed toward analgesic therapy if pain is present. The second question is typically "is the patient agitated?," with therapy focused on sedative medications. Importantly, most algorithms include medication de-escalation parameters and directives. Several algorithms have extended these principles to include patient-ventilator synchrony,[59] detailed examination of pain and agitation,[45] and delirium.[60] De Jonghe and colleagues[59] used the ATICE tool that includes five scales (awakeness, comprehension, calmness, ventilator synchrony, and facial relaxation) and structured management to address over-sedation, pain,

Table 1
Prospective clinical trials that test sedation protocols, algorithms, and guidelines

RCTs

Author, Year, References	Key Components of Protocol	Analgesic and Sedative Medications	Patients and Settings	Study Design	Inclusion/Exclusion Criteria	Major Findings	Comment
Brook, 1999[46]	Nursing-directed protocol that emphasizes using intermittent therapy, primarily with fentanyl and lorazepam RSS	A: Fentanyl, morphine S: Lorazepam, propofol	321 MV MICU patients, US University Hospital	RCT: Protocol-directed sedation vs non-protocol-directed sedation (control)	I: MV, age >17 y E: Surgical patient temporarily "boarding" in the MICU	Protocol group had: - shorter duration MV (56 h vs 117 h, $P = .008$) - shorter ICU LOS (5.7 d vs 7.5 d, $P = .013$) - shorter hospital LOS (14.0 d vs 19.9 d, $P = .003$) - lower tracheostomy rate (6.2% vs 13.2%, $P = .038$)	
Kress, 2000[47]	Daily interruption of sedation and analgesia continuous iv infusions RSS	A: Morphine S: Midazolam, propofol	128 MV MICU patients, US university hospital	RCT: 2×2 factorial design. 1. Intervention (DIS) vs standard care (control) 2. Midazolam vs propofol	I: MV E: Pregnancy; s/p cardiac resuscitation	Intervention (DIS) group had: - shorter duration MV (4.9 d vs 7.3 d, $P = .004$) - shorter ICU LOS (6.4 d vs 9.9 d, $P = .02$) - fewer diagnostic tests for changes in mental status (9% vs 27%, $P = .02$)	No difference in major outcomes for midazolam vs propofol. DIS resulted in less midazolam but not propofol

Study	Intervention	Population	Design	Inclusion/Exclusion	Results
Breen, 2005[57]	Titration of analgesic (remifentanil, fentanyl, or morphine) and sedative (midazolam) drugs to goal target SAS and pain intensity scale	A: Remifentanil A: Morphine or fentanyl S: Midazolam	105 MV medical-surgical ICU patients, 10 European centers	10-center RCT: analgesic (remifentanil) vs sedative (midazolam) based	I: Long-term MV (expected greater than 96 h) E: History of AOD, pregnancy, neuromuscular blockade	Analgesic-based group had: - shorter time from weaning to extubation (0.9 h vs 27.5 h, $P<.001$) - shorter duration MV (94 h vs 147.5 h, $P = .033$)
Carson, 2006[64]	DIS was performed in both groups, continuous infusion propofol compared with intermittent lorazepam RSS	A: Morphine S: Lorazepam vs propofol	132 MV sedated MICU patients, 2 US university hospitals	RCT: Lorazepam by intermittent bolus, or propofol by continuous infusion	I: Anticipated MV > 48 h, continuous sedation or 6 or more doses of lorazepam in 24 h E: Benzodiazepine dependence, high risk for EtOH withdrawal, pancreatitis, pregnancy, head trauma	Continuous infusion propofol group had: - shorter duration MV (5.8 d vs 8.4 d, $P = .04$) - trend for more ventilator-free survival (18.5 d vs 10.2 d, $P = .06$)

(continued on next page)

Table 1
(continued)

Author, Year, References	Key Components of Protocol	Analgesic and Sedative Medications	Patients and Settings	Study Design	Inclusion/Exclusion Criteria	Major Findings	Comment
Richman, 2006[56]	Nurse-implemented sedation protocol using benzodiazepine vs benzodiazepine with an opiate. RSS	A: Fentanyl S: Midazolam	30 MV MICU patients, US university hospital	RCT: Sedation with benzodiazepine, or cosedation with benzodiazepine + opiate	I: MV anticipated for > 48 h and need continuous infusion of sedation E: Need scheduled opiates, neuromuscular blockade, refractory shock, dialysis, ileus	Co-sedation group had: - fewer hours with "off-target" sedation (4.2 h vs 9.1 h, P<.002) - fewer episodes of patient-ventilator asynchrony (0.4/h vs 1.0/h, P<.05)	- small sample size. - trend for more ileus with co-sedation. - duration of MV not reported - AOD history noted
Bucknall, 2008[48]	Nursing-directed sedation algorithm SAS	A: Morphine, fentanyl S: Midazolam, propofol	312 MV patients, general ICU, Australian teaching hospital	RCT: Sedation algorithm vs usual care (no algorithm)	I: MV E: Postcardiac surgery (because of brief ICU stay)	Protocol group had: - no difference in duration of MV (control 58 h, protocol 79 h, P = .2) - no difference in ICU LOS(88 h vs 94 h, P = .58) - no difference in ICU survival (80% control vs 79% protocol, P = .89)	1:1 nursing ratio

de Wit, 2008[76]	Nursing-directed sedation algorithm vs DIS and usual care RASS	A: Fentanyl and morphine S: Midazolam, propofol, lorazepam	74 MV MICU patients, US university hospital	RCT: DIS vs sedation algorithm	I: MV E: Neuromuscular blockade, severe neurocognitive dysfunction, tracheostomy	Study terminated early by data safety monitoring board DIS group had: - increased duration of MV by 2.8 d (6.7 d vs 3.9 d, P = .0003) - increased ICU LOS (15 d vs 8 d, P<.0001 - increased mortality	Query whether higher percentage of AOD in this patient population
Girard, 2008[21]	Daily SBT paired with DIS SAT vs standard patient targeted sedation and a daily SBT Sedative and analgesic medications left up to each institution's standard practice RASS and CAM-ICU for delirium	A: Varied per institution S: Varied per institution	336 MV MICU patients. Multicenter US university hospitals	4-center RCT: DIS with SBT vs standard protocol sedation with daily SBT	I: MV > 12 h E: Profound neurologic deficits, s/p cardiac resuscitation, already MV > 2 wk	Intervention group (SAT + SBT) had: - increased days of breathing without assistance (in 28d) (14.7 d vs 11.6 d, P = .02) fewer ICU days (9.1 vs 12.9, P = .01) - fewer hospital days	More liberal SBT criteria 2 patients with diagnosis of EtOH withdrawal

(continued on next page)

Table 1
(continued)

Author, Year, References	Key Components of Protocol	Analgesic and Sedative Medications	Patients and Settings	Study Design	Inclusion/Exclusion Criteria	Major Findings	Comment
						(14.9 vs 19.2, $P = .04$) - increased self-extubation rate (16 episodes vs 6 episodes, $P = .04$)	
Mehta, 2008[70]	Protocolized sedation with or without DIS SAS	A: Morphine, fentanyl if renal failure S: Midazolam	65 MV, 3 Canadian university medical-surgical ICUs	RCT: Sedation protocol with DIS vs sedation protocol alone	I: MV > 48 h, continuous infusion sedation, age > 18 y E: NMBA, drug allergy, alcohol/analgesic abuse, psychiatric illness, neurologic dysfunction, postcardiac arrest, DNR, near death, estimated 6 mo mortality >50%, non-English speaking, sedative infusion >24 h at other hospital	Sedation protocol with DIS group had: - less midazolam ($P<.05$) - no difference in ventilator days (10.5 d vs 8 d) - no difference in ICU LOS (13 d vs 10 d) - no difference in hospital LOS (20 d vs 14 d)	Not powered adequately because of slow patient recruitment. >90% of patients had medical problems

2-Phase studies

Costa, 1994[43]	"Controlled" sedation, use of sedation scale (modified Cook sedation scale)	Midazolam	40 ICU patients, Spanish hospital	Randomized, crossover: "controlled" vs "empiric"		Controlled sedation had: - lower mean midazolam dose - lower sedation cost - fewer hours of oversedation
MacLaren, 2000[49]	Evidence-based sedation and analgesia protocol. Modified RSS; modified visual analog pain scale	A: Morphine, fentanyl, (codeine if frequent neuro checks required) S: Propofol, midazolam	158 MV patients in medical-surgical-neurologic Canadian ICU	Prospective 2-phase study: empiric before/ protocol after	I: Continuous IV sedation for >6 h E: Receiving analgesics only	Protocol group had: - less "discomfort" (11% vs 22.4%, $P<.001$) - less pain (5.9% vs 9.6%, $P<.05$) - lower hourly sedation cost (C\$5.68 vs C\$7.69, $P<.01$) - trend for longer sedation duration (122.7 h vs 88.0 h, $P<.1$) - trend for longer duration MV (61.6 h vs 39.1 h, $P = .13$)	Protocol adherence = 83.7%

(continued on next page)

Table 1
(continued)

Author, Year, References	Key Components of Protocol	Analgesic and Sedative Medications	Patients and Settings	Study Design	Inclusion/Exclusion Criteria	Major Findings	Comment
Mascia, 2000[50]	Guidelines based upon "rational cost-effective use of drugs" including sedation, analgesia, and neuromuscular blockade RSS	A: Morphine, meperidine, fentanyl S: Propofol <24 h, midazolam or lorazepam >24 h	158 MV medical and surgical ICU patients, US tertiary care university hospital	Prospective 2-phase study: baseline before/guidelines after	I: Continuous infusion of sedative E: None mentioned	Guideline group had: - lower direct drug costs - shorter duration MV (167 h vs 317 h)[a] - shorter ICU LOS (9.2 d vs 19.1 d)[a] - shorter hospital LOS (19.1 d vs 34.3 d)[a]	
Brattebo, 2004[51]	Small scale rapid cycle improvement model; protocol, sedation scale Motor activity sedation scale	A: Morphine S: Midazolam	285 MV surgical ICU patients, Norwegian university hospital	Prospective observational 2-phase study: baseline before/guideline after	I: MV > 24 h E: None mentioned	Protocol group had: - shorter duration MV (5.3 d vs 7.4 d)[a] - trend for shorter ICU LOS (8.3 d vs 9.3 d)[a]	

Study	Intervention	Population	Design	Criteria	Results
de Jonghe, 2005[59]	Algorithm: regular assessment of consciousness and tolerance to ICU environment with goal of tolerance and high level of consciousness. ATICE sedation/analgesia algorithm	A: Fentanyl S: Midazolam	102 MV MICU patients, French university-affiliated hospital	Prospective 2-phase study: control before/algorithm after	I: MV > 24 h E: Acute brain injury, cardiac arrest, tracheostomy	Algorithm group had: - shorter time to arousal (2 d vs 4 d, $P = .006$) - shorter duration MV (4.4 d vs 10.3 d, $P = .014$)
Chanques, 2006[45]	Protocol emphasis on systematic evaluation of pain and agitation using BPS, NRS, and RASS	A: Fentanyl or morphine S: Midazolam, propofol	MV medical-surgical ICU patients, French university hospital	Prospective 2-phase study: Control before/protocol after	I: ICU admission > 24 h E: Brain injury limiting communication	Protocol group had: - lower incidence of pain (42% vs 63%, $P = .002$) - lower incidence of agitation (12% vs 29%, $P = .002$) - shorter duration MV (65 h vs 120 h, $P<.05$) - fewer nosocomial infections (8% vs 17%, $P<.05$)

(continued on next page)

Table 1
(continued)

Author, Year, References	Key Components of Protocol	Analgesic and Sedative Medications	Patients and Settings	Study Design	Inclusion/Exclusion Criteria	Major Findings	Comment
Elliott, 2006[52]	Nursing-directed sedation algorithm patterned after Brook.[65] RSS	A: Fentanyl S: Midazolam	322 MV patients, general ICU, Australian tertiary care hospital	2-Phase study: pre-post sedation algorithm	I: MV E: Neuromuscular disease, high spinal cord injury	Algorithm group had: - no difference in duration of MV (Pre-4.8 d, post-5.6 d, $P = .99$) - increased ICU LOS (pre-7.06d vs post-8.16d, $P = .04$) - trend toward increased tracheostomy (pre-21 vs post-30, $P = .22$)	1:1 nursing ratio ETIC-7

| Quenot, 2007[53] | Nurse-implemented sedation protocol to evaluate effect on incidence of VAP. MV weaning protocols same in both groups. Same standard VAP prevention in both time periods (chlorhexidine mouth care, head of bed >45°, orogastric tubes, etc) Cambridge scale | A: No analgesics used S: Midazolam or propofol | 423 MV MICU patients French university hospital | Prospective 2-phase study. control before/algorithm after | I: MV > 48 h E: Use of analgesics with sedative, peripheral nervous system disorder, postcardiac arrest | Protocol group had: - decreased VAP (6% vs 15%, $P = .005$) - decreased duration MV (4.2 vs 8 d, $P = .001$) - decreased extu bation failure (6% vs 13%, $P = .01$) - decreased ICU LOS (5 vs 11 d, $P = .004$) - decreased hospital LOS (17 vs 21 d, $P = .003$) - trend toward increased self-extubation (10.7% vs 7%, $P = .09$) - no change in mortality | Excluded patients receiving analgesics Nursing compliance with protocol not measured |

(continued on next page)

Table 1
(continued)

Author, Year, References	Key Components of Protocol	Analgesic and Sedative Medications	Patients and Settings	Study Design	Inclusion/Exclusion Criteria	Major Findings	Comment
Arias-Rivera, 2008[54]	Nursing implemented sedation protocol to evaluate weaning outcome on MV patients deemed ready to wean Cook sedation scoring system	A: Morphine S: Midazolam or propofol	356 MV medical-surgical ICU patients Spanish university hospital	Prospective 2-phase study; control before/ algorithm after	I: MV > 48 h E: MV < 48 h tracheostomy; neuromuscular blockade	Protocol group had: - increased vent free days (19 vs 17 d, P = .02) - trend toward decreased days intubated (8 vs 10 d, P = .07) - decreased morphine use (15 mg vs 40 mg, P = <.001) - no change in sedative use, ICU LOS or ICU mortality	Does not appear to have any vent weaning algorithm in place NEMS

Study	Intervention	Drugs	Population	Design	Inclusion/Exclusion	Results	Comments
Marshall, 2008[22]	Active pharmacist input to existing sedation protocol SAS	Midazolam, lorazepam, propofol, fentanyl	156 MV MICU patients US university hospital	2-phase study: Sedation guidelines both groups retrospective—(control) no pharmacist intervention; prospective—pharmacist intervention	I: MV; continuous infusion sedation E: age <18 y	Intervention group had: - reduced duration of MV (178 h vs 338 h, $P<.001$ - decreased ICU LOS (238 h vs 380 h, $P = .001$ - decreased hospital LOS (369 h vs 537 h, $P = .001$	
Muller, 2008[55]	First phase "standard care" with benzo and opiate algorithm. Sedation depth not measured, no pain scale Second phase used propofol-remifentanil, nurse-implemented algorithm using RSS	Phase 1 A: fentanyl, sufentanil S: Flunitrazepam, midazolam Phase 2 A: Remifentanil S: Propofol	85 MV medical-surgical ICU patients French ICU	Prospective 2-phase study	I: ICU, MV > 24 h E: Neurologic and neuromuscular disease; postcardiac arrest; uncontrolled dyslipidemia	Second phase group had: - decreased time to extubation after cessation of sedation (10 h vs 92 h, $P \leq 0001$ - no change in duration of MV, ICU LOS or mortality	Phase 1 dose of fentanyl seems high (125 µg to 500 µg/h)

Prospective clinical trials are listed in order of publication within two groups. The first group consists of randomized controlled trials, and the second group prospective 2-phase (before-after) trials.

Abbreviations: A, Analgesic; AOD, alcohol and other drugs disorder; ATICE, adaption to intensive care environment; BPS, behavioral pain scale; DIS, daily interruption of sedation; DNR, do not resuscitate; E, exclusion criteria; ETIC-7, experience after treatment in intensive care 7 item scale; EtOH, ethyl alcohol; I, inclusion criteria; ICU, intensive care unit; LOC, level of consciousness; LOS, length of stay; MICU, medical intensive care unit; MV, mechanical ventilation; NEMS, nine equivalents of nurse manpower score; NMBA, neuromuscular blocking agent; NRS, numerical rating scale; RASS, Richmond agitation sedation scale; RCT, randomized controlled trial; RSS, Ramsay sedation scale; S, sedative; SAS, sedation agitation scale; SBT, spontaneous breathing trial; US, United States; VAP, ventilator-associated pneumonia.

^a P values not reported.

patient-ventilator synchrony, and indirectly, patient agitation. After introduction of the algorithm, a reduction in duration of mechanical ventilation compared with a baseline period was seen.

Chanques and coworkers[45] introduced a more rigorous management strategy for pain and agitation. Pain was assessed using NRS and BPS[26] and agitation using RASS.[32] Extensive education of caregivers and detailed guidelines for assessing the risk-benefit for analgesic and psychoactive drug administration and emphasis on de-escalation of therapy were included. Reductions in the incidence of pain and agitation and a shorter duration of mechanical ventilation were seen. Robinson and colleagues[60] showed that for patients in surgical ICU implementation of an "analgesia-delirium-sedation protocol" led to shorter duration of mechanical ventilation and other favorable outcomes. Pain was measured with a visual/objective pain assessment scale, agitation with RASS[32] and delirium with CAM-ICU.[38] The protocol included identifying patients at high risk for delirium and also detected delirium using CAM-ICU, with haloperidol recommended for treatment. Haloperidol was not used in a significantly higher percentage of patients nor at an elevated total dose following implementation of the protocol.

Use of a structured algorithm or protocol for managing sedation and analgesia is supported by multiple controlled trials that typically compare these interventions to "usual care" with favorable or equivalent results, but with no evidence of harm. Conclusions about the optimal structure are not very clear, given the wide variety of protocol designs; however, a common practice is to reduce the likelihood of oversedation. These algorithms vary considerably in terms of complexity; however, implementation concerns favor as simple an approach as is feasible.

Daily Interruption of Sedation

In 2000, Kress and coworkers[47] showed that temporarily stopping sedative (midazolam or propofol) and analgesic (morphine) infusions until the patient was able to follow three or four simple tasks or was agitated led to significant reductions in duration of mechanical ventilation, shorter ICU LOS, and use of fewer diagnostic tests (such as head CT or lumbar puncture) for unexplained changes in mental status.[47] Once awakening was shown, sedative and analgesic infusions were restarted at half the original dose and titrated to clinical targets. The study was designed as a 2 × 2 factorial study with patients also randomized to propofol or midazolam. The outcomes were nearly identical for patients who received propofol and for those who received midazolam. This is despite administration of a significantly lower total dose of midazolam and morphine to the midazolam subgroup who received DIS, whereas there was no decrement in total doses of propofol or morphine with DIS in the propofol subgroup. This observation that DIS is linked to more rapid resolution of respiratory failure may be related to several factors: (a) reduced accumulation of sedative drugs and their metabolites resulting in faster recovery of mental status sufficiently alert for effective ventilator weaning and (b) the additional opportunities for clinicians to recognize that the patient is actually capable of breathing independently when they undergo interruption of sedation, so-called "wake up and breathe."[61] This hypothesis was recently tested by comparing the combination of DIS plus an SBT—the key test in many weaning protocols[62]—with a protocol of SBT without structured sedation management.[21]

The awakening and breathing controlled study published in 2008 was the first multicenter trial that tested the combination of protocolized and mandatory DIS followed by SBT versus a strategy that used targeted sedation combined with SBTs.[21] This study, covered in detail in another article (by Hooper and Girard) in this issue of the *Clinics*, showed significant reduction in benzodiazepine and opiate administration, reduction in time on mechanical ventilation, and reduction in ICU and hospital LOS, although twice as many self-extubations occurred with DIS + SBT. A significant reduction in all-cause mortality at 1 year (but not 28-day mortality) in the DIS group was observed.[21]

Kress and colleagues have performed additional studies that examine the potential benefits and risks of DIS. In a retrospective review of data from patients who were prospectively enrolled, significantly fewer complications of critical care were found among patients randomized to DIS, compared with usual management.[63] This appears to be primarily the result of shorter duration of mechanical ventilation. Carson and colleagues[64] performed a two-center RCT, comparing propofol infusion to intermittent therapy using lorazepam. Patients in both groups received morphine sulfate for pain and DIS of sedative drugs. Patients randomized to receive propofol with DIS had shorter duration of mechanical ventilation and a trend for more ventilator-free survival. A potential confounding factor was the presence of dialysis-requiring renal failure in twice as many patients randomized to lorazepam (20% vs 10%)—this may be important since renal failure can lead to longer duration of sedation from accumulation of the morphine-6-glucuronide, the active metabolite of morphine.[65] In a post hoc evaluation of the relative costs of continuous propofol infusion with DIS versus intermittent lorazepam with DIS, total costs were significantly reduced with propofol plus DIS, despite the higher acquisition cost.[66] This reflects the cost savings of shorter time on mechanical ventilation and shorter ICU and hospital LOS.

Concerns have been raised regarding the safety of withdrawing all sedatives and analgesics until the patient is either alert or agitated.[67] Readily apparent effects of DIS might include agitated behavior that can be accompanied by self-removal of critical tubes and catheters or other forms of interference with provision of care, increased patient-ventilator asynchrony, and violence toward caregivers.[68,69] Reassuringly, most investigations found no significant increase in the incidence of such events,[47,64,70] although Girard and colleagues[21] reported more self-extubations with DIS. An additional concern has been that the repeated rather abrupt awakening of DIS might be alarming to the patient[67] and perhaps have long-term consequences for mental health. Yet in a follow-up study, DIS was actually associated with fewer signs of PTSD and trends for a decreased incidence of PTSD and better adjustment to the residual effects of critical illness when tested 6 months or more after hospitalization.[71] This is encouraging; however, the relationship between awakening from sedation, developing agitation, and long-term psychological health is complicated. Some investigators have correlated greater number of episodes of being alert or agitated with a higher incidence of having delusional memories of the ICU experience.[72] The use of physical restraints without sedation—which might be a surrogate for agitation—has been linked to subsequent PTSD.[73] The "quality" of the periods of relative alertness may be important since a higher likelihood of having post-ICU PTSD was seen among patients who had hallucination and nightmares, whereas those with better recall for factual events, ie, concrete memories, had less PTSD.[74] This topic is addressed elsewhere in this issue of the *Clinics*. Additional work in this interesting area is warranted.

Awakening during the withholding of sedatives and/or analgesics in DIS is associated with increases in heart rate and blood pressure and several-fold increases in circulating catecholamines.[75] Despite this adrenergic surge, in an observational study of patients with risk factors for coronary artery disease, the DIS-related stress response resulted in no increase in the proportion of patients who had cardiac ischemia as reflected by increased cardiac enzymes or ST-segment changes on continuous ECG recording.[75] Further work is needed before DIS can be endorsed for patients in whom the stress response may carry greater risk—such as those who have ongoing hypertensive emergency or acute myocardial infarction.[61]

Daily interruption has been recently examined in two smaller RCTs, in both cases in comparison to protocolized sedation. In a pilot study by Mehta and colleagues,[70] all 65 patients who enrolled were managed with a sedation protocol in which midazolam and morphine infusions (or fentanyl infusions if renal failure) were titrated according to sedation scale measurements. In addition, one group had daily interruption of sedation and analgesic infusions, whereas the other group had no scheduled interruption. DIS resulted in decreased total doses of midazolam but not of opioids. There were no differences in duration of mechanical ventilation, or ICU or hospital LOS. The authors reported their results as pilot data and acknowledged inadequate power to detect important outcomes; slow enrollment was cited.

De Wit and colleagues[76] compared "usual care" plus DIS to a sedation algorithm that included preferences for intermittent therapy in 74 patients from a MICU. In contrast to earlier studies, no differences in total sedative or analgesic doses were found. Randomization to the sedation algorithm group was associated with favorable outcomes including shorter duration of mechanical ventilation, shorter hospital and ICU LOS, and more rapid recovery of organ dysfunction. Hospital mortality was higher in the DIS group, although analyses could discern no causal connection between DIS and increased mortality. This unexpected finding contrasts sharply with other investigations of DIS in which no difference in hospital mortality was noted.[47,64,70] If one pools the results from four studies, including that by de Wit, hospital mortality was 39% for 198 patients who were randomized to DIS and 40% for 194 patients randomized to no DIS.[47,64,70,76] Girard and colleagues did not present hospital mortality data but reported similar 28-day mortality (28% with DIS vs 35% with no DIS, $P = .2$) but significantly lower 1-year mortality in the DIS group (44% vs 58%, $P = .01$).[21] What could account for these differences? de Wit and colleagues noted a high rate of alcohol and other drug use disorders among patients admitted to the ICU, whereas such patients were excluded[64,70] or rare[21] in other studies. One hypothesis is that DIS could repeatedly provoke brief episodes of more intense withdrawal from drugs or alcohol in patients with high risk. Patients with alcohol and other drug use disorders require higher doses of sedatives and opioids.[77] Changes in blood pressure, heart rate, and evoked potentials, and overshoot of blood levels of endorphins suggest that withdrawal from opioids and sedatives can occur within 6 hours of discontinuing infusions of short-acting drugs like sufentanil, midazolam, and propofol.[78] It is plausible that DIS in patients with alcohol and drug use disorders is potentially harmful and alternative strategies should be considered in this subset of patients until additional research is performed.

Despite some variability among results, the weight of evidence favors DIS as a safe method to reduce oversedation and increase the speed of recovery from respiratory failure for many critically ill patients. It is important to recognize, however, that some form of safety screening is crucial to avoid subjecting at-risk patients to potential harm. In the study by Girard and colleagues,[21] for example, their safety screen required that a patient did not receive a sedative infusion for active seizures or alcohol withdrawal, did not receive escalating sedative doses due to ongoing agitation, did not receive neuromuscular blockers, had no evidence of active myocardial ischemia in the previous 24 hours, and had no evidence of increased intracranial pressure, before proceeding to DIS. Close observation during DIS is required to reduce the risk of self-extubation and other consequences of agitation. More work is needed to clarify the most optimal approach to patient selection and actual performance of DIS.

IMPLEMENTATION OF SEDATION ALGORITHMS

Development, implementation, and successful continuation of complex decision-making tools such as sedation algorithms is a daunting task. Historically, sedation scales have been used in fewer than half of the ICUs.[24] The more recent surveys are 5–8 years old, but provide some perspective. In a 2004 survey of French ICUs, only about 50% of patients who were receiving active sedative or analgesic treatment had a sedation or pain scale in use, a guideline or protocol was in place in 36% of ICUs, and no ICU reported using DIS.[9] In a 2001 survey of Canadian ICU workers, a sedation scale was used in 49%, and a sedation protocol, guideline, or care-set was used in 29%, but surprisingly, 40% of respondents used DIS.[40] In a German survey conducted in 2002, sedation monitoring was performed in 30% of hospitals and 21% used a written sedation/analgesia guideline.[79] Although there is no accurate real-time measure of current penetration of sedation algorithms, or even the use of a sedation scale, in sedation practice, the surge in published reports addressing aspects of sedation management is encouraging for greater awareness and hopefully wider use of structured approaches. For details regarding international surveys related to sedation and analgesic practices, we refer you to the article by Dr Mehta in this issue of the *Clinics*.

Translating clinical science findings into routine daily patient care is challenging, and slow adoption of new therapies is widely recognized.[80] Work by Pun and colleagues suggests that widespread implementation of sedation and delirium assessment tools (RASS and CAM-ICU) is achievable.[81] In a survey of their nurses, the most often-cited difficulties for implementing CAM-ICU were inadequate time and lack of physician "buy-in." Studies on difficulties of implementation of other ICU interventions reveal similar patterns of insufficient time and resources, and skepticism regarding value.[82,83] These activities require a substantial investment of time and effort by clinicians and ICU staff, so trade-offs in time spent performing other patient-care and administrative activities must be considered. Involving key ICU staff—physicians, nurses, and pharmacists—in the design and implementation may help to address concerns about validity. A common concern with any protocolized approach is that each patient is unique and may have characteristics that do not fit well with the underlying assumptions regarding intended patient populations when the protocol was developed. There is often tension between competing priorities of simplicity and generalizability with any protocol, and this should be considered. The consideration of inclusion and exclusion criteria to the supporting studies and consideration of a safety screen can help address this issue. The emerging "science of implementation"[80] should help define better means of adopting new practices such as structured sedation management. Experts argue that the ICU is an ideal environment to examine new approaches to implementation since it is geographically compact, staff are familiar with measuring quantitative outcomes, multidisciplinary practice is common, and there are numerous logical target conditions and illnesses.[80]

SUMMARY

Protocolized target-based sedation and analgesia is central to effective management of sedation. Important components include identifying goals and specific targets, using valid and reliable tools to measure pain, agitation, and sedation, and titrating a logically selected combination of sedatives and analgesics to defined end-points. A variety of approaches to structured management have been tested in controlled trials with major categories of (1) sedation algorithms and protocols and (2) daily interruption of sedation. Although not all studies that compare new interventions to "usual care" document dramatic improvements, many studies show that by reducing oversedation, using a structured approach, faster recovery from respiratory failure may ensue. The somewhat discrepant results illustrate, however, that various approaches, such as DIS, may not be optimal for all patients. Further research will be necessary to define these patients and examine alternative strategies. Finally, implementation of structured approaches to sedation management is a challenging, time-consuming process for clinicians that must be supported with sufficient resources to be successful.

REFERENCES

1. Sessler CN, Varney K. Patient-focused sedation and analgesia in the ICU. Chest 2008;133(2):552–65.
2. Jacobi J, Fraser GL, Coursin DB, et al. Clinical practice guidelines for the sustained use of sedatives and analgesics in the critically ill adult. Crit Care Med 2002;30(1):119–41.
3. Kress JP, Hall JB. Sedation in the mechanically ventilated patient. Crit Care Med 2006;34(10):2541–6.
4. Morandi A, Watson PL, Trabucchi M, et al. Advances in sedation for critically ill patients. Minerva Anestesiol 2009;75(6):385–91.
5. Fraser GL, Riker RR. Sedation and analgesia in the critically ill adult. Curr Opin Anaesthesiol 2007;20(2):119–23.
6. Sessler CN, Grap MJ, Brophy GM. Multidisciplinary management of sedation and analgesia in critical care. Semin Respir Crit Care Med 2001;22(2):211–25.
7. Schweickert WD, Kress JP. Strategies to optimize analgesia and sedation. Crit Care 2008;12(Suppl 3):S6.
8. Aitken LM, Marshall AP, Elliott R, et al. Critical care nurses' decision making: sedation assessment and management in intensive care. J Clin Nurs 2009; 18(1):36–45.
9. Payen JF, Chanques G, Mantz J, et al. Current practices in sedation and analgesia for mechanically ventilated critically ill patients: a prospective multicenter patient-based study. Anesthesiology 2007;106(4):687–95.
10. Weinert CR, Calvin AD. Epidemiology of sedation and sedation adequacy for mechanically ventilated patients in a medical and surgical intensive care unit. Crit Care Med 2007;35(2):393–401.
11. Kollef MH, Levy NT, Ahrens TS, et al. The use of continuous i.v. sedation is associated with prolongation of mechanical ventilation. Chest 1998;114(2):541–8.
12. Devlin JW. The pharmacology of oversedation in mechanically ventilated adults. Curr Opin Crit Care 2008;14(4):403–7.
13. Ramachandran V, Jo Grap M, Sessler CN. Protocol-directed weaning: a process of continuous performance improvement. Crit Care 2005;9(2):138–40.
14. Ely EW, Baker AM, Dunagan DP, et al. Effect on the duration of mechanical ventilation of identifying patients capable of breathing spontaneously. N Engl J Med 1996;335(25):1864–9.
15. Grap MJ, Strickland D, Tormey L, et al. Collaborative practice: development, implementation, and evaluation of a weaning protocol for patients receiving mechanical ventilation. Am J Crit Care 2003;12(5):454–60.
16. Marelich GP, Murin S, Battistella F, et al. Protocol weaning of mechanical ventilation in medical and surgical patients by respiratory care practitioners and nurses: effect on weaning time and incidence of ventilator-associated pneumonia. Chest 2000;118(2):459–67.

17. Krishnan JA, Moore D, Robeson C, et al. A prospective, controlled trial of a protocol-based strategy to discontinue mechanical ventilation. Am J Respir Crit Care Med 2004;169(6):673–8.
18. Salam A, Tilluckdharry L, Amoateng-Adjepong Y, et al. Neurologic status, cough, secretions and extubation outcomes. Intensive Care Med 2004;30(7):1334–9.
19. Kollef MH, Shapiro SD, Silver P, et al. A randomized, controlled trial of protocol-directed versus physician-directed weaning from mechanical ventilation. Crit Care Med 1997;25(4):567–74.
20. Caruso P, Carnieli DS, Kagohara KH, et al. Trend of maximal inspiratory pressure in mechanically ventilated patients: predictors. Clinics 2008;63(1):33–8.
21. Girard TD, Kress JP, Fuchs BD, et al. Efficacy and safety of a paired sedation and ventilator weaning protocol for mechanically ventilated patients in intensive care (Awakening and Breathing Controlled trial): a randomised controlled trial. Lancet 2008;371(9607):126–34.
22. Marshall J, Finn CA, Theodore AC. Impact of a clinical pharmacist-enforced intensive care unit sedation protocol on duration of mechanical ventilation and hospital stay. Crit Care Med 2008;36(2):427–33.
23. Erstad B, Gilbert H, Grap MJ, et al. Management of pain in the ICU. Chest 2009; 135(4):1075–86.
24. Sessler CN, Jo Grap M, Ramsay MA. Evaluating and monitoring analgesia an sedation in the intensive care unit. Crit Care 2008;12(Suppl 3):S2.
25. Puntillo K, Pasero C, Li D, et al. Evaluation of ICU patients with pain. Chest 2009; 135(4):1069–74.
26. Payen JF, Bru O, Bosson JL, et al. Assessing pain in critically ill sedated patients by using a behavioral pain scale. Crit Care Med 2001;29(12):2258–63.
27. Gelinas C, Fillion L, Puntillo KA, et al. Validation of the critical-care pain observation tool in adult patients. Am J Crit Care 2006;15(4):420–7.
28. Ahlers SJ, van Gulik L, van der Veen AM, et al. Comparison of different pain scoring systems in critically ill patients in a general ICU. Crit Care 2008;12(1): R15.
29. Gelinas C, Harel F, Fillion L, et al. Sensitivity and specificity of the critical-care pain observation tool for the detection of pain in intubated adults after cardiac surgery. J Pain Symptom Manage 2009;37(1):58–67.
30. Li D, Puntillo K, Miaskowski C. A review of objective pain measures for use with critical care adult patients unable to self-report. J Pain 2008;9(1):2–10.
31. Ramsay MA, Savege TM, Simpson BR, et al. Controlled sedation with alphax-alone-alphadolone. Br Med J 1974;2(920):656–9.
32. Sessler CN, Gosnell MS, Grap MJ, et al. The Richmond agitation-sedation scale: validity and reliability in adult intensive care unit patients. Am J Respir Crit Care Med 2002;166(10):1338–44.
33. De Jonghe B, Cook D, Griffith L, et al. Adaptation to the Intensive Care Environment (ATICE): development and validation of a new sedation assessment instrument. Crit Care Med 2003;31(9):2344–54.
34. Riker RR, Picard JT, Fraser GL. Prospective evaluation of the sedation-agitation scale for adult critically ill patients. Crit Care Med 1999;27(7):1325–9.
35. Devlin JW, Boleski G, Mlynarek M, et al. Motor activity assessment scale: a valid and reliable sedation scale for use with mechanically ventilated patients in an adult surgical intensive care unit. Crit Care Med 1999;27(7):1271–5.
36. Sessler CN. Sedation scales in the ICU. Chest 2004;126(6):1727–30.
37. Girard TD, Pandharipande PP, Ely EW. Delirium in the intensive care unit. Crit Care 2008;12(Suppl 3):S3.

38. Ely EW, Inouye SK, Bernard GR, et al. Delirium in mechanically ventilated patients: validity and reliability of the confusion assessment method for the intensive care unit (CAM-ICU). JAMA 2001;286(21):2703–10.
39. Bergeron N, Dubois MJ, Dumont M, et al. Intensive care delirium screening checklist: evaluation of a new screening tool. Intensive Care Med 2001;27(5):859–64.
40. Mehta S, Burry L, Fischer S, et al. Canadian survey of the use of sedatives, analgesics, and neuromuscular blocking agents in critically ill patients. Crit Care Med 2006;34(2):374–80.
41. Van Eijk MM, Kesecioglu J, Slooter AJ. Intensive care delirium monitoring and standardised treatment: a complete survey of Dutch intensive care units. Intensive Crit Care Nurs 2008;24(4):218–21.
42. Ely EW, Stephens RK, Jackson JC, et al. Current opinions regarding the importance, diagnosis, and management of delirium in the intensive care unit: a survey of 912 healthcare professionals. Crit Care Med 2004;32(1):106–12.
43. Costa J, Cabre L, Molina R, et al. Cost of ICU sedation: comparison of empirical and controlled sedation methods. Clin Intensive Care 1994;5(5 Suppl):17–21.
44. Botha JA, Mudholkar P. The effect of a sedation scale on ventilation hours, sedative, analgesic and inotropic use in an intensive care unit. Crit Care Resusc 2004;6(4):253–7.
45. Chanques G, Jaber S, Barbotte E, et al. Impact of systematic evaluation of pain and agitation in an intensive care unit. Crit Care Med 2006;34(6):1691–9.
46. Brook AD, Ahrens TS, Schaiff R, et al. Effect of a nursing-implemented sedation protocol on the duration of mechanical ventilation. Crit Care Med 1999;27(12):2609–15.
47. Kress JP, Pohlman AS, O'Connor MF, et al. Daily interruption of sedative infusions in critically ill patients undergoing mechanical ventilation. N Engl J Med 2000;342(20):1471–7.
48. Bucknall TK, Manias E, Presneill JJ. A randomized trial of protocol-directed sedation management for mechanical ventilation in an Australian intensive care unit. Crit Care Med 2008;36(5):1444–50.
49. MacLaren R, Plamondon JM, Ramsay KB, et al. A prospective evaluation of empiric versus protocol-based sedation and analgesia. Pharmacotherapy 2000;20(6):662–72.
50. Mascia MF, Koch M, Medicis JJ. Pharmacoeconomic impact of rational use guidelines on the provision of analgesia, sedation, and neuromuscular blockade in critical care. Crit Care Med 2000;28(7):2300–6.
51. Brattebo G, Hofoss D, Flaatten H, et al. Effect of a scoring system and protocol for sedation on duration of patients' need for ventilator support in a surgical intensive care unit. Qual Saf Health Care 2004;13(3):203–5.
52. Elliott R, McKinley S, Aitken L. Adoption of a sedation scoring system and sedation guideline in an intensive care unit. J Adv Nurs 2006;54(2):208–16.
53. Quenot JP, Ladoire S, Devoucoux F, et al. Effect of a nurse-implemented sedation protocol on the incidence of ventilator-associated pneumonia. Crit Care Med 2007;35(9):2031–6.
54. Arias-Rivera S, Sanchez-Sanchez Mdel M, Santos-Diaz R, et al. Effect of a nursing-implemented sedation protocol on weaning outcome. Crit Care Med 2008;36(7):2054–60.
55. Muller L, Chanques G, Bourgaux C, et al. Impact of the use of propofol remifentanil goal-directed sedation adapted by nurses on the time to extubation in

mechanically ventilated ICU patients: the experience of a French ICU. Ann Fr Anesth Reanim 2008;27(6):481, e1–8.

56. Richman PS, Baram D, Varela M, et al. Sedation during mechanical ventilation: a trial of benzodiazepine and opiate in combination. Crit Care Med 2006;34(5): 1395–401.

57. Breen D, Karabinis A, Malbrain M, et al. Decreased duration of mechanical ventilation when comparing analgesia-based sedation using remifentanil with standard hypnotic-based sedation for up to 10 days in intensive care unit patients: a randomised trial [ISRCTN47583497]. Crit Care 2005;9(3):R200–10.

58. Muellejans B, Lopez A, Cross MH, et al. Remifentanil versus fentanyl for analgesia based sedation to provide patient comfort in the intensive care unit: a randomized, double-blind controlled trial [ISRCTN43755713]. Crit Care 2004; 8(1):R1–11.

59. De Jonghe B, Bastuji-Garin S, Fangio P, et al. Sedation algorithm in critically ill patients without acute brain injury. Crit Care Med 2005;33(1):120–7.

60. Robinson BR, Mueller EW, Henson K, et al. An analgesia-delirium-sedation protocol for critically ill trauma patients reduces ventilator days and hospital length of stay. J Trauma 2008;65(3):517–26.

61. Sessler CN. Wake up and breathe. Crit Care Med 2004;32(6):1413–4.

62. MacIntyre NR. Evidence-based ventilator weaning and discontinuation. Respir Care 2004;49(7):830–6.

63. Schweickert WD, Gehlbach BK, Pohlman AS, et al. Daily interruption of sedative infusions and complications of critical illness in mechanically ventilated patients. Crit Care Med 2004;32(6):1272–6.

64. Carson SS, Kress JP, Rodgers JE, et al. A randomized trial of intermittent lorazepam versus propofol with daily interruption in mechanically ventilated patients. Crit Care Med 2006;34(5):1326–32.

65. Barr J, Donner A. Optimal intravenous dosing strategies for sedatives and analgesics in the intensive care unit. Crit Care Clin 1995;11(4):827–47.

66. Cox CE, Reed SD, Govert JA, et al. Economic evaluation of propofol and lorazepam for critically ill patients undergoing mechanical ventilation. Crit Care Med 2008;36(3):706–14.

67. Heffner JE. A wake-up call in the intensive care unit. N Engl J Med 2000;342(20): 1520–2.

68. Mion LC, Minnick AF, Leipzig R, et al. Patient-initiated device removal in intensive care units: a national prevalence study. Crit Care Med 2007;35(12):2714–20.

69. Woods JC, Mion LC, Connor JT, et al. Severe agitation among ventilated medical intensive care unit patients: frequency, characteristics and outcomes. Intensive Care Med 2004;30(6):1066–72.

70. Mehta S, Burry L, Martinez-Motta JC, et al. A randomized trial of daily awakening in critically ill patients managed with a sedation protocol: a pilot trial. Crit Care Med 2008;36(7):2092–9.

71. Kress JP, Gehlbach B, Lacy M, et al. The long-term psychological effects of daily sedative interruption on critically ill patients. Am J Respir Crit Care Med 2003; 168(12):1457–61.

72. Samuelson K, Lundberg D, Fridlund B. Memory in relation to depth of sedation in adult mechanically ventilated intensive care patients. Intensive Care Med 2006; 32(5):660–7.

73. Jones C, Backman C, Capuzzo M, et al. Precipitants of post-traumatic stress disorder following intensive care: a hypothesis generating study of diversity in care. Intensive Care Med 2007;33(6):978–85.

74. Jones C, Griffiths RD, Humphris G, et al. Memory, delusions, and the development of acute posttraumatic stress disorder-related symptoms after intensive care. Crit Care Med 2001;29(3):573–80.

75. Kress JP, Vinayak AG, Levitt J, et al. Daily sedative interruption in mechanically ventilated patients at risk for coronary artery disease. Crit Care Med 2007; 35(2):365–71.

76. de Wit M, Gennings C, Jenvey WI, et al. Randomized trial comparing daily interruption of sedation and nursing-implemented sedation algorithm in medical intensive care unit patients. Crit Care 2008;12(3):R70.

77. de Wit M, Wan SY, Gill S, et al. Prevalence and impact of alcohol and other drug use disorders on sedation and mechanical ventilation: a retrospective study. BMC Anesthesiol 2007;7(3).

78. Korak-Leiter M, Likar R, Oher M, et al. Withdrawal following sufentanil/propofol and sufentanil/midazolam Sedation in surgical ICU patients: correlation with central nervous parameters and endogenous opioids. Intensive Care Med 2005;31(3):380–7.

79. Martin J, Parsch A, Franck M, et al. Practice of sedation and analgesia in German intensive care units: results of a national survey. Crit Care 2005;9(2):R117–23.

80. Weinert CR, Mann HJ. The science of implementation: changing the practice of critical care. Curr Opin Crit Care 2008;14(4):460–5.

81. Pun BT, Gordon SM, Peterson JF, et al. Large-scale implementation of sedation and delirium monitoring in the intensive care unit: a report from two medical centers. Crit Care Med 2005;33(6):1199–205.

82. Carlbom DJ, Rubenfeld GD. Barriers to implementing protocol-based sepsis resuscitation in the emergency department—results of a national survey. Crit Care Med 2007;35(11):2525–32.

83. Rubenfeld GD, Cooper C, Carter G, et al. Barriers to providing lung-protective ventilation to patients with acute lung injury. Crit Care Med 2004;32(6):1289–93.

Sedation and Weaning from Mechanical Ventilation: Linking Spontaneous Awakening Trials and Spontaneous Breathing Trials to Improve Patient Outcomes

Michael H. Hooper, MD[a,*], Timothy D. Girard, MD, MSC[a,b]

KEYWORDS

• Weaning • Sedation • Spontaneous awakening
• Interruption of sedation • Wake-up and breathe

Mechanical ventilation is a lifesaving intervention used to treat hundreds of thousands of critically ill patients each year. Among the many goals of care in these patients is safe, early liberation from the ventilator. Traditionally, critical care physicians attempted to minimize the duration of mechanical ventilation and improve clinical outcomes by manipulating ventilator modes and parameters to slowly decrease mechanical support and allow the resumption of spontaneous, unassisted ventilation. Clinical trials conducted in the 1990s, reviewed in this article, compared multiple approaches to ventilator weaning and produced results that established the efficacy of a daily spontaneous breathing trial for expediting liberation from mechanical ventilation.

In addition to manipulation of ventilator parameters, recent research has revealed that management of patients' sedation, which almost universally accompanies the acute use of mechanical ventilation, affects the duration of mechanical ventilation

A version of this article appeared in the 25:3 issue of *Critical Care Clinics*.
[a] Division of Allergy, Pulmonary, and Critical Care Medicine, Department of Medicine, Center for Health Services Research, Vanderbilt University School of Medicine, 6th Floor MCE, #6100, Nashville, TN 37232-8300, USA
[b] Tennessee Valley Geriatric Research, Education and Clinical Center (GRECC), Department of Veterans Affairs Medical Center, Tennessee Valley Healthcare System, 1310 24th Avenue South, Nashville, TN 37212-2637, USA
* Corresponding author.
E-mail address: michael.hooper@vanderbilt.edu

Anesthesiology Clin 29 (2011) 651–661
doi:10.1016/j.anclin.2011.09.005   anesthesiology.theclinics.com
1932-2275/11/$ – see front matter © 2011 Elsevier Inc. All rights reserved.

and other patient outcomes. This research has led to the use of patient-targeted sedation protocols and spontaneous awakening trials as tools to improve patient outcomes.

By focusing on seminal clinical trials, this review highlights the progressive changes in the management of mechanical ventilation and sedation that have occurred during the last 2 decades. The interdependence of these aspects of critical care is also discussed.

WEANING FROM MECHANICAL VENTILATION AND THE EMERGENCE OF SPONTANEOUS BREATHING TRIALS

The decision to intubate and mechanically ventilate a critically ill patient obligates a physician to later decide when it is appropriate to allow spontaneous, unassisted ventilation and to proceed with extubation. Delays in this process are associated with significant increases in hospital costs, morbidity, and mortality.[1–4] The benefits of shortening the duration of mechanical ventilation have long been suspected, and, historically, this led many physicians to develop methods for "weaning" their patients from mechanical ventilation. The term "weaning" arose because of the assumption that patients who required the use of mechanical ventilation gradually regained the strength and ability to breathe spontaneously as the etiologies of their respiratory failure abated. Many clinicians believed that gradually decreasing ventilator support (ie, weaning the ventilator) was the most appropriate method for assisting patients on their path toward unassisted ventilation and extubation. This concept of weaning the ventilator was intuitive and led to widespread use of various modes of ventilation and methods for gradually decreasing the amount of ventilator support provided to patients, including the reduction of inspiratory pressure in pressure support ventilation, the reduction of controlled breaths in intermittent mandatory ventilation (IMV), or the gradual lengthening of periods of spontaneous breathing by T-piece trials.

In the 1990s, two pivotal, randomized clinical trials were conducted to compare different strategies for weaning of mechanical ventilation. Brochard and colleagues[5] compared gradual reductions in pressure support ventilation to gradual reductions in ventilator support with synchronized IMV or progressively longer T-piece trials (which some referred to as spontaneous breathing trials despite important differences when compared with spontaneous breathing trials used in later studies). Of 456 patients who met weaning criteria, only 109 patients failed a 2-hour trial of spontaneous breathing and were enrolled in the study. Among these 109 patients, the use of gradually decreasing pressure support ventilation resulted in a reduction in the duration of weaning compared with the other weaning methods. In another seminal trial, Esteban and colleagues[6] compared once-daily spontaneous breathing trials (defined as up to 2 hours—depending on patient tolerance—of spontaneous breathing through a T-tube circuit or with <5 cm H_2O of continuous positive airway pressure) with intermittent spontaneous breathing trials, gradually reducing pressure support ventilation, and gradually reducing ventilator support in IMV. In Esteban's trial, once-daily and intermittent spontaneous breathing trials proved superior, reducing time to successful weaning compared with the approaches that gradually weaned ventilator support in IMV or pressure support ventilation modes.

In both these trials, approximately 75% of patients screened for enrollment met criteria for extubation (ie, tolerated a 2-hour spontaneous breathing trial) and did not require any additional weaning, indicating that physicians failed to identify a significant number of patients who were ready for extubation. Ely and colleagues[7] conducted a randomized, controlled trial that showed respiratory care-driven weaning protocols using spontaneous breathing trials led to a significantly shorter time to extubation when compared with physician-driven weaning. The data generated by these trials established the use of a weaning protocol based on the spontaneous breathing trial as an effective tool to achieve safe and early liberation from mechanical ventilation in critically ill patients. This type of approach has thus been widely recommended as a standard of care in the intensive care unit (ICU).[8–10]

SEDATION AND WEANING FROM MECHANICAL VENTILATION

Minimizing patient pain and discomfort is among the many goals of health providers in the ICU. With limitations on communication, intubated patients in the ICU are at especially high risk for experiencing prolonged, untreated pain or psychological distress.[11] Thus, pharmacologic agents that produce sedation or analgesia are commonly used to alleviate perceived pain or distress in these patients. In patients with altered mental status and agitation, the same agents are often used to chemically restrain patients for their own protection. The need for pharmacologic agents to provide sedation or analgesia in the ICU is widely accepted by medical professionals; however, as discussed in previous articles in this review series, the specifics of how sedation is administered can substantially impact the clinical outcomes for mechanically ventilated ICU patients. Kollef and colleagues,[12] for example, showed that patients receiving continuous intravenous (IV) sedation spent more time on the ventilator than those receiving sedation by way of intermittent boluses (this analysis was adjusted for potential confounders such as severity of illness, use of chemical paralysis, presence of a tracheostomy, and others). Patients sedated continuously also had worse outcomes in other areas, including ICU and hospital length of stay, organ system failure, and reintubation.

In the past 10 years, concern over the deleterious effects of oversedation has prompted the investigation of ways to safely deliver the appropriate level of sedation to patients without delaying extubation or adversely affecting other outcomes. Two specific concepts that were developed to achieve this goal were patient-targeted sedation protocols and spontaneous awakening trials. The former was reviewed in detail in an earlier article by Dr Sessler, elsewhere in this issue the authors discuss the latter herein.

Spontaneous Awakening Trials

Just as spontaneous breathing trials are used to determine when a patient is ready for unassisted breathing, spontaneous awakening trials are used to determine a patient's need for sedation by a careful assessment conducted when the patient's pharmacologic sedation has been discontinued. The spontaneous awakening trial—originally referred to as daily interruption of sedatives—was first introduced into the literature by Kress and colleagues[13] in a single-center trial that enrolled 128 mechanically ventilated patients receiving continuous IV sedation. In this randomized trial, compared with usual care, a sedation strategy involving daily interruption of sedative infusions (until patients were awake) significantly reduced duration of mechanical ventilation (**Fig. 1** and **Table 1**) and ICU length of stay. This benefit came without the cost of significant increases in the rate of adverse events. Specifically, 2 of 68 patients in the intervention group self-extubated, whereas 4 of 60 patients in the control group self-extubated ($P = .88$).

Further analysis of this study was published by Schweickert and colleagues,[14] who investigated the benefits of spontaneous awakening trials. They reviewed the clinical trial data to identify hospital complications, including ventilator-associated

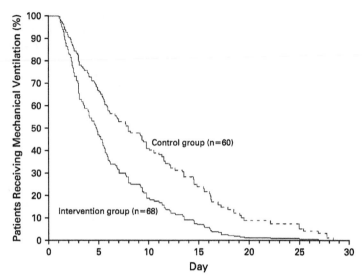

Fig. 1. Effect of daily interruption of sedative infusions on the duration of mechanical ventilation in medical ICU patients receiving sedatives. After adjustment for age, sex, weight, acute physiology and chronic health enquiry II (APACHE II) score, and type of respiratory failure, mechanical ventilation was discontinued earlier in the intervention group than in the control group (relative risk of extubation, 1.9; 95% confidence interval [CI], 1.3–2.7; P<.001). (*From* Kress JP, Pohlman AS, O'Connor MF, et al. Daily interruption of sedative infusions in critically ill patients undergoing mechanical ventilation. N Engl J Med 2000;342(20):1474; with permission.)

pneumonia, upper gastrointestinal hemorrhage, bacteremia, barotrauma, venous thromboembolic disease, cholestasis, and sinusitis. The overall rate of complications was 2.8% in the intervention group versus 6.2% in the control group (P = .04). This blinded, retrospective evaluation suggested that complications related to a longer stay in the ICU and to mechanical ventilation were significantly decreased when daily spontaneous breathing trials were used, thus providing further support for their use when caring for mechanically ventilated critically ill patients.

Despite the data supporting inclusion of spontaneous awakening trials as part of standard sedation strategy, their routine implementation in ICUs has been limited. Surveys have indicated that less than 40% of ICUs use this strategy regularly.[15–18] To understand the infrequent use of this sedation strategy, Tanios and colleagues[19] identified barriers to the use of spontaneous awakening trials in a 2004 survey of 904 Society of Critical Care Medicine members.[20] The most frequently reported reasons for not using regular spontaneous awakening trials included concerns regarding patient safety, patient comfort, and self-extubation. Other barriers expressed included concern that the supporting data arose from a single-center trial that did not include a standardized ventilator weaning protocol. Additionally, it was postulated that a patient-targeted sedation protocol would deliver equivalent results without mandating complete interruption of sedation,[21] which some believed would precipitate a traumatic psychological experience for critically ill patients.[22,23]

In a follow-up study, Kress and coworkers[24] sought to address concern of psychological harm attributable to spontaneous awakening trials by interviewing patients enrolled in their original 128-person trial and additional patients not enrolled in the original trial but recruited at the same time. Each patient underwent a detailed

Table 1
Improvements in patient outcomes after implementation of management strategies for mechanical ventilation and sedation

	SBT[a]			DIS[b]			Wake-up-and-Breathe Protocol[c]		
	SBTs	No SBTs	P Value	DIS	Usual Care	P Value	SAT + SBT	SBT Alone	P Value
Days of mechanical ventilation	4.5	6	0.003	4.9	7.3	0.004	n/a	n/a	—
Ventilator-free days	n/a	n/a	—	n/a	n/a	—	14.7[d]	11.6[d]	0.02
Mortality[e]	38%	40%	0.63	36%	46%	0.25	44%	58%	0.01
Tracheostomy	9%	15%	0.1	18%	27%	0.31	13%	20%	0.06
Self-extubation	1%	3%	0.25	4%	7%	0.88	10%[f]	4%	0.03
Reintubation	4%	10%	0.04	18%	30%	0.17	14%	13%	0.73

Abbreviations: DIS, daily interruption of sedation; SAT, spontaneous awakening trial; SBT, spontaneous breathing trial.

[a] *Data from* Ely EW, Baker AM, Dunagan DP, et al. Effect on the duration of mechanical ventilation of identifying patients capable of breathing spontaneously. N Engl J Med 1996;335(25):1864–9.

[b] *Data from* Kress JP, Pohlman AS, O'Connor MF, et al. Daily interruption of sedative infusions in critically ill patients undergoing mechanical ventilation. N Engl J Med 2000;342(20):1471–7.

[c] *Data from* Girard TD, Kress JP, Fuchs BD, et al. Efficacy and safety of a paired sedation and ventilator weaning protocol for mechanically ventilated patients in intensive care (Awakening and Breathing Controlled trial): a randomised controlled trial. Lancet 2008;371(9607):126–34.

[d] *Data from* this study was reported in ventilator-free days (during a 28-day period). Patients who died during the study were assigned zero ventilator-free days.

[e] *Data for* "spontaneous breathing trials" and "daily interruption of sedation" expressed as in-hospital mortality. Data for the "wake-up-and-breathe protocol" is 1-year mortality.

[f] The rate of self-extubations requiring reintubation was 3% in the intervention (SAT + SBT) group. The rate of self-extubations requiring reintubation in the control group was 2%. There was not a statistically significant difference (P = .47).

psychological evaluation by a clinical psychologist blinded to details of the patient's ICU stay, including use of spontaneous awakening trials. The evaluation included validated assessments for symptoms of posttraumatic stress disorder (PTSD), a determination of the diagnosis of PTSD (when warranted according to the criteria set forth in the *Diagnostic and Statistical Manual of Mental Disorders*, 4th edition), and assessments of overall perceived health and psychological well-being, anxiety, and depression. The results of this follow-up study showed a decrease in signs of PTSD among the 13 patients who were managed with daily spontaneous awakening trials compared with the 19 patients managed with usual care sedation strategies. No patient in the intervention group was diagnosed with PTSD, whereas six patients (32%) in the control group demonstrated criteria for this diagnosis ($P = .06$). No difference was found between the groups in terms of anxiety or depression. These data, combined with the demonstrated safety benefit in terms of outcomes and complications, suggested that spontaneous awakening trials (ie, daily interruption of sedatives) can safely and dramatically improve care for mechanically ventilated critically ill patients.

The Wake-up and Breathe Protocol

Seeking to enhance the efficacy of daily spontaneous breathing trials and to address some limitations of Kress and colleagues' seminal trial, Girard and coworkers[25] conducted a multicenter, randomized controlled trial to evaluate a protocol that paired spontaneous awakening trials with spontaneous breathing trials. In the awakening and breathing controlled (ABC) trial, the wake-up and breathe protocol used in the intervention group was designed to focus the benefit of spontaneous awakening by temporally associating it with the process of evaluating a patient's need for continued mechanical ventilation. In total, 336 patients were enrolled and randomized; all were analyzed but one withdrew shortly after enrollment, before management with trial protocols (intervention group, 167; control group, 168). The intervention group in this trial was managed with the wake-up and breathe protocol, consisting of protocolized spontaneous awakening trials and spontaneous breathing trials. An overview of the protocol is shown in **Fig. 2**. The control group, also managed with protocolized spontaneous breathing trials, received patient-targeted sedation according to "usual care;" sedative doses were titrated to achieve the level of sedation ordered by the ICU team. For the monitoring and ordering of sedation, validated sedation scales were routinely used in both groups. Notably, physicians were permitted to interrupt sedation as part of their usual practice in the control population. Sedatives were stopped before at least one spontaneous breathing trial in 31% of the patients in the control group but cessation of sedation was not conducted on a daily basis for any patients in the control group.

To ensure that spontaneous awakening trials were not inappropriately conducted on days when clinical circumstances dictated an absolute need for sedation, a spontaneous awakening trial safety screen was performed each day for patients in the intervention group. This prevented a spontaneous awakening trial from being performed on patients who were receiving sedation for seizures, alcohol withdrawal, ongoing agitation, or neuromuscular blockade. The safety screen also prevented spontaneous awakening trials in patients with evidence for myocardial ischemia (within the previous 24 hours) or evidence of increased intracranial pressure. Implementation of these screens led to 10% of the patients in the intervention group never receiving a spontaneous awakening trial. Patients who failed the safety screen were rescreened the next day.

Each patient in the intervention group underwent a spontaneous awakening trial on every day they passed the spontaneous awakening trial safety screen. Sedatives and

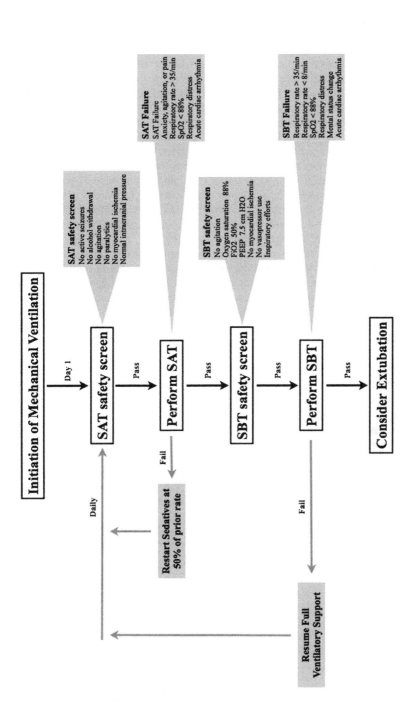

Fig. 2. Overview of a wake-up and breathe protocol. Includes criteria for passing the safety screens that were implemented before spontaneous awakening trials and spontaneous breathing trials. Also includes criteria for failing a spontaneous awakening trial or spontaneous breathing trial.

any analgesics being used for sedation were interrupted, and patients were monitored for predefined criteria that indicated passage or failure of the spontaneous awakening trial. Patients failed the trial if they had sustained anxiety, agitation, pain, respiratory rate greater than 35 times/min for five consecutive minutes, an SpO_2 of less than 88% for five consecutive minutes, cardiac dysrhythmia, or other signs of respiratory distress. Patients passed the trial when they opened their eyes to verbal stimuli or tolerated sedative interruption for 4 hours without exhibiting failure criteria; 94% of all spontaneous awakening trials were passed by patients, whereas only 5% (42 of 895) were failed because of signs of anxiety, agitation, or pain. The very low incidence of spontaneous awakening trial failure indicates that the safety screen was effective in identifying patients at high risk for failing a spontaneous awakening trial.

Each day they passed a spontaneous awakening trial, patients in the intervention group were managed with the spontaneous breathing trial portion of the wake-up-and-breathe protocol (see **Fig. 2**). A spontaneous breathing trial protocol was applied daily to patients in the control group. The spontaneous breathing trial protocol included a safety screen followed by a 2-hour spontaneous breathing trial by either T-piece circuit or minimal pressure support ventilation.

The predetermined primary endpoint of the trial, ventilator-free days (defined as the number of days patients were breathing without assistance during the 28-day study period), was significantly improved for patients in the intervention group. Patients managed with a daily wake-up-and-breathe protocol had an average of 3.1 more ventilator-free days than patients in the control group ($P = .02$). This improvement was seen despite the fact that the time to first passage of a spontaneous breathing trial was equivalent in the intervention and control groups. The patients in the intervention group, however, were significantly more awake than patients in the control group at the time they first passed a spontaneous breathing trial; thus, patients in the intervention group were also much more likely to be extubated at that time. This suggests that the mechanism for improvement in ventilator-free days was not a change in respiratory function but an improvement in level of sedation.

Multiple secondary endpoints were also improved by the wake-up-and-breathe protocol (**Table 2**), including length of stay in the ICU and hospital (both reduced by 4 days) and duration of coma. Of particular note, the secondary endpoint of 1-year survival was significantly improved in the intervention group (**Fig. 3**). Management with the wake-up-and-breathe protocol resulted in a 14% absolute reduction in the risk for death up to 1 year after enrollment, possibly because of a decrease in ICU

Table 2
Spontaneous breathing trials and spontaneous awakening trials

	SBT	SAT
Treatment interrupted	Mechanical ventilation	Pharmacologic sedation
Safety screens passed	65%[a]	82%[a]
Desired outcome	Stable patient breathing without assistance ≥ 2 h	Calm, awake patient
Trials passed	52%[a]	94%[a]
Most common cause for failure	Tachypnea (37% of all trials)[a]	Anxiety, agitation, pain (5% of all trials)[a]

[a] *Data from* Girard TD, Kress JP, Fuchs BD, et al. Efficacy and safety of a paired sedation and ventilator weaning protocol for mechanically ventilated patients in intensive care (Awakening and Breathing Controlled trial): a randomised controlled trial. Lancet 2008;371(9607):126–34.

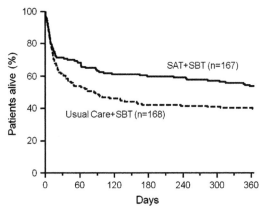

Fig. 3. Effect of paired sedation and ventilator weaning protocol on 1-year survival in medical ICU patients receiving mechanical ventilation. An unadjusted Cox proportional hazard analysis showed that patients in the SAT + SBT group were 32% less likely to die at any instant during the year after enrollment than patients in the usual care + SBT group (hazard ratio for death, 0.68; 95% CI, 0.50–0.92; P = .01). (*From* Girard TD, Kress JP, Fuchs BD, et al. Efficacy and safety of a paired sedation and ventilator weaning protocol for mechanically ventilated patients in intensive care (Awakening and Breathing Controlled trial): a randomised controlled trial. Lancet 2008;371(9607):131; with permission.)

complications as described by Schweickert and colleagues,[14] though this hypothesis was not tested in the ABC trial.

These results confirmed the benefit of daily spontaneous awakening trials first shown by Kress and colleagues[13] and extended their benefit by pairing spontaneous awakening trials with spontaneous breathing trials in a protocol that improved multiple outcomes, including 1-year survival, compared with usual care. Notably, "usual care" represented standard practices based on strong evidence, including titration of sedative doses based on Richmond agitation-sedation scale (RASS) assessments and physician-ordered target RASS scores as well as a spontaneous breathing trial weaning protocol. Thus, the ABC trial and the seminal trial by Kress and colleagues in 2000 established the efficacy and safety of spontaneous awakening trials and the wake-up-and-breathe protocol for the management of mechanically ventilated critically ill patients.

SUMMARY

The use of sedation has long been integrated into critical care. Because pain, discomfort, anxiety, and agitation are commonly experienced by critically ill patients, the use of medications to alleviate and control these symptoms will continue; however, data showing that prolonged use of sedating medications imparts harm to patients obligate physicians to use agents and methods of sedation that minimize these negative side effects. Numerous observational studies and clinical trials have proven that decisions in sedation management play a crucial role in determining outcomes for mechanically ventilated ICU patients, and recent evidence supports the use of protocols that streamline efforts to discontinue sedation and mechanical ventilation in a safe and parallel fashion. Regardless of choice of sedating agent, and even when patient-targeted sedation protocols are used to minimize oversedation, the use of spontaneous awakening trials dramatically improves patient outcomes for critically ill patients.

Intensive care physicians must continue to study the delivery of sedation in efforts to maximize patient comfort while minimizing patient harm.

REFERENCES

1. Zilberberg MD, Luippold RS, Sulsky S, et al. Prolonged acute mechanical ventilation, hospital resource utilization, and mortality in the United States. Crit Care Med 2008;36(3):724–30.
2. Rashid A, Sattar KA, Dar MI, et al. Analyzing the outcome of early versus prolonged extubation following cardiac surgery. Ann Thorac Cardiovasc Surg 2008;14(4):218–23.
3. Cook DJ, Walter SD, Cook RJ, et al. Incidence of and risk factors for ventilator-associated pneumonia in critically ill patients. Ann Intern Med 1998;129(6):433–40.
4. Pinhu L, Whitehead T, Evans T, et al. Ventilator-associated lung injury. Lancet 2003;361(9354):332–40.
5. Brochard L, Rauss A, Benito S, et al. Comparison of three methods of gradual withdrawal from ventilatory support during weaning from mechanical ventilation. Am J Respir Crit Care Med 1994;150(4):896–903.
6. Esteban A, Frutos F, Tobin MJ, et al. A comparison of four methods of weaning patients from mechanical ventilation. Spanish Lung Failure Collaborative Group. N Engl J Med 1995;332(6):345–50.
7. Ely EW, Baker AM, Dunagan DP, et al. Effect on the duration of mechanical ventilation of identifying patients capable of breathing spontaneously. N Engl J Med 1996;335(25):1864–9.
8. MacIntyre NR, Cook DJ, Ely EW Jr, et al. Evidence-based guidelines for weaning and discontinuing ventilatory support: a collective task force facilitated by the American College of Chest Physicians; the American Association for Respiratory Care; and the American College of Critical Care Medicine. Chest 2001;120(6 Suppl):375S–95S.
9. Dellinger RP, Levy MM, Carlet JM, et al. Surviving Sepsis Campaign: international guidelines for management of severe sepsis and septic shock. Crit Care Med 2008;36(1):296–327.
10. Boles JM, Bion J, Connors A, et al. Weaning from mechanical ventilation. Eur Respir J 2007;29(5):1033–56.
11. Turner JS, Briggs SJ, Springhorn HE, et al. Patients' recollection of intensive care unit experience. Crit Care Med 1990;18(9):966–8.
12. Kollef MH, Levy NT, Ahrens TS, et al. The use of continuous i.v. sedation is associated with prolongation of mechanical ventilation. Chest 1998;114(2):541–8.
13. Kress JP, Pohlman AS, O'Connor MF, et al. Daily interruption of sedative infusions in critically ill patients undergoing mechanical ventilation. N Engl J Med 2000;342(20):1471–7.
14. Schweickert WD, Gehlbach BK, Pohlman AS, et al. Daily interruption of sedative infusions and complications of critical illness in mechanically ventilated patients. Crit Care Med 2004;32(6):1272–6.
15. Martin J, Franck M, Sigel S, et al. Changes in sedation management in German intensive care units between 2002 and 2006: a national follow up survey. Crit Care 2007;11(6):R124.
16. Mehta S, Burry L, Fischer S, et al. Canadian survey of the use of sedatives, analgesics, and neuromuscular blocking agents in critically ill patients. Crit Care Med 2006;34(2):374–80.

17. Payen JF, Chanques G, Mantz J, et al. Current practices in sedation and anal-gesia for mechanically ventilated critically ill patients: a prospective multicenter patient-based study. Anesthesiology 2007;106(4):687–95.
18. Patel RP, Gambrell M, Speroff T, et al. Delirium and sedation in the intensive care unit: survey of behaviors and attitudes of 1384 healthcare professionals. Crit Care Med 2009;37(3):825–32.
19. Tanios MA, deWit M, Epstein SK, et al. Perceived barriers to the use of sedation protocols and daily sedation interruption: A multidisciplinary survey. J Crit Care 2009;24:66–73.
20. Devlin JW, Tanios MA, Epstein SK. Intensive care unit sedation: waking up clini-cians to the gap between research and practice. Crit Care Med 2006;34(2):556–7.
21. Hong JJ, Mazuski JE, Shapiro MJ. Daily interruption of sedative infusions in crit-ically ill patients. N Engl J Med 2000;343(11):814–5.
22. Heffner JE. A wake-up call in the intensive care unit. N Engl J Med 2000;342(20):1520–2.
23. Riker RR. Neuromuscular blockade at the end of life. N Engl J Med 2000;342:1921–2.
24. Kress JP, Gehlbach B, Lacy M, et al. The long-term psychological effects of daily sedative interruption on critically ill patients. Am J Respir Crit Care Med 2003;168(12):1457–61.
25. Girard TD, Kress JP, Fuchs BD, et al. Efficacy and safety of a paired sedation and ventilator weaning protocol for mechanically ventilated patients in intensive care (Awakening and Breathing Controlled trial): a randomised controlled trial. Lancet 2008;371(9607):126–34.

Altering Intensive Care Sedation Paradigms to Improve Patient Outcomes

Richard R. Riker, MD, FCCM[a,b,]*, Gilles L. Fraser, PharmD, FCCM[a,c]

KEYWORDS

• Sedation • Critical care • Adults • Analgesia
• Delirium • Outcomes

SEDATION ALGORITHMS: A HISTORY

The clinical approach to sedation for intensive care unit (ICU) patients has evolved significantly during the last 30 years, as new medications have emerged, and clinicians have embraced systematic and evidence-based approaches to care. One of the first studies to address this issue was published in 1974 by Ramsay and colleagues; it was a report ahead of its time in many ways: sedation was titrated to a scale, a subset of patients was monitored with electroencephalography, sedation medication was interrupted, and a relatively light level of sedation was targeted (Ramsay scale of 2–4).[1] Reports describing different approaches to ICU sedation began to appear in the 1980s and early 1990s. Although highly variable, they generally reported deep levels of sedation, frequent use of neuromuscular blockade, and no standard approach to medication selection or strategy for administration.[2] Simpson and colleagues[3] reported the advantages of lorazepam relative to the lasting effects of diazepam, and continuous infusion etomidate initially gained popularity, until it was recognized not to be as safe as originally believed.[4,5] Patient perceptions and recall of the ICU experience were a novel consideration,[6] and the impact of organ dysfunction on drug and metabolite elimination was described.[7] Early reports of continuous sedation with midazolam and propofol appeared,[8,9] and innovative approaches to avoid prolonged sedation from continuous infusions were proposed.[10] Reports of lingering

A version of this article appeared in the 25:3 issue of *Critical Care Clinics*.
[a] Tufts University School of Medicine, Boston, MA, USA
[b] Departments of Medicine and Neurocritical Care, Maine Medical Center, 22 Bramhall Street, Portland, ME 04102, USA
[c] Departments of Medicine and Pharmacy, Maine Medical Center, 22 Bramhall Street, Portland, ME 04102, USA
* Corresponding author. Departments of Medicine and Neurocritical Care, Maine Medical Center, 22 Bramhall Street, Portland, ME 04102.
E-mail address: rikerr@mmc.org

Anesthesiology Clin 29 (2011) 663–674
doi:10.1016/j.anclin.2011.09.006   anesthesiology.theclinics.com
1932-2275/11/$ – see front matter © 2011 Elsevier Inc. All rights reserved.

neuromuscular dysfunction after prolonged ICU neuromuscular blockade first appeared in 1990, leading to a reevaluation of that approach.[11]

As attention to the practice of sedation and analgesia for ICU patients grew, the Society of Critical Care Medicine published the first sedation practice guideline in 1995, summarized in a five-page document with 13 references.[12] A follow-up report published in 2002 (but reflecting literature published up to 2000) was a much-expanded effort, encompassing 23 pages, 235 references, and 28 recommendations.[13] A revision to the 2002 sedation guidelines has been completed and is currently undergoing peer review. The document is entitled "Clinical practice guidelines for the management of pain, agitation, and delirium in adult patients in the intensive care unit." This title reflects a patient centered approach and emphasizes the identification, prevention, and management (utilizing both pharmacologic and nonpharmacologic strategies) of these common clinical issues. These new guidelines reflect an almost exponential growth in published data to guide care for the ICU patient, as shown in **Fig. 1**.

SHOULD WE CHANGE STANDARD PRACTICE?

As additional clinical research results have accumulated, the quality of research has varied, results have often conflicted (even among seemingly similar studies), diagnostic and treatment approaches have been inconsistent, and many important areas have not been studied. Many significant findings have been identified, several with consistent results in multiple research reports. It is apparent that changes in the clinical practice of ICU sedation are warranted. Before listing these proposed changes (which the author's are not defining as comprehensive), it is important to describe the existing approach to sedation, if possible.

Sedation practice depends on several factors, including geographic location, approved and available drugs within that region, and the type of ICU patient population served. Given these multiple factors, the few available reports, and the many different approaches used, a common pattern for ICU sedation is difficult to construct, but several observations can be made. Various surveys of practice have been completed in the United States,[14–16] Germany,[17,18] Australia,[19] and Canada.[20–22]

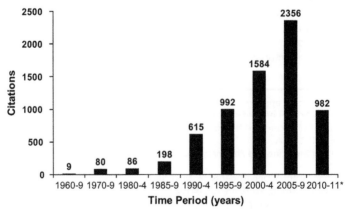

Fig. 1. PubMed citations (accessed September 26, 2011) for (sedation OR analgesia OR delirium) AND (intensive OR critical) care, grouped by specific publication dates. Note that the first 2 periods are 10-year intervals, and the last period (2010–11) is less than 2 years.

Although sedation protocols and sedation scales (21% vs 46%) are being incorporated in care protocols more frequently, more than half the responders still do not use these tools. When used, the Ramsay scale,[1] Sedation-Agitation Scale (SAS),[23] and Richmond Agitation and Sedation Scale (RASS)[24] appear to be the most common sedation assessment tools. Across all time frames of sedation (short [<24 hours], intermediate [24–72 hours], and long [>72 hours]), the gamma-aminobutyric acid (GABA) agonists remain the most commonly prescribed sedatives, essentially limited to midazolam (Versed), lorazepam (Ativan), and propofol (Diprivan). Daily sedation interruptions are incorporated by roughly a third of responders, and less than half the clinicians routinely assess pain and delirium (most commonly with the Confusion Assessment Method for the ICU [CAM-ICU][25,26] or the Intensive Care Delirium Screening Checklist [ICDSC][27,28]).

Several important breakthroughs have been made in the last 10 years that should guide future practice in the ICU. These are summarized in **Box 1**.

Analgesia

As part of the American Association of Critical Care Nurses Thunder II project, Puntillo and colleagues[29] assessed the level of pain during six ICU procedures in 6000 adults. Their findings were surprising in that patients reported the greatest level of discomfort with the simple procedures that occur frequently in the ICU, such as suctioning and repositioning. This fits well with earlier data that 90% of patients have unpleasant recall of their ICU experience, including pain.[58] Despite many years of focused attention on pain as an important clinical issue in the ICU, the desired outcomes have not yet been attained. Gélinas[30] reported that 64% of open heart surgery patients experienced moderate or severe pain, similar to earlier data from 17 years earlier.

Caring for critically ill patients who cannot verbalize their analgesic needs remains a common clinical problem. In the absence of patient self-report of pain, behavioral indicators have traditionally been used to assess analgesic needs and response to therapy. Two reliable and valid pain assessment tools based on these behaviors, in conjunction with other patient features (such as compliance with mechanical ventilation), have now

---

Box 1
Important research findings that should guide ICU sedation practice

1. Routine daily ICU care procedures are among the most painful or stressful events reported by patients[29,30]

2. Providing analgesia before sedation may reduce sedation requirements and shorten ventilator time[31–35]

3. Lighter sedation and early mobilization appear to be associated with improved outcomes[36–38]

4. Dangerous adverse effects associated with sedative medications are better understood, including prolonged effects of midazolam,[39,40] propylene glycol toxicity with lorazepam,[41,42] delirium with benzodiazepines,[43–45] propofol infusion syndrome,[46–48] and bradycardia associated with dexmedetomidine[43,49]

5. Dexmedetomidine reduces the incidence of delirium,[49,50] shortens ventilator time,[49,51] and appears cost-effective, relative to the GABA agonists[52,53]

6. New monitoring tools help detect ICU delirium[25–28] and better define pain among nonverbal ICU patients[54,55]

7. Cognitive sequelae among critical illness survivors are beginning to be characterized[56,57]

been validated. Although the Critical Care Pain Observation Tool[54] and the Behavioral Pain Scale[55] represent significant improvements for monitoring pain in these challenging patients, data linking these scores with patient self-report of pain severity and improved outcomes have yet to be published. Of note however, patients with documented assessment of the presence or absence of pain on day 2 of their ICU stay appear to have shorter ICU stays and be liberated from mechanical ventilation faster.[59]

Several papers have focused on improving the approach to ICU sedation by employing a strategy we call "analgesia-first" or "A1."[31–35,60] This strategy, in which sedating medications are given only after aggressive analgesic strategies have been used, compares favorably to traditional propofol or benzodiazepine-based regimens for sedation. Patients receiving A1 therapy consistently achieve comfort goals, and less than 50% require sedating medications. There are no overwhelming data to support use of one analgesic over another, but the extremely short half-life of remifentanil may be beneficial for patients requiring frequent neurologic evaluations. Breen and colleagues[31] randomized patients to either remifentanil first (supplemented by midazolam as needed: an A1 approach) or midazolam first, supplemented by fentanyl or morphine. The A1 approach reduced the time of mechanical ventilation by 54 hours and the time from start of weaning to extubation by 27 hours. An open-label study by Rozendaal and colleagues[34] randomized medical and surgical ICU patients to remifentanil-based sedation (with propofol as required) versus a GABA-based regimen supplemented with fentanyl or morphine. Patients treated with the A1 approach weaned from mechanical ventilation faster, and they were almost twice as likely to be extubated and discharged from the ICU during the first 3 days. Dahaba and colleagues[32] randomized patients to two different medications, both using an A1 strategy (remifentanil or morphine), with midazolam supplementation as needed to maintain a SAS of four. This sedation target was attained more commonly in patients in the remifentanil group (78.3% vs 66.5%), who also spent less time on ventilators and left the ICU sooner after extubation. Mullejeans and colleagues[33] similarly randomized patients to remifentanil or fentanyl, with propofol supplementation as needed. Optimal sedation approached 90% in both groups, and less than 40% of patients required propofol. The rapid offset of analgesia when remifentanil was stopped was associated with a slightly greater incidence of pain. Similarly, Spies and colleagues[60] randomized patients to receive remifentanil or fentanyl, stopping the study early for futiity when a similar percentage of patients maintained analgesia scores in the target range.

Sedation

The benzodiazepines, midazolam and lorazepam, are among the most commonly used ICU sedative drugs in the United States.[14,16] The major adverse effects specific to these two medications, prolonged sedative effect for midazolam and propylene glycol toxicity with lorazepam, are now better understood. Midazolam has a rapid onset and short duration of action with single dose administration, and it is recommended because it works quickly. It is not recommended for sustained sedation because prolonged administration results in extended pharmacologic activity, caused by accumulation of parent drug, especially in patients who are obese, have low serum albumin, or have renal impairment.[40] Prolonged sedative activity from midazolam may also be related to accumulation of its active metabolite, alpha-hydroxymidazolam, especially in patients with renal insufficiency.[39] In addition, because it is metabolized by cytochrome P450 3A4, this drug is subject to significant interactions with several inhibitors and substrates of this enzyme system, including fluconazole, fentanyl, and propofol.[61]

Propylene glycol is used as a diluent in many medications, but parenteral formulations of lorazepam contain a substantial amount that can accumulate and cause toxicity in patients receiving large lorazepam doses. Although initially thought to accumulate only with very high lorazepam doses in the 15 to 25 mg/h range,[62–64] data suggest that total daily lorazepam doses (including infusion and bolus administration) as low as 1 mg/kg are associated with toxic propylene glycol concentrations and adverse effects such as acute kidney injury and metabolic acidosis.[41] These clinical features of propylene glycol toxicity occur frequently from other causes in critically ill patients, and it is easy to overlook that lorazepam administration may cause these events. Because most hospitals do not have the ability to quickly measure propylene glycol concentrations, the serum osmol gap has been used as a reliable screening and surveillance tool. An osmol gap greater than 10 to 12 may help identify patients accumulating this toxic substance, and some physicians have recommended screening patients at least every other day when lorazepam doses approximate 1 mg/kg/d.[41]

The other major GABA agonist commonly used to provide ICU sedation is propofol.[14,16] Popular for its quick onset of sedation and rapid elimination when discontinued, propofol has several adverse effects that are well defined and expected, including hypotension, respiratory depression, hypertriglyceridemia, and pancreatitis.[46] The least understood, least predictable, and most dangerous adverse effect is the propofol infusion syndrome (PRIS). Possible mechanisms for this life-threatening syndrome include inhibition of enzymes in the mitochondrial respiratory chain, impaired fatty acid oxidation, diversion of carbohydrate metabolism to fat substrates, and metabolite accumulation.[47]

The associated signs and symptoms of PRIS vary by report but generally include worsening metabolic acidosis (sometimes specifically identified as lactic acidosis), triglyceride elevations, worsening hypotension and pressor requirements, and arrhythmias (tachycardia, bradycardia, and bundle branch block), with variable inclusion of renal failure, hyperkalemia, rhabdomyolysis, and liver dysfunction.[46–48] An analysis of more than 1100 cases (including 342 fatalities) suggested that death was more likely if patients were younger than 18 years, or if cardiac symptoms, hypotension, rhabdomyolysis, renal dysfunction, or metabolic acidosis were present.[48] Although usually associated with prolonged, high-dose administration greater than 70 μg/kg/min, several cases have been reported with short duration and lower doses, including surgical anesthesia or sedation for nonoperative cardiac procedures.[65,66] Early recognition of possible PRIS is of critical importance, and management remains empiric but must include stopping propofol. Additional treatment options include supporting the hemodynamic and cardiac dysfunction with fluids and pressors or inotropes and even extracorporeal devices, and consideration for hemodialysis or hemofiltration.

The alpha-2 agonists clonidine and dexmedetomidine represent the major alternative to the GABA-agonist drug class for ICU sedation. Clonidine is available for intravenous use in many countries. Dexmedetomidine, first approved in 1999 by the FDA, is the only intravenous alpha-2 agonist available in the United States. Both medications bind to noradrenergic receptors in the brain, spinal cord, and throughout the body. Distinct from GABA agonists, alpha-2 agonists provide analgesic effects and sedation, with little or no respiratory depression. The analgesic component of dexmedetomidine provides patient comfort simultaneously with sedation, possibly similar to the A1 philosophy, although this has not been directly studied. Sympatholytic effects lower heart rate and blood pressure, which may be beneficial (reducing tachycardia and hypertension) or undesirable (hypotension and bradycardia).

Several randomized studies have compared the benzodiazepines (lorazepam or midazolam) or propofol to dexmedetomidine.[43,49–51,67] The major benefits with dexmedetomidine include a reduction in the incidence of delirium, a reduction in time on mechanical ventilation, and a reduction in tachycardia and hypertension. The incidence of delirium was reduced with dexmedetomidine in three of the four studies reporting this outcome, complementing earlier data that benzodiazepines may be deliriogenic in the dose range commonly used among adult ICU patients.[44] The pilot study that did not show a delirium reduction[51] compared dexmedetomidine with standard care rather than a protocol-controlled comparator medication, and it used a composite definition of delirium (**Fig. 2**). The incidence of adverse effects varied between studies, but hypotension appeared to be similar between benzodiazepines and dexmedetomidine. Tachycardia and hypertension were more frequent with benzodiazepines, whereas bradycardia was more common with dexmedetomidine. The definitions for bradycardia varied by study, but treatment for the bradycardia was rarely required. Two studies allowed clinicians to select different sedation target goals for their patients[43,51]; post hoc analysis suggested that deep sedation levels may be attained less easily with dexmedetomidine than with benzodiazepines.

The 2 blinded, randomized controlled studies that compared dexmedetomidine with benzodiazepines (Maximizing Efficacy of Targeted Sedation and Reducing Neurological Dysfunction [MENDS] and Safety and Efficacy of Dexmedetomidine Compared With Midazolam [SEDCOM]) showed similar findings.[43,49] The MENDS study compared dexmedetomidine (in doses up to 1.5 μg/kg/h) and lorazepam infusions (in doses up to 10 mg/h) among 106 medical and surgical ICU patients at two centers for up to 5 days.[43] Target sedation levels were defined by the clinical team for each patient. Patients who received dexmedetomidine had a higher number of days alive without delirium or coma and were within their target sedation range more often. The SEDCOM multicenter study compared dexmedetomidine (in doses up to 1.4 μg/kg/h) and midazolam infusions (in doses up to 0.1 mg/kg/h) among 375 medical and surgical ICU patients for up to 30 days[49] with a common light sedation target for all patients (RASS of −2 to +1) and a required daily arousal assessment. Patients receiving dexmedetomidine had a lower prevalence of delirium (54% vs 76.6%, P<.001) and a shorter duration of ventilatory support (3.7 days vs 5.6 days, P = .01). Regardless of which sedative agent is selected, a strategy to provide lighter sedation consistently reduces length of stay in the ICU and reduces duration of mechanical ventilation.[36,68–70] Daily interruption of sedation (63 kress) and providing a protocol to down-titrate sedative agents (rather than interrupt)[69] appear similarly effective in a pilot study.[70] A larger study to compare these strategies is nearing completion.[71]

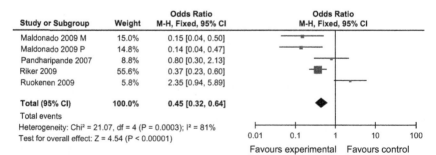

Fig. 2. Forest plot showing the incidence of delirium in 4 randomized studies that compared dexmedetomidine with midazolam or propofol after cardiac surgery, with lorazepam, with midazolam, or with standard care. The cumulative odds ratio shows a dramatic reduction (0.45) of delirium with dexmedetomidine use. (*Data from* Refs.[43,49–51])

Delirium

A major advancement in patient monitoring during the last decade includes the development and validation of delirium-screening tools. ICU delirium is a clinically important, but commonly undetected, problem affecting as many as 80% of critically ill patients. Underrecognition may relate to the complex nature of this syndrome, to the variability of symptoms, and to the fact that the most common form of delirium, the hypoactive subtype, is easy to overlook unless routine assessment is performed.[72] Two assessment tools were published in 2001 to facilitate recognition of delirium: CAM-ICU and the ICDSC.[25–28] These tools have improved identification of ICU delirium, but it is not yet confirmed that these tools improve outcomes, nor how best to treat delirium. These questions remain the next challenges for clinical researchers. A recent multidimensional ICU protocol howed reductions in subsyndromal delirium.[73]

Cognitive Sequelae

After surviving their stay in the ICU, many patients will suffer from cognitive deficits, such as memory impairments, difficulty maintaining attention or concentrating, reduced processing speed, and general intellectual decline.[56,57] The prevalence of these impairments varies from 25% to 78% and they are a major determining factor in whether patients return to work and regain productivity.[56] More subtle cognitive impairments can affect driving, money management, the ability to perform activities of daily living, and family interactions. There is growing data that the sedation approach clinicians choose in the ICU is associated with these outcomes.[56]

RECOMMENDATIONS FOR CHANGES IN PRACTICE

Based on the above evidence, several important changes supported in multiple studies can now be recommended when providing sedation for ICU patients. These are summarized in **Box 2**.

Consider providing analgesia first before initiating sedative therapy, guided by patient self-report or validated pain tools, such as the Critical-Care Pain Observation Tool or the Behavioral Pain Scale. Analgesics such as remifentanil, fentanyl, morphine, and dexmedetomidine may allow patient comfort and wakefulness to coexist. Many ICU patients can remain awake or lightly sedated if they are comfortable. If lightly sedated but pain-free patients are still not able to tolerate their care, additional sedation may be needed. Consider dexmedetomidine because of its beneficial effects to reduce delirium and duration of mechanical ventilation, and its cost-effectiveness.[52,53] There is no evidence to identify which patients require deep sedation (SAS of 1 or 2, RASS of −4 or −5, Ramsay of 4–6), but if patients remain intolerant of their care despite analgesia and light or moderate sedation, dexmedetomidine may require supplementation. If GABA agonists, such as midazolam, lorazepam, or propofol, are added or substituted, avoid prolonged sedation with daily awakenings or dose-reduction strategies, especially with the benzodiazepines. A multicenter study showed reductions in duration of mechanical ventilation, ICU time, and mortality when daily awakening is linked to spontaneous breathing trials.[74]

When using the GABA agonists, understand the common adverse effects that can occur and the less common but life-threatening adverse effects. Many of these are dose-related, so strategies to reduce sedative doses may reduce the incidence of adverse effects. Avoid midazolam accumulation by dose-reduction protocols or daily awakening.[49,68,69] Avoid propylene glycol toxicity with lorazepam dosing by monitoring the osmol gap serially as daily doses approach or exceed 1 mg/kg.[41] Recognize the signs of PRIS associated with death (age <18 years, dysrhythmias, hypotension,

---

Box 2
A recommended approach for ICU sedation

1. Provide analgesia first, with remifentanil, fentanyl, morphine, or possibly dexmedetomidine. Monitor analgesia adequacy with patient self-report if possible, or, if not possible, with a validated assessment tool.

2. Propofol and dexmedetomidine may be beneficial compared with benzodiazepines, if a sedative is needed. Consider dexmedetomidine for ICU patients because of its beneficial effects on delirium, cost-effectiveness, and mechanical ventilation, unless

   A. Deep sedation or an amnestic condition is required

   B. The patient has bradycardia or severe left ventricular dysfunction

3. Avoid the adverse effects commonly associated with standard sedative medications.

   A. Avoid midazolam accumulation by limiting the duration of use; practice at least daily interruption of drug or awakening the patient, and targeting the lightest level of sedation possible.

   B. If lorazepam is used, avoid continuous infusion if possible; monitor the serum osmol gap if daily doses approach 1 mg/kg. If lorazepam is infused continuously, interrupt drug or awaken the patient at least daily, and target the lightest level of sedation possible.

   C. If propofol is used, avoid prolonged use or doses greater than 70 mg/kg/min, and monitor triglycerides, creatine kinase, arterial blood gases, liver and renal function, and electrocardiogram. Be aware of the signs of PRIS, and discontinue propofol if these appear.

4. Monitor all patients for delirium, even those who are calm and not agitated.

5. Before hospital discharge, assess cognitive function in patients, and consider neuropsychiatric follow-up for anyone who needs it.

---

rhabdomyolysis, renal dysfunction, or metabolic acidosis) and substitute other medications for propofol if these develop or progress.[48] Finally, routine monitoring of all patients for delirium using the CAM-ICU or ICDSC allows clinicians to identify patients with delirium and to develop specific treatment plans for this disorder.[25–28] This may identify a cohort of patients at very high risk for prolonged cognitive impairments for whom neuropsychiatric testing and counseling may be beneficial, although even non-delirious patients may suffer from these cognitive sequelae.[75]

SUMMARY

Providing sedation and comfort for intensive care patients has evolved in the last 30 years but remains difficult for clinicians. As research has focused on this challenging area, the authors have identified ways to improve practice, including providing analgesia before sedation, strategies to help recognize dangerous adverse effects associated with the medications that are used, and better ways to monitor pain and delirium in patients. Dexmedetomidine and propofol have become the preferred sedatives for many ICU situations, and creative ways to administer them, such as linking awakening and breathing trials, are emerging. Finally, screening survivors for cognitive impairments may allow clinicians to refer them for the focused rehabilitation they require.

REFERENCES

1. Ramsay MA, Savege TM, Simpson BR, et al. Controlled sedation with alphax-alone-alphadolone. Br Med J 1974;2(5920):656–9.

2. Merriman HM. The techniques used to sedate ventilated patients. A survey of methods used in 34 ICUs in Great Britain. Intensive Care Med 1981;7(5):217–24.
3. Simpson PJ, Eltringham RJ. Lorazepam in intensive care. Clin Ther 1981;4(3): 150–63.
4. Edbrooke DL, Newby DM, Mather SJ, et al. Safer sedation for ventilated patients. A new application for etomidate. Anaesthesia 1982;37(7):765–71.
5. Ledingham IM, Watt I. Influence of sedation on mortality in critically ill multiple trauma patients. Lancet 1983;1(8336):1270.
6. Parker MM, Schubert W, Shelhamer JH, et al. Perceptions of a critically ill patient experiencing therapeutic paralysis in an ICU. Crit Care Med 1984;12(1):69–71.
7. Ball M, McQuay HJ, Moore RA, et al. Renal failure and the use of morphine in intensive care. Lancet 1985;1(8432):784–6.
8. Shapiro JM, Westphal LM, White PF, et al. Midazolam infusion for sedation in the intensive care unit: effect on adrenal function. Anesthesiology 1986;64(3): 394–8.
9. Grounds RM, Lalor JM, Lumley J, et al. Propofol infusion for sedation in the intensive care unit: preliminary report. Br Med J (Clin Res Ed) 1987;294(6569): 397–400.
10. Geller E, Halpern P, Barzelai E, et al. Midazolam infusion and the benzodiazepine antagonist flumazenil for sedation of intensive care patients. Resuscitation 1988; 16(Suppl):S31–9.
11. Segredo V, Matthay MA, Sharma ML, et al. Prolonged neuromuscular blockade after long-term administration of vecuronium in two critically ill patients. Anesthesiology 1990;72(3):566–70.
12. Shapiro BA, Warren J, Egol AB, et al. Practice parameters for intravenous analgesia and sedation for adult patients in the intensive care unit: an executive summary. Crit Care Med 1995;23(9):1596–600.
13. Jacobi J, Fraser GL, Coursin DB, et al. Clinical practice guidelines for the sustained use of sedatives and analgesics in the critically ill adult. Crit Care Med 2002;30(1):119–41.
14. Rhoney DH, Murry KR. National survey of the use of sedating drugs, neuromuscular blocking agents, and reversal agents in the intensive care unit. J Intensive Care Med 2003;18(3):139–45.
15. Patel RP, Gambrell M, Speroff T, et al. Delirium and sedation in the intensive care unit: survey of behaviors and attitudes of 1384 healthcare professionals. Crit Care Med 2009;37(3):825–32.
16. Wunsch H, Kahn JM, Kramer AA, et al. Use of intravenous infusion sedation among mechanically ventilated patients in the United States. Crit Care Med 2009;37(12):3031–9.
17. Martin J, Franck M, Sigel S, et al. Changes in sedation management in German intensive care units between 2002 and 2006: a national follow-up survey. Crit Care 2007;11(6):R124.
18. Martin J, Franck M, Fischer M, et al. Sedation and analgesia in German intensive care units: how is it done in reality? Results of a patient-based survey of analgesia and sedation. Intensive Care Med 2006;32(8):1137–42.
19. Shehabi Y, Botha JA, Boyle MS, et al. Sedation and delirium in the intensive care unit: an Australian and New Zealand perspective. Anaesth Intensive Care 2008; 36:1–9.
20. Mehta S, Burry L, Fischer S, et al. Canadian survey of the use of sedatives, analgesics, and neuromuscular blocking agents in critically ill patients. Crit Care Med 2006;34(2):374–80.

21. Mehta S, Meade MO, Hynes P, et al. A multicenter survey of Ontario intensive care unit nurses regarding the use of sedatives and analgesics for adults receiving mechanical ventilation. J Crit Care 2007;22(3):191–6.
22. Mehta S, McCullagh I, Burry L. Current sedation practices: lessons learned from international surveys. Crit Care Clin 2009;25(3):471–88.
23. Riker RR, Picard JT, Fraser GL. Prospective evaluation of the sedation-agitation scale in adult ICU patients. Crit Care Med 1999;27:1325–9.
24. Sessler CN, Gosnell MS, Grap MJ, et al. The Richmond Agitation-Sedation Scale: validity and reliability in adult intensive care unit patients. Am J Respir Crit Care Med 2002;166(10):1338–44.
25. Ely EW, Margolin R, Francis J, et al. Evaluation of delirium in critically ill patients: validation of the confusion assessment method for the intensive care unit (CAM-ICU). Crit Care Med 2001;29(7):1370–9.
26. Ely EW, Inouye SK, Bernard GR, et al. Delirium in mechanically ventilated patients: validity and reliability of the confusion assessment method for the intensive care unit (CAM-ICU). JAMA 2001;286(21):2703–10.
27. Bergeron N, Dubois MJ, Dumont M, et al. Intensive Care Delirium Screening Checklist: evaluation of a new screening tool. Intensive Care Med 2001;27(5): 859–64.
28. Devlin JW, Fong JJ, Schumaker G, et al. Use of a validated delirium assessment tool improves the ability of physicians to identify delirium in medical intensive care unit patients. Crit Care Med 2007;35(12):2721–4.
29. Puntillo KA, White C, Morris AB, et al. Patients' perceptions and responses to procedural pain: results from Thunder Project II. Am J Crit Care 2001;10(4):238–51.
30. Gélinas C. Management of pain in cardiac surgery ICU patients: have we improved over time? Intensive Crit Care Nurs 2007;23(5):298–303.
31. Breen D, Karabinis A, Malbrain M, et al. Decreased duration of mechanical ventilation when comparing analgesia-based sedation using remifentanil with standard hypnotic-based sedation for up to 10 days in intensive care unit patients: a randomised trial. Crit Care 2005;9(3):R200–10.
32. Dahaba AA, Grabner T, Rehak PH, et al. Remifentanil versus morphine analgesia and sedation for mechanically ventilated critically ill patients: a randomized double blind study. Anesthesiology 2004;101(3):640–6.
33. Muellejans B, Lopez A, Cross MH, et al. Remifentanil versus fentanyl for analgesia based sedation to provide patient comfort in the intensive care unit: a randomized double-blind controlled trial. Critical Care 2004;8:R1–11.
34. Rozendaal FW, Spronk PE, Snellen FF, et al. Remifentanil-propofol analgosedation shortens duration of ventilation and length of ICU stay compared to a conventional regimen: a centre randomised, cross-over, open-label study in the Netherlands. Intensive Care Med 2008;35:291–8.
35. Muellejans B, Matthey T, Scholpp J, et al. Sedation in the intensive care unit with remifentanil/propofol versus midazolam/fentanyl: a randomized, open-label, pharmacoeconomic trial. Critical Care 2006;10:R91.
36. Treggiari MM, Romand JA, Yanez ND, et al. Randomized trial of light versus deep sedation on mental health after critical illness. Crit Care Med 2009;37(9):2527–34.
37. Schweickert WD, Pohlman MC, Pohlman AS, et al. Early physical and occupational therapy in mechanically ventilated, critically ill patients: a randomised controlled trial. Lancet 2009;373(9678):1874–82.
38. Strøm T, Martinussen T, Toft P. A protocol of no sedation for critically ill patients receiving mechanical ventilation: a randomised trial. Lancet 2010;375(9713): 475–80.

39. Bauer TM, Ritz R, Haberthür C, et al. Prolonged sedation due to accumulation of conjugated metabolites of midazolam. Lancet 1995;346(8968):145–7.
40. Spina SP, Ensom MH. Clinical pharmacokinetic monitoring of midazolam in critically ill patients. Pharmacotherapy 2007;27(3):389–98.
41. Yahwak JA, Riker RR, Fraser GL, et al. Determination of a lorazepam dose threshold for using the osmol gap to monitor for propylene glycol toxicity. Pharmacotherapy 2008;28:984–91.
42. Nelsen JL, Haas CE, Habtemariam B, et al. A prospective evaluation of propylene glycol clearance and accumulation during continuous-infusion lorazepam in critically ill patients. J Intensive Care Med 2008;23(3):184–94.
43. Pandharipande PP, Pun BT, Herr DL, et al. Effect of sedation with dexmedetomidine vs lorazepam on acute brain dysfunction in mechanically ventilated patients: the MENDS randomized controlled trial. JAMA 2007;298(22):2644–53.
44. Pandharipande P, Shintani A, Peterson J, et al. Lorazepam is an independent risk factor for transitioning to delirium in intensive care unit patients. Anesthesiology 2006;104(1):21–6.
45. Pandharipande P, Cotton BA, Shintani A, et al. Prevalence and risk factors for development of delirium in surgical and trauma intensive care unit patients. J Trauma 2008;65(1):34–41.
46. Mallow Corbett S, Montoya ID, Moore FA. Propofol-related infusion syndrome in intensive care patients. Pharmacotherapy 2008;28(2):250–8.
47. Kam PCA, Cardone D. Propofol infusion syndrome. Anaesthesia 2007;62:690–701.
48. Fong JJ, Sylvia L, Ruthazer R, et al. Predictors of mortality in patients with suspected propofol infusion syndrome. Crit Care Med 2008;36:2281–7.
49. Riker RR, Shehabi Y, Bokesch PM, et al. Dexmedetomidine vs midazolam for sedation of critically ill patients: a randomized trial. JAMA 2009;301(5):489–99.
50. Maldonado J, Wysong A, van der Starre P, et al. Dexmedetomidine and the reduction of postoperative delirium after cardiac surgery. Psychosomatics, in press.
51. Ruokonen E, Parviainen I, Jakob SM, et al. Dexmedetomidine versus propofol/midazolam for long-term sedation during mechanical ventilation. Intensive Care Med 2009;35(2):282–90.
52. Dasta JF, Kane-Gill SL, Pencina M, et al. A cost-minimization analysis of dexmedetomidine compared to midazolam for long-term sedation in the ICU. Crit Care Med 2010;38(1):497–503.
53. Dasta JF, Jacobi J, Sesti AM, et al. Addition of dexmedetomidine to standard sedation regimens after cardiac surgery: an outcomes analysis. Pharmacotherapy 2006;26(6):798–805.
54. Gélinas C, Fillion L, Puntillo KA, et al. Validation of the critical-care pain observation tool in adult patients. Am J Crit Care 2006;15(4):420–7.
55. Payen JF, Bru O, Bosson JL, et al. Assessing pain in critically ill sedated patients by using a behavioral pain scale. Crit Care Med 2001;29(12):2258–63.
56. Hopkins RO, Jackson JC. Long-term neurocognitive function after critical illness. Chest 2006;130(3):869–78.
57. Milbrandt EB, Angus DC. Bench-to-bedside review: critical illness-associated cognitive dysfunction–mechanisms, markers, and emerging therapeutics. Crit Care 2006;10(6):238.
58. Bergbom-Engberg I, Haljamäe H. Assessment of patients' experience of discomforts during respiratory therapy. Crit Care Med 1989;17(10):1068–72.
59. Payen JF, Bosson JL, Chanques G, et al. Pain assessment is associated with decreased duration of mechanical ventilation in the intensive care unit: a post Hoc analysis of the DOLOREA study. Anesthesiology 2009;111(6):1308–16.

60. Spies C, Macguill M, Heymann A, et al. A prospective, randomized, double-blind, multicenter study comparing remifentanil with fentanyl in mechanically ventilated patients. Intensive Care Med 2011;37(3):469–76.
61. Kanazawa H, Okada A, Igarashi E, et al. Determination of midazolam and its metabolite as a probe for cytochrome P450 3A4 phenotype by liquid chromatography-mass spectrometry. J Chromatogr A 2004;1031(1-2):213–8.
62. Laine GA, Hossain SM, Solis RT, et al. Polyethylene glycol nephrotoxicity secondary to prolonged high-dose intravenous lorazepam. Ann Pharmacother 1995;29(11):1110–4.
63. Seay RE, Graves PJ, Wilkin MK. Comment: possible toxicity from propylene glycol in lorazepam infusion. Ann Pharmacother 1997;31(5):647–8.
64. Reynolds HN, Teiken P, Regan ME, et al. Hyperlactatemia, increased osmolar gap, and renal dysfunction during continuous lorazepam infusion. Crit Care Med 2000;28(5):1631–4.
65. Merz TM, Regli B, Rothen HU, et al. Propofol infusion syndrome–a fatal case at a low infusion rate. Anesth Analg 2006;103(4):1050.
66. Chukwuemeka A, Ko R, Ralph-Edwards A. Short-term low-dose propofol anaesthesia associated with severe metabolic acidosis. Anaesth Intensive Care 2006; 34(5):651–5.
67. Herr DL, Sum-Ping STJ, England M. ICU sedation after coronary artery bypass graft surgery: dexmedetomidine-based versus propofol-based sedation regimens. J Cardiothorac Vasc Anesth 2003;17(5):576–84.
68. Kress JP, Pohlman AS, O'Connor MF, et al. Daily interruption of sedative infusions in critically ill patients undergoing mechanical ventilation. N Engl J Med 2000; 342(20):1471–7.
69. Brook AD, Ahrens TS, Schaiff R, et al. Effect of a nursing-implemented sedation protocol on the duration of mechanical ventilation. Crit Care Med 1999;27(12): 2609–15.
70. Mehta S, Burry L, Martinez-Motta JC, et al. A randomized trial of daily awakening in critically ill patients managed with a sedation protocol: a pilot trial. Crit Care Med 2008;36(7):2092–9.
71. Study NCT00675363. Available at: Clintrials.gov. Accessed September 23, 2011.
72. Peterson JF, Pun BT, Dittus RS, et al. Delirium and its motoric subtypes: a study of 614 critically ill patients. J Am Geriatr Soc 2006;54(3):479–84.
73. Skrobik Y, Ahern S, Leblanc M, et al. Protocolized intensive care unit management of analgesia, sedation, and delirium improves analgesia and subsyndromal delirium rates. Anesth Analg 2010;111(2):451–63.
74. Girard TD, Kress JP, Fuchs BD, et al. Efficacy and safety of a paired sedation and ventilator weaning protocol for mechanically ventilated patients in intensive care (Awakening and Breathing Controlled trial): a randomised controlled trial. Lancet 2008;371(9607):126–34.
75. Jones C, Griffiths RD, Slater T, et al. Significant cognitive dysfunction in non-delirious patients identified during and persisting following critical illness. Intensive Care Med 2006;32(6):923–6.

Sedation and Sleep Disturbances in the ICU

Gerald L. Weinhouse, MD[a],*, Paula L. Watson, MD[b]

KEYWORDS

• Sedation • Sleep • Critically ill • Intensive care unit • Outcomes

Critically ill patients are often given sedating medications to facilitate their treatment and to increase their comfort. These medications enable some patients to tolerate mechanical ventilation, serve as an adjunct to pain management, and help many patients cope with the psychosocial stresses of critical illness. They have also been believed to facilitate sleep; however, the relationship between sedation and sleep is complex. Patients under the influence of sedation may appear to be asleep; however, sedation differs from sleep physiologically and clinically. This relationship may be important because it has become apparent that intensive care unit (ICU) patients sleep poorly and that this poor sleep is associated with poor ICU outcomes.[1]

Sleep disturbances experienced by ICU patients are common and consistent across different types of ICUs. Decades of research has confirmed that the sleep of ICU patients is disrupted by ICU environmental factors, medical illness, diagnostic testing, and treatment-related factors.[2–9] Medications, in particular the sedatives and analgesics, have been implicated in some of the adverse effects on sleep observed in critically ill patients; however, sedatives may also promote sleep.

This article reviews (1) the common ICU sleep disturbances, (2) the relationship between sedation and sleep, and (3) the effects of commonly used sedatives on natural sleep, by their acute effects and by withdrawal.

SLEEP DISTURBANCES IN THE ICU

The sleep characteristic of critically ill patients differs from that of healthy individuals in its distribution during the course of a day and the percentage of time spent in the different sleep stages, that is, sleep architecture. Critically ill patients, especially those on mechanical ventilation, have severely fragmented sleep (**Fig. 1**).[3,6,7] Although many studies have shown that the total number of sleep hours may be normal over 24 hours, they are distributed across day and night in short periods.[3,4,6] A disproportionate

A version of this article appeared in the 25:3 issue of *Critical Care Clinics*.
[a] Department of Medicine, Harvard Medical School, 75 Francis Street, Boston, MA 02115, USA
[b] Department of Medicine, Vanderbilt University School of Medicine, 6th Floor MCE 6115, 21st Avenue South, Nashville, TN 37232-8300, USA
* Corresponding author.
E-mail address: gweinhouse@partners.org

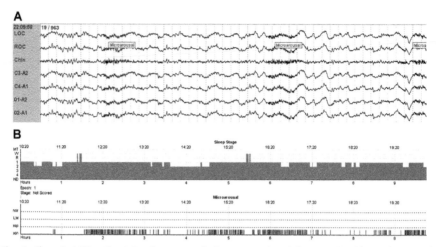

Fig. 1. Sleep in ICU patients is often severely fragmented and characterized by an increase in light sleep and a paucity of slow wave and REM sleep. (*A*) Polysomnography tracing from a critically ill, sedated patient, demonstrating sleep fragmentation with microarousals noted approximately every 10 s. (*B*) Sleep histogram from the same patient showing a predominance of stage I sleep with frequent microarousals.

amount of time is spent in light sleep (non–rapid eye movement [NREM] sleep stages I and II) and wakefulness and a relatively small percentage of time in deep sleep (slow wave sleep [SWS], formerly referred to as NREM stages III and IV) and rapid eye movement (REM) sleep.[3,5,7,8,10,11]

Experimental models of sleep fragmentation and sleep stage deprivation have demonstrated many of the same consequences as with periods of total sleep deprivation, but controlled studies have not been done in the critically ill.[12,13] It is clear, however, that problems with sleep have had a profound effect on patients who consistently recall their ICU sleep problems as disturbing.[14–18] Many continue to have difficulty sleeping long after surviving their critical illness.[17] In addition, this model of experimental sleep loss may be associated with neurocognitive effects with clinical and physiologic similarities to delirium and has effects on many biologic, immunologic, and metabolic functions that could be important to patients' recovery.[19–26]

RELATIONSHIP BETWEEN SEDATION AND SLEEP

Natural sleep is an active process that occurs when neurons located in the hypothalamus coordinate the inhibition of the arousal pathways located in the brainstem and hypothalamus and those in the thalamus.[27] The transition from wakefulness to NREM sleep occurs when these γ-aminobutyric acid (GABA) and galananin-containing inhibitory neurons become activated. Sedatives intersect with these pathways at various points, leading to the observed similarities and differences between states.

Sleep and sedation lead to a decrease in responsiveness to external stimuli, reduction in muscle tone, and respiratory depression. Positron emission tomography has demonstrated patterns of regional change in cerebral metabolism similar between the two states.[28] It is known that patients respond to anesthetic agents differently when sleep-deprived than when allowed to sleep, and animal models further suggest that there may be a genetic relationship between sleep and sedation.[29,30] Ultimately, because the functions of sleep are not known, it is not possible to determine if the essential benefits of sleep are recovered during sedation. However, at least one of the phenotypic characteristics of sleep loss, the clinical signs of sleepiness, may be improved during sedation (to be further discussed in a later section).

Although the similarities between sleep and sedation are compelling, the differences are numerous. Sleep is an essential biologic function necessary for life and easily reversed by external stimuli. It is influenced by circadian rhythmicity and characterized by cyclic progression of stages defined by well-established electroencephalographic (EEG) criteria. Sedation has none of these characteristics. The effects of sedation on the EEG are medication-specific and dose-dependent rather than cyclic. The effects of these medications and of the underlying illness itself on the EEG may lead to atypical patterns that cannot be classified by normal sleep staging criteria (**Fig. 2**). A recent study calls into question whether multichannel polysomnography, which is the traditional method of measuring sleep and depends on EEG recording, can even be considered the diagnostic standard in the sedated, mechanically ventilated critically ill.[31] Previous investigators have also found EEG anomalies in the sedated critically ill, which made it difficult to interpret the studies.[7]

It is clear, therefore, that the differences between sleep and sedation are at least as important as the similarities, but it is less clear whether sedation is directly responsible for the adverse outcomes associated with the poor sleep of the critically ill. Sedatives have effects that may overall serve to benefit some patients' sleep. As with other medications, it may be the case that the overall benefits of the medication to the primary problem might outweigh the direct negative effects on sleep architecture. Asthma medications, for example, may directly worsen sleep by their sympathomimetic effects; however, they improve patients' dyspnea and therefore have been shown to improve sleep overall.[32] For those patients whose anxiety and stress might lead to significant sleep disruption, therefore, sedatives may be beneficial overall to their sleep.

Sedatives do have some direct beneficial effects on sleep in healthy individuals. They shorten the time to sleep latency and increase total time asleep by EEG criteria.[33] Some sedatives also have an amnestic effect and may benefit those patients who might otherwise recall unpleasant ICU experiences. Sedatives, therefore, may have positive and negative effects on patients' sleep and ICU quality of life.

THE EFFECTS OF SEDATIVE MEDICATIONS ON NATURAL SLEEP

The two classes of medications most commonly used for ICU sedation include those that interact with the GABA receptor to enhance central nervous system (CNS) inhibition and those that bind to α-2-receptors in locus ceruleus to decrease noradrenergic innervation. Other classes of medications are often used by clinicians to capitalize on

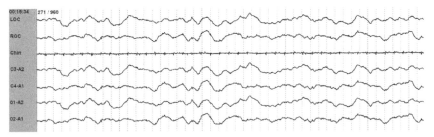

Fig. 2. A30-s epoch showing polymorphic delta activity in a sedated, critically ill patient. Atypical EEG characteristics such as these are seen in critically ill patients and often make it difficult to characterize sleep stages using standard sleep staging criteria.

sedation as a side effect of the drug, but they are not in the sedative class; these medications include antipsychotics and opioids. What is known of the effects of these medications on natural sleep has been reviewed.

GABA Agonists

GABA agonists, which include benzodiazepines and propofol, are the medications recommended as first-line sedation in the ICU.[34] Benzodiazepines, as well as barbiturates and ethanol, activate the α subunit of the GABA receptor, thus enhancing the most potent CNS inhibitory system and leading to the psychomotor depression seen clinically.[27] They exert their sedative effect on the α-1-GABA$_A$ receptor subunit; however, they may exert their hypnotic effect on subunits other than the α-1-GABA$_A$ receptor subunit and affect targets of the ventrolateral preoptic area (VLPO) of the hypothalamus to suppress arousal.[35] At higher doses, they have a more generalized CNS inhibitory effect.

Their effect on the EEG is to induce a dose-dependent increase in EEG characteristics of NREM sleep, a mild reduction of REM sleep, a potent suppression of SWS, and an increase in spindle activity (an EEG hallmark of stage II NREM sleep) but with subtle qualitative differences from those seen with natural sleep.[35–37] Their effect at the more downstream targets of the natural sleep pathway leaves norepinephrine release, decreased during natural sleep, unaffected. In addition, regional cerebral blood flow after a dose of benzodiazepine has been shown to differ from that during natural sleep.[38]

Propofol is believed to bind to the GABA$_A$ receptor at a site distinct from the benzodiazepines' binding site where it allosterically enhances activity of the receptor.[39] Similar to the benzodiazepines, propofol suppresses SWS but has no definite effect on REM sleep.

Blood concentration of propofol is negatively correlated with EEG frequency to the point where high enough doses cause a burst-suppression pattern (**Fig. 3**).[40,41] Its effect on cerebral perfusion is also somewhat distinct from that of the benzodiazepines with a more global effect seen on imaging of glucose metabolism. Propofol titrated just to the point of loss of consciousness causes a 55% reduction in overall cerebral glucose metabolism compared with a 23% reduction during NREM sleep.[28] There are also regional differences with propofol having a greater effect on cortical than subcortical regions, which is consistent with previous observations of higher benzodiazepine receptor density in cortical compared with subcortical regions.

There have been a limited number of clinical studies in humans on the effects of these agents on sleep. Diurnal sedation has been achieved with propofol in some critically ill patients in one study.[42] Treggiari-Venzi and colleagues[43] found that there was a trend toward improved patient perception of sleep under the influence of both midazolam and propofol, which was independent of their effect on anxiety and depression. And in a small study of healthy volunteers, propofol given to subjects from 2 PM to 3 PM was associated with a delayed sleep onset latency.[44] This study could reflect an overlapping function between sleep and sedation with propofol because a similar delay in sleep latency would occur if natural sleep were allowed to occur

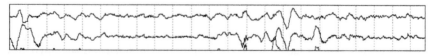

Fig. 3. Burst-suppression EEG pattern may be seen in association with heavy sedation.

during the day. More study, however, would be necessary to reach any conclusion about the relationship between sleep and sedation with benzodiazepines and propofol.

It is the animal studies of the clinical effects of propofol on sleep that are most provocative. Tung and colleagues[45] found that rats sedated with propofol during their normal sleep time did not demonstrate clinical signs of sleep deprivation. They concluded that sedation with propofol is compatible with a restorative process similar to that occurring during natural sleep but could only speculate whether this is a direct effect of the drug or whether propofol facilitated natural sleep. They followed their investigation to determine if recovery from sleep deprivation can occur during sedation with propofol. Using the same rat model, they found that after 24 hours of imposed total sleep deprivation, recovery sleep was no different under the influence of 6 hours of propofol compared with normal recovery sleep, suggesting that the normal homeostatic control of sleep may occur during sedation with propofol.[46] These data may not be enough to guide clinical practice but should serve to encourage further study.

α-2-Agonist

In the United States, dexmedetomidine is the only parenteral agent in this class of sedatives available for use. It binds to receptors in locus ceruleus, which reduces norepinephrine release and thereby disinhibits the VLPO neurons that inhibit the arousal pathways.[47] Its effects on the EEG are to induce a dose-dependent slowing, a decrease in percentage of REM, an increase in percentage of SWS, and an increase in percentage of stage II based on an increase in spindle activity. The spindles observed under sedation with dexmedetomidine are similar qualitatively to those during natural sleep but have a longer duration.[48] In addition, functional magnetic resonance imaging has demonstrated similar patterns under dexmedetomidine and natural sleep.[49]

Clinically, sedation under dexmedetomidine more closely resembles natural sleep than sedation under the GABA agonists. Patients sedated with α-agonists are more easily aroused and more cognitively intact when aroused.[50,51] In summary, it interacts with the natural sleep pathway at a site farther upstream than the GABA agonists and leads to a state with clinical features similar to natural sleep. Unfortunately, these theoretical advantages have not been demonstrated to improve patients' perception of their sleep in the ICU. In fact, a survey of patients who underwent elective coronary artery bypass surgery reported that patients believed they had more difficulty resting or sleeping when sedated with dexmedetomidine compared with propofol.[52] The role of dexmedetomidine in improving sleep in the critically ill remains to be defined, and further studies are underway.

Antipsychotics

The "typical" and "atypical" antipsychotics are used in the ICU for their sedative effects, especially given the association between conventional sedation and delirium and respiratory depression.[53] The most commonly used typical antipsychotic, haloperidol, has been associated with increased sleep efficiency and stage II sleep with little effect on SWS in healthy volunteers.[54] In a randomized, controlled prospective trial of pediatric burn patients, haloperidol increased total sleep time and stage II sleep compared with control nights but did not restore a normal quantity of sleep over a 6-night study period.[55]

The atypical antipsychotics, such as olanzapine and risperidone, increase total sleep time, sleep efficiency, and SWS in healthy volunteers and schizophrenic patients.[54] Subjective sleep quality has been correlated with SWS.[56] These medications have been prescribed with increasing frequency in the ICU for their sedating effects beyond those of haloperidol. The adverse effect and safety profiles of all antipsychotics, however, argue for their use with caution.

Opioids

Opioids are analgesics often used in conjunction with sedatives and occasionally titrated for their sedative effect. They exert their sedative/hypnotic effect on the ponto-thalamic arousal pathway most active in REM generation rather than the hypo-thalamic pathway more affected by the GABA agonists.[27,57] As a result, they have a potent, dose-dependent REM-suppressive effect mediated by the mu receptor.[58] In addition, they also decrease SWS and increase stage II NREM sleep by EEG criteria. A single low dose of an opioid was associated with a 30% to 50% reduction in SWS in healthy adult volunteers.[59]

Sleep disturbances are common for individuals with pain and occur in 50% to 70% of chronic pain patients.[60,61] Poor sleep may also increase patients' perception of pain.[61] After surgery, pain may be the most important impediment to sleep; analgesia may be an effective intervention despite its effects on sleep architecture.[62] In a large randomized, placebo-controlled, double-blind trial in patients with osteoarthritis pain, opioids were found to improve several subjective measures of sleep quality, including subjects' overall perception of sleep quality.[63] In a small study of the contribution of opioids to postoperative sleep disturbance, investigators randomized subjects to receive either fentanyl or bupivacaine through an epidural and found no statistically significant differences between subjects' sleep quality.[64] They concluded that although there were minor effects of the opioids on SWS, the profound sleep disturbance observed postoperatively occurs independent of the medication. Therefore, the adverse effects of opioids on the sleep architecture of healthy, pain-free subjects may be counterbalanced by their beneficial effects, especially in the postoperative period.

MEDICATION WITHDRAWAL ON SLEEP

When individuals are deprived of sleep, they begin to build up pressure to recover the lost sleep. The EEG characteristics of recovery sleep depend on the characteristics of the lost sleep. If, for example, a patient is deprived of REM sleep, the recovery sleep could be expected to have a disproportionately high percentage of REM sleep, that is, REM rebound. When medications are withdrawn, a similar phenomenon may be observed. Withdrawal of REM-suppressive medications, such as opiates and benzo-diazepines, may be associated with sleep characterized by a high percentage of REM sleep.[65] REM is the sleep stage associated with the greatest cardiac and respiratory variability; therefore, critically ill patients vulnerable to these changes may be at greater risk during recovery sleep if it is characterized by a high REM percentage. These effects may be clinically undetectable if the medications are withdrawn gradually.

Acute medication withdrawal syndromes, however, may be underestimated in the ICU. In a study of patients requiring mechanical ventilation more than 7 days, 32% of the 28 patients developed an acute withdrawal syndrome potentially attributable to the management of the sedation or analgesic medications given.[66] A similar incidence (40%) of sedative withdrawal was found in a retrospective study of children who required sedation for mechanical ventilation.[67] Even clinically apparent withdrawal from haloperidol has been reported in ICU patients.[68] It behooves clinicians, therefore, to wean these medications slowly and to be aware of the clinical signs of medication withdrawal.

EFFECT OF SEDATION ON PREEXISTING SLEEP DISORDERS

Sleep disorders are extremely prevalent in the community and may be relevant to the care of the critically ill patient. Sedating medications may, in some cases, worsen these preexisting conditions. Obstructive sleep apnea, for example, may be worsened by benzodiazepines and opiates, which may increase upper airway obstruction in a nonintubated patient.[69–71] Periodic limb movements and restless leg syndrome may be worsened by dopamine antagonists such as the neuroleptics.[72] A history of these conditions would argue for judicious use of sedation.

THE SLEEP-FRIENDLY SEDATION PROTOCOL

Despite the proliferation of sedation protocols, there has never been a sedation algorithm studied specifically for its effects on sleep. A patient-focused approach with attention to the potential causes of sleep disruption should be undertaken for each patient. A thorough search for the specific causes of ICU sleep disruption (anxiety, pain, depression, noise, patient-care activities, and so on) should be undertaken with medication tailored to the perceived needs of the patient.

Sleep in the ICU should first be allowed to occur naturally by providing a hospitable environment. Noise, light, and patient-care interactions should be minimized to the extent possible before considering the need for pharmacologic intervention. If nonpharmacologic measures have been implemented and specific causes of sleep disruption have been adequately addressed, that is, pain, anxiety, and so on, then hypnotics may be offered as an adjunct.

Nonintubated patients with difficulty sleeping may be able to sleep with the aid of a short-acting hypnotic such as zolpidem; however, short-acting benzodiazepines and the benzodiazepine-receptor agonists may cause delirium. Sedating antidepressants such as trazodone and mirtazapine and sedating antipsychotics such as olanzapine have been used off-label to promote sleep because they are generally well-tolerated and not associated with respiratory depression. These medications have not been tested in the critically ill. Melatonin, however, has had limited success in clinical trials in critically ill patients.[73,74] Intubated patients, however, are likely to require more aggressive pharmacologic sedation and analgesia.

Unfortunately, monitoring sleep in the ICU is expensive and labor-intensive. The best method for monitoring sleep in the ICU is still to be determined. Further investigation may facilitate this process and make it easier to measure the success of any sedation strategy with regard to its effects on sleep.

SUMMARY

Sedation in the ICU is, paradoxically, both a cause and a potential treatment for the sleep disruption almost universally observed in the critically ill. A patient-focused sedation strategy that minimizes unnecessary medication, avoids medication withdrawal, addresses the specific impediments to sleep, and serves as an adjunct to attentive environmental control may ultimately serve patients best.

REFERENCES

1. Salas RE, Gamaldo CE. Adverse effects of sleep deprivation in the ICU. Crit Care Clin 2008;24:461–76.

2. Freedman N, Kotzer N, Schwab R. Patient perception of sleep quality and etiology of sleep disruption in the intensive care unit. Am J Respir Crit Care Med 1999;159:1155–62.

3. Freedman NS, Gazendam J, Levan L, et al. Abnormal sleep/wake cycles and the effect of environmental noise on sleep disruption in the intensive care unit. Am J Respir Crit Care Med 2001;163:451–7.

4. Gabor J, Cooper A, Crombach S, et al. Contribution of the intensive care unit environment to sleep disruption in mechanically ventilated patients and healthy subjects. Am J Respir Crit Care Med 2003;167:708–15.

5. Meyer TJ, Eveloff SE, Bauer MS, et al. Adverse environmental conditions in the respiratory and medical ICU settings. Chest 1994;105:1211–6.

6. Aurell J, Elmqvist D. Sleep in the surgical intensive care unit: continuous polygraphic recording of sleep in nine patients receiving postoperative care. BMJ 1985;290:1029–32.

7. Cooper AB, Thornley KS, Young GB, et al. Sleep in critically ill patients requiring mechanical ventilation. Chest 2000;117:809–18.

8. Broughton R, Baron R. Sleep patterns in the intensive care unit and on the ward after acute myocardial infarction. Electroencephalogr Clin Neurophysiol 1978;45: 348–60.

9. Bentley S, Murphy F, Dudley H. Perceived noise in surgical wards and an intensive care area: an objective analysis. Br Med J 1977;2:1503–6.

10. Richards KC, Bairnsfather L. A description of night sleep patterns in the critical care unit. Heart Lung 1988;17:35–42.

11. Orr WC, Stahl ML. Sleep disturbances after open heart surgery. Am J Cardiol 1977;39:196–201.

12. Landis CA. Partial and sleep-state selective deprivation. In: Kushida CA, editor. Sleep deprivation: basic science, physiology, and behavior. New York: Marcel Dekker; 2005. p. 81–102.

13. Bonnet MH. Sleep fragmentation. In: Kushida CA, editor. Sleep deprivation: basic science, physiology, and behavior. New York: Marcel Dekker; 2005. p. 103–20.

14. Novaes MA, Knobel E, Bork AM, et al. Stressors in ICU: perception of the patient, relatives and health care team. Intensive Care Med 1999;25:1421–6.

15. Rotondi AJ, Lakshmipathi C, Sirio C, et al. Patients' recollections of stressful experiences while receiving prolonged mechanical ventilation in an intensive care unit. Crit Care Med 2002;30:746–52.

16. Nelson JE, Meier DE, Oei EJ, et al. Self-reported symptom experience of critically ill cancer patients receiving intensive care. Crit Care Med 2001;29:277–82.

17. Eddleston JM, White P, Guthrie E. Survival, morbidity, and quality of life after discharge from intensive care. Crit Care Med 2000;28:2293–9.

18. Simini B. Patients' perceptions of intensive care. Lancet 1999;354:571–2.

19. Harrison Y, Horne JA. One night of sleep loss impairs innovative thinking and flexible decision making. Organ Behav Hum Decis Process 1999;78:128–45.

20. Killgore WD, Killgore DB, Day LM, et al. The effects of 53 hours of sleep deprivation on moral judgement. Sleep 2007;30:345–52.

21. Benca R, Quintans J. Sleep and host defenses: a review. Sleep 1997;20:1027–37.

22. Dinges D, Douglas SD, Hamarman S, et al. Sleep deprivation and human immune function. Adv Neuroimmunol 1995;5:97–110.

23. Spiegel K, Sheridan JF, Cauter EV. Effect of sleep deprivation on response to immunization. JAMA 2002;288:1471–2.

24. Spiegel K, Leproult R. Impact of sleep debt on metabolic and endocrine function. Lancet 1999;354:1435–9.

25. Bonnet MH, Berry RB, Arand DL. Metabolism during normal, fragmented, and recovery sleep. J Appl Physiol 1991;71:1112–8.

26. Vondra K, Brodan V, Bass A, et al. Effects of sleep deprivation on the activity of selected metabolic enzymes in skeletal muscle. Eur J Appl Physiol 1981;47: 41–6.

27. Saper CB, Scammell TE, Lu J. Hypothalamic regulation of sleep and circadian rhythms. Nature 2005;437:1257–63.

28. Alkire MT, Haier RJ, Barker SJ, et al. Cerebral metabolism during propofol anesthesia in humans studied with positron emission tomography. Anesthesiology 1995;82:393–403.

29. Tung A, Szafran MJ, Bluhm B, et al. Sleep deprivation potentiates the onset and duration of loss of righting reflex induced by propofol and isoflurane. Anesthesiology 2002;97:906–11.

30. Weber B, Rohlfs M, Voler S, et al. Isoflurane sensitivity in Drosophila minisleep mutants [abstract: A1101]. Anesthesiology 2006;105:A1101.

31. Ambrogio C, Koebnick J, Quan SF, et al. Assessment of sleep in ventilator-supported critically ill patients. Sleep 2008;31:1559–68.

32. Wiegand L, Mende CN, Zaidel G, et al. Salmeterol vs theophylline: sleep and efficacy outcomes in patients with nocturnal asthma. Chest 1999;115:1525–32.

33. Mendelson WB. Human sleep: research and clinical care. New York: Plenum Press; 1987.

34. Jacobi J, Gilles LF, Coursin DB, et al. Clinical practice guidelines for the sustained use of sedatives and analgesics in the critically ill adult. Crit Care Med 2002;30:119–41.

35. Tobler I, Kopp C, Deboer T, et al. Diazepam-induced changes in sleep: role of the $\alpha 1$ GABA$_A$ receptor subtype. Proc Natl Acad Sci U S A 2001;98:6464–9.

36. Feshchenko VA, Veselis RA, Reinsel RA. Comparison of the EEG effects of midazolam, thiopental, and propofol: the role of underlying oscillatory systems. Neuropsychobiology 1997;35:211–20.

37. Veselis RA, Reinsel R, Marino P, et al. The effect of midazolam on the EEG during sedation of critically ill patients. Anaesthesia 1993;48:463–70.

38. Kajimura N, Nishikawa M, Uchiyama M, et al. Deactivation by benzodiazepine of the basal forebrain and amygdala in normal humans during sleep: a placebo-contolled [^{15}O]H$_2$O PET study. Am J Psychiatry 2004;161:748–51.

39. Hales TG, Lambert JJ. The actions of propofol on inhibitory amino acid receptors of bovine adrenomedullary chromaffin cells and rodent central neurons. Br J Pharmacol 1991;104:619–28.

40. Herregods L, Rolly G, Mortier E, et al. EEG and SEMG monitoring during induction and maintenance of anaesthesia with propofol. Int J Clin Monit Comput 1989; 6:67–73.

41. Billard V, Gambus PL, Chamoun N, et al. A comparison of spectral edge, delta power, and bispectral index as EEG measures of alfentanil, propofol, and midazolam drug effect. Clin Pharmacol Ther 1997;61:45–58.

42. McLeod G, Wallis C, Dick J, et al. Use of 2% propofol to produce diurnal sedation in critically ill patients. Intensive Care Med 1997;23:428–34.

43. Treggiari-Venzi M, Borgeat A, Fuchs-Buder T, et al. Overnight sedation with midazolam or propofol in the ICU: effects on sleep quality, anxiety and depression. Intensive Care Med 1996;22:1186–90.

44. Ozone M, Itoh H, Wataru Y, et al. Changes in subjective sleepiness, subjective fatigue and nocturnal sleep after anaesthesia with propofol. Psychiatry Clin Neurosci 2000;54:317–8.

45. Tung A, Lynch JP, Mendelson WB. Prolonged sedation with propofol in the rat does not result in sleep deprivation. Anesth Analg 2001;92:1232–6.
46. Tung A, Bergmann BM, Herrara S, et al. Recovery from sleep deprivation occurs during propofol anesthesia. Anesthesiology 2004;100:1419–26.
47. Nelson LE, Lu J, Guo T, et al. The α_2-adrenoceptor agonist dexmedetomidine converges on an endogenous sleep-promoting pathway to exert its sedative effects. Anesthesiology 2003;98:428–36.
48. Huupponen E, Maksimow A, Lapinlampi P, et al. Electroencephalogram spindle activity during dexmedetomidine sedation and physiological sleep. Acta Anaesthesiol Scand 2008;52:289–94.
49. Coull JT, Jones MEP, Egan TD, et al. Attentional effects of noradrenaline vary with arousal level: selective activation of thalamic pulvinar in humans. Neuroimage 2004;22:315–22.
50. Hall JE, Uhrich TD, Barney JA, et al. Sedative, amnestic, and analgesic properties of small-dose dexmedetomidine infusions. Anesth Analg 2000;90:699–705.
51. Hall JE, Uhrich TD, Ebert TJ, et al. Sedative, analgesic and cognitive effects of clonidine infusions in humans. Br J Anaesth 2001;86:5–11.
52. Corbett SM, Rebuck JA, Greene CM, et al. Dexmedetomidine does not improve patient satisfaction when compared with propofol during mechanical ventilation. Crit Care Med 2005;33:940–5.
53. Pandharipande P, Shintani A, Truman Pun B, et al. Lorazepam is an independent risk factor for transitioning to delirium in intensive care unit patients. Anesthesiology 2006;104:21–6.
54. Gimenez S, Clos S, Romero S, et al. Effects of olanzapine, risperidone and haloperidol on sleep after a single oral morning dose in healthy volunteers. Psychopharmacology 2007;190:507–16.
55. Armour A, Gottschlich MM, Khoury J, et al. A randomized, controlled prospective trial of zolpidem and haloperidol for use as sleeping agents in pediatric burn patients. J Burn Care Res 2008;29:238–47.
56. Akerstedt T, Hume K, Minors D, et al. Good sleep-its timing and physiological sleep characteristics. J Sleep Res 1997;6:221–9.
57. Keifer JC, Baghdoyan HA, Lydic R. Sleep disruption and increased apneas after pontine microinjection of morphine. Anesthesiology 1992;77:973–82.
58. Cronin A, Keifer JC, Baghdoyan HA, et al. Opioid inhibition of rapid eye movement sleep by a specific mu receptor agonist. Br J Anaesth 1995;74:188–92.
59. Dimsdale JE, Norman D, DeJardin D, et al. The effect of opioids on sleep architecture. J Clin Sleep Med 2007;3:33–6.
60. Cohen MJM, Menefee LA, Doghramji K, et al. Sleep in chronic pain: problems and treatments. Int Rev Psychiatry 2000;12:115–27.
61. Pilowsky I, Crettenden I, Townley M. Sleep disturbance in pain clinic patients. Pain 1985;23:27–33.
62. Close SJ. Patients' night-time pain, analgesic provision and sleep after surgery. Int J Nurs stud 1992;29:381–92.
63. Caldwell JR, Rapoport RJ, Davis JC, et al. Efficacy and safety of a once-daily morphine formulation in chronic, moderate-to-severe osteoarthritis pain: results from a randomized, placebo-controlled, double-blind trial and an open-label extension trial. J Pain Symptom Manage 2002;23:278–91.
64. Cronin AJ, Keifer JC, Davies MF, et al. Postoperative sleep disturbance: influences of opioids and pain in humans. Sleep 2001;24:39–44.
65. Novak M, Shapiro CM. Drug-induced sleep disturbances: focus on nonpsychotropic medications. Drug Saf 1997;16:133–49.

66. Cammarano WB, Pittet JF, Weitz S, et al. Acute withdrawal syndrome related to the administration of analgesic and sedative medications in adult intensive care unit patients. Crit Care Med 1998;26:676–84.
67. Fonsmark L, Rasmussen YH, Carl P. Occurrence of withdrawal in critically ill sedated children. Crit Care Med 1999;27:196–9.
68. Riker RR, Fraser GL, Richen P. Movement disorders associated with withdrawal from high-dose intravenous haloperidol therapy in delirious ICU patients. Chest 1997;111:1778–81.
69. Dolly FR, Block AJ. Effect of flurazepam on sleep-disordered breathing and nocturnal desaturation in asymptomatic subjects. Am J Med 1982;73:239–43.
70. Mendelson WB, Garnett D, Gillin JC. Flurazepam-induced sleep apnea syndrome in a patient with insomnia and mild sleep-related respiratory changes. J Nerv Ment Dis 1981;160:261–4.
71. Robinson RW, Zwillich CW, Bixler EO, et al. Effects of oral narcotics on sleep-disordered breathing in healthy adults. Chest 1987;91:197–203.
72. Salin-Pascual RJ, Galicia-Polo L, Drucker-Colin R. Sleep changes after 4 consecutive days of venlafaxine administration in normal volunteers. J Clin Psychiatry 1997;58:348–50.
73. Bourne RS, Mills GH, Minelli C. Melatonin therapy to improve nocturnal sleep in critically ill patients: encouraging results from a small randomized controlled trial. Crit Care 2008;12:R52.
74. Ibrahim MG, Bellomo R, Hart GK, et al. A double-blind placebo-controlled randomized pilot study of nocturnal melatonin in tracheostomised patients. Crit Care Resusc 2006;8:187–91.

Sedation & Immunomodulation

Robert D. Sanders, BSc, MBBS, FRCA[a,b,*], Tracy Hussell, BSc, PhD[b],
Mervyn Maze, MBChB, FRCP, FRCA, FMedSci[a]

KEYWORDS

- Infection • Sepsis • Morphine • Benzodiazepine • Propofol
- Dexmedetomidine

Sedatives exert profound effects on the central nervous system yet their effects on other organ systems are potentially underappreciated. The immunologic effects of sedation fall into this latter category. These effects are important as immune responses are intrinsically involved in the mechanisms of critical illness. For example, systemic sepsis accounts for 30% of intensive care admissions and has an incumbent mortality of 30% to 45%.[1–3] Of even more relevance is the morbidity and mortality that occurs due to secondary infections in critically ill patients.[3] The effects of sedative-induced immunomodulation could alter the course of other inflammatory processes, such as acute respiratory distress syndrome,[4] acute renal failure,[5] and delirium,[6] as well as cross talk with other processes including the coagulation cascade. Due to the high prevalence of sedative and analgesic use in critically ill patients, it is important that the effects of sedatives on the immune response are fully understood. The immune system is a complicated balance of effectors from the innate and adaptive systems. In this article the known effects of sedatives on each of these systems are discussed, followed by discussion of potential applications in clinical sepsis.

THE INNATE IMMUNE SYSTEM

Innate immunity comprises a series of host defenses including barrier function, cytokines, complement, phagocytes, natural killer (NK) cells, and gamma-delta ($\gamma\delta$) T cells to provide the initial (nonspecific) response to a pathogen or injury. These responses are phylogenetically ancient and have been developed to cope with pathogens that

A version of this article appeared in the 25:3 issue of *Critical Care Clinics*.
Conflict of Interest: Prof Maze has been a consultant for Abbott Laboratories, Abbott Park, Illinois, to facilitate registration of dexmedetomidine in the United States.
[a] Magill Department of Anaesthetics, Intensive Care and Pain Medicine, Imperial College London, Chelsea and Westminster Hospital, 369 Fulham Road, SW10 9NH, London, UK
[b] National Heart & Lung Institute, Imperial College London, Sir Alexander Fleming building, South Kensington Campus, SW7 2AZ, London, UK
* Corresponding author.
E-mail address: robert.sanders@imperial.ac.uk

Anesthesiology Clin 29 (2011) 687–706
doi:10.1016/j.anclin.2011.09.008
1932-2275/11/$ – see front matter © 2011 Elsevier Inc. All rights reserved.

are encountered regularly but that rarely cause disease. Unlike the adaptive (specific) immune system, responses are generic and leave no memory; nonetheless the innate immune system functions effectively to keep organisms healthy. Indeed a failing in innate immunity is hypothesized to contribute to secondary infections in critical illness and death in sepsis.[3,7]

Stimulation of the active components of the innate immune system occurs by way of pathogen-associated molecular pattern (PAMP) receptors or damage-associated molecular pattern (DAMP) receptors. PAMPs are recognized by membrane bound or vesicular pathogen recognition receptors (PRRs) including the Toll-like receptors (TLRs), nucleotide binding oligomerization domain (NOD)-like receptors, and RIG-I-like receptors. Bacteria stimulate these PRRs to activate various intracellular signaling cascades, leading to a proinflammatory response. For example, the gram-negative bacterial endotoxin, lipopolysaccharide, binds to TLR 4, whereas the gram-positive peptidoglycan binds to TLR 2. In the setting of tissue damage from an infection or trauma, DAMPs activate the innate immune system through these PRRs. Indeed there is significant overlap in mechanisms stimulated by PAMPs and DAMPs. As sedatives are frequently administered during infection and surgery, investigation of their immune effects on these mechanisms of immune stimulation would seem prudent.

Many different immunologic cells express PRRs to facilitate recognition of invading pathogens or tissue damage. Phagocytes (predominantly macrophages and neutrophils) become activated early in the response, migrate (by chemotaxis) to the required site, and produce an inflammatory milieu, subsequently activating other immune cells and the adaptive immune response.

Phagocyte literally means 'eating cell', engulfing pathogens or particles forming an endosome that fuses with a lysosome (containing enzymes in an acidic environment) to digest pathogens. The generation of reactive oxygen species (by way of a 'respiratory burst') is central to the killing mechanisms of macrophages and neutrophils. Dendritic cells are a further type of phagocyte which, along with resident macrophages, are situated in tissues. They phagocytose pathogens and act with their fellow phagocytes to act as antigen-presenting cells. When pathogens are ingested by phagocytes they become trapped in a phagosome, which fuses with a lysosome; thereafter enzymes and toxic peroxides digest the pathogen. Some bacteria, such as mycobacteria, have developed some resistance to this mechanism of injury. Macrophages will then act as antigen-presenting cells to activate the adaptive immune response.

Circulating complement proteins are activated by pathogens to stimulate an amplifying cascade to produce opsonization and lysis of bacteria, chemotaxis of immune effectors, mast cell activation, coagulation, and inflammatory responses by the classic, alternative, and mannose binding protein pathways. The end product, the membrane attack complex, damages the cell membrane to facilitate osmotic lysis of the pathogen.

THE ADAPTIVE IMMUNE SYSTEM

Adaptive or acquired immunity differs from the innate response as it is specific, has an element of memory, and is unique to vertebrates. The humoral component involves the proliferation of antigen-stimulated B lymphocytes into antibody-secreting plasma cells.

The cellular component is mediated by T lymphocytes, the predominant cell types being helper T cells (Th) and cytotoxic T cells. Recently, regulatory T cells that likely dampen the immune response have been identified. T cells recognize antigens bound to major histocompatibility complex (MHC) proteins by way of T cell receptors that are antigen specific. Th lymphocytes act through secretion of cytokines to elaborate and prime the immune response. This action includes inducing immunoglobin class switching of B cells, activation of Tc, and optimization of bactericidal capacity of phagocytes. Th lymphocytes are characterized by expression of CD4 proteins and are activated when MHC type II molecules, expressed on professional antigen-presenting cells (dendritic cells, macrophages, and B cells), activate the specific T cell receptor.

Th1 cells are regarded as "proinflammatory," secreting cytokines such as inter-feron-γ and interkeukin (IL)-12, and stimulate macrophage function and cytotoxic T cell function. Th2 cells have an "anti-inflammatory" phenotype and secrete cytokines such as IL-4 and IL-10, acting cooperatively to activate B cells. Further, Th cells include the regulatory T cells that act to dampen the immune response and the Th17 class that modulates neutrophil function. A shift from Th1 to Th2 cells has been observed in the latter stages of sepsis, possibly induced by the apoptotic cell death of lymphocytes, and the subsequent anti-inflammatory phenotype has been associated with secondary infections in these patients.[3]

Cytotoxic T (Tc) cells can induce death in somatic or tumor cells after stimulation by MHC type 1 related signaling by releasing the cytotoxins perforin and granulysin, which form pores in the target cell membrane to allow entrance of granzymes. Granzymes are serine proteases that activate a series of enzymes to induce apoptosis. Alternatively, Tc expression of Fas ligand can activate the extrinsic apoptotic cascade to induce cell death. NK cells are a form of cytotoxic lymphocyte that play a role in the innate immune response; they attack host cells that have been infected by pathogens and are involved in the clearance of cancerous cells. $\gamma\delta$ T cells are a further lymphocyte that seems to play a role in mucosal defense as part of the innate immune system.

KNOWN EFFECTS OF SEDATIVES ON IMMUNE RESPONSES

The immune effects of sedatives used in critical care have undergone preliminary investigations only. The studies to date predominantly suggest the sedatives have anti-inflammatory effects and may increase susceptibility to infection (**Table 1**). The possible exception to this generalization is the α_2-adrenoceptor agonist class of drugs that may improve immune function and outcomes, including mortality, in sepsis.[8] Dex-medetomidine sedation showed significant neurocognitive advantages over loraze-pam in the recent MENDS study,[9] but was particularly effective in septic patients.[8] In the future, consideration of the immune effects of sedatives may play a role in their selection, and their use may be tailored toward therapeutic manipulation of the immune response.

Table 1
Summarized effects of sedatives on the innate and adaptive immune response ($\downarrow$ represents immunodepression; $\uparrow$ represents immune potentiation; $-$, unknown effect)

Drug Class	Innate Immune Response	Adaptive Immune Response
Propofol	$\downarrow$	$-$
Benzodiazepines	$\downarrow$	$-$
Opioids	$\downarrow$	$\downarrow$
α_2-Adrenoceptor agonists	$\uparrow$	$-$

The sedative profile of the different agents may also play a role as sleep deprivation is a currently a major problem in the critically ill and may contribute to the immune dysfunction encountered in these patients. Differences have been noted in the sedative profiles of the different agents. In patients, GABAergic agents (such as propofol and midazolam) and opioids reduce the amount of nonrapid eye movement sleep. The electroencephalogram and pattern of cerebral blood flow show greater similarity to natural sleep with dexmedetomidine than with benzodiazepines.[10,11] Therefore the use of dexmedetomidine may improve the burden of sleep deprivation in the intensive care unit (ICU) compared with benzodiazepines, and this is under investigation at present. Thus, it is possible that sedatives may affect the immune system through direct and indirect mechanisms.

Stimulation of the autonomic nervous system also suppresses immune responses; the available data have particularly associated immune dysfunction with activation of the sympathetic nervous system (SNS).[12,13] Thus, suppression of SNS activity by appropriate or sympatholytic sedation (such as with an α_2-adrenoceptor agonist) may exert certain benefits to the immune system. Thus, multiple lines of evidence converge to suggest that sedatives affect immune responses by direct effects on immune cells or indirect effects through neural-immune interactions.

PROPOFOL

Propofol (2-6 di-iso-propyl phenol) is an intravenous sedative/anesthetic agent that is commonly employed for induction and maintenance of general anesthesia, and procedural and critical care sedation. At present it is prepared with intralipid, which may contribute to immunosuppressant effects,[14,15] although a water-soluble preparation (Aquavan, fospropofol disodium, MGI Pharma) will soon be available that may show an altered immune profile. Indeed propofol's use for long-term sedation is currently hindered by the intralipid preparation as triglyceride accumulation can lead to a metabolic acidosis.

Propofol exhibits anti-inflammatory effects in various in vitro and in vivo animal models that may in part be related to its antioxidant properties.[14,15] Propofol inhibits the generation of reactive oxygen species[14,16] in vitro, correlating with evidence of reduced free radical generation in cardiac surgery in humans.[17] This antioxidant effect may contribute to the observed impaired neutrophil phagocytosis of Escherichia coli and Staphylococcus aureus from whole blood in vitro.[18,19]

Macrophage Function

Impaired macrophage chemotaxis, oxidative burst, and phagocytosis of E coli have been reported with propofol administration.[18,20] These effects may be related to the loss of mitochondrial membrane potential and a reduction in macrophage ATP levels.[20] Propofol suppresses lipopolysaccharide (LPS)-induced nitric oxide formation by inhibition of inducible nitric oxide synthase (iNOS).[21–23] Propofol's antioxidant effects may have contributed to the prevention of nitric oxide induced apoptosis in macrophages.[21] Propofol also suppresses the formation of LPS-stimulated production of interferon-γ,[20] tumor necrosis factor (TNF)-α, IL-1β, and IL-6.[23] Comparison of propofol and isoflurane anesthesia in humans showed that propofol suppressed proinflammatory cytokine (TNF-α, IL-1β, interferon [IFN]-γ, and IL-8) expression in alveolar macrophages to a greater extent than isoflurane.[24] Thus, propofol's immune suppressive effects stem in part from inhibition of macrophage and neutrophil function.

Neutrophil Function

Impaired phagocytosis of *E coli* by neutrophils was also noted with propofol administration[18,19] in vitro, and this may be secondary to reduced intracellular calcium concentrations.[16] The evidence for impaired phagocytosis of *S aureus* is less clear, with two conflicting reports in the literature.[19,25] When ex vivo neutrophils were compared between patients sedated in the neuro-ICU with propofol or methohexital, no differences in immune function were apparent.[26] A further study of ex vivo human neutrophils found that propofol decreased neutrophilic respiratory burst without affecting phagocytic responses in comparison with isoflurane.[27] Reduced hydrogen peroxide production from septic rat ex vivo neutrophils was also observed with propofol or midazolam treatment although propofol suppressed this response by a greater degree. Neither sedative affected CD11b/c adhesion molecule expression.[28] Propofol, again similar to midazolam, suppresses LPS-induced release of the chemotactic and activating factor IL-8 from isolated neutrophils.[29] Propofol also inhibits neutrophil polarization and chemotaxis[16,30] that may be related to impaired mitogen-activated protein kinase (MAPK) activity.[31]

Lymphocyte Function

During anesthesia the use of propofol preserves Th1/Th2 subsets[32] and does not alter lymphocyte proliferative responses[33,34]; however, ex vivo testing of lymphocytes showed that propofol reduced proliferative responses in critically ill patients more so than in healthy controls.[33] Propofol can inhibit lymphocyte potassium channels, therefore there is a mechanism for this attenuation of lymphocyte activation and proliferation.[35] Propofol also induces lymphocyte apoptosis at high concentrations[36]; any synergism with other apoptogens such as LPS should be sought, as lymphocyte and enterocyte apoptosis is an important pathogenic mechanism in immune failure in sepsis.[3] Investigation of whether all sedatives contribute to this apoptotic mechanism of immunosuppression is required.

Systemic Immune Response

The in vivo anti-inflammatory effects of propofol have been demonstrated after high-dose endotoxin administration to rats. Propofol attenuates the consequent increase in plasma TNF-α and IL-6 levels whether given immediately, or 1 or 2 hours after endotoxin administration.[37,38] In this model baseline sedation was provided by baseline pentobarbital sodium (which may have affected immune responses) and the rats were ventilated with 100% oxygen. Takemoto addressed the dose response of this propofol effect and found that, whereas 10 mg^{-1} kg^{-1} h^{-1} and 20 mg^{-1} kg^{-1} h^{-1} reduced IL-6 levels, only 10 mg^{-1} kg^{-1} h^{-1} reduced TNF-α levels.[39] Propofol (5 mg^{-1} kg^{-1} h^{-1}) also reduced endotoxin-induced increases in TNF-α, IL-6, IL-1β, and IL-10 levels in conscious rats when given immediately after endotoxin challenge.[40]

Perhaps critically, propofol (20 mg^{-1} kg^{-1} h^{-1}) impairs bacterial clearance from the lung and spleen in rabbits injected with *E coli* in vivo (compared with saline with baseline ketamine/xylazine anesthesia).[41] Whereas some of the immune effects of propofol are likely related to its lipid vehicle intralipid,[41] the pharmacodynamic actions of propofol itself also help to reduce bacterial clearance.[19] The advent of Aquavan (water-soluble propofol) will help dissect these two mechanisms of immunosuppression. In contrast to the extensive preclinical evidence, the data from one unpowered clinical study suggests propofol may have a proinflammatory effect[42] 48 hours after enrollment. Whether confounding factors have produced this finding or this merely represents an inferior anti-inflammatory effect of propofol compared with its sedative comparator, midazolam, is currently unclear.

Propofol Summary

Significant in vitro and in vivo data suggest that propofol has anti-inflammatory effects due to impairments of the innate immune response. Little functional information is available as to any effects of propofol on the adaptive immune response. Propofol may have a therapeutic application for attenuation of sterile inflammation; however, in the presence of infection the impaired clearance of bacteria may prove a significant problem.

BENZODIAZEPINES

Benzodiazepines are one of the most abundant hypnotic agents used for critical care sedation and interestingly they exhibit a similar immune-suppressant profile to propofol. Unfortunately evidence from preclinical studies suggests that this affect may be detrimental with benzodiazepines increasing mortality from infections in animals (**Table 2**).

Macrophage

Midazolam also possesses anti-inflammatory actions against the innate immune system. Midazolam significantly inhibited LPS-induced up-regulation of cyclooxygenase 2 and inducible nitric oxide synthase in a macrophage cell line (RAW264.7 cells). IκB-α degradation, NF-κB transcriptional activity, phosphorylation of p38 mitogen-activated protein kinase, and superoxide production induced by lipopolysaccharide were also suppressed by the midazolam.[43] Impaired oxidative burst and S aureus phagocytosis by macrophages and neutrophils have also been demonstrated with midazolam treatment in horses.[44] Midazolam also suppressed LPS-induced TNF-α activity in macrophages; this effect was blocked by the peripheral benzodiazepine receptor antagonist PK 11195.[45]

Neutrophils

In contrast to other findings,[43–45] one study showed that an acute dose of diazepam had a proinflammatory effect, improving neutrophil function. However, chronic dosing produces a consistent immune depressant effect[46,47] with depression of polymorphonuclear cell phagocytosis, adherence, and chemotaxis.[47] Further in vitro studies suggest that midazolam and diazepam suppress neutrophil oxidative burst by action at the peripheral benzodiazepine receptor.[48–50]

Lymphocytes

The interaction of benzodiazepines with lymphocyte function requires further investigation although preliminary evidence shows impairment of humoral responses following long-term (60 days or greater) dosing in mice.[46] In this study the doses given were significantly lower than sedative doses, thus it is possible that higher doses may produce a more acute effect. With this low-dose treatment the benzodiazepines improved stimulated lymphocyte proliferation over the first 7 to 15 days of treatment and then decreased the proliferation with longer treatment times.

Systemic Immune Response

The effects of benzodiazepines on responses to systemic LPS have not been studied in as much detail as those of propofol. However, the similarities between propofol and midazolam in vitro suggest that both possess anti-inflammatory effects. A head-to-head in vivo comparison is required.

Preliminary data show impaired in vivo *Salmonella typhimurium* clearance with infra-sedative dosing of benzodiazepines for 7 days or greater.[46] Treatment for longer than 15 days of low-dose benzodiazepines increased mortality from this infection (see **Table 2**). Data published 25 years ago showed that 3 days of treatment with diazepam reduced resistance to systemic *Klebsiella pneumoniae*, increasing mortality (see **Table 2**).[51] Furthermore, prenatal treatment with benzodiazepines affects the development of the immune system,[63] impairing immune defenses in adulthood. Human epidemiologic data have reported benzodiazepine use as a risk factor for complicated community-acquired lower respiratory tract infection.[64] Further preclinical and clinical studies are required to probe the effects of other benzodiazepines in this setting.

Benzodiazepines Summary

Similar to propofol, benzodiazepines induce suppression of the innate immune response. This response is unsurprising given the identification of the peripheral benzodiazepine receptor as the target of benzodiazepines in immune cells.[65] Increased mortality in animal infection models correlates with this impairment of the innate immune response; studies probing effects on adaptive immunity are required. As discussed in more detail later, the authors have recently associated lorazepam sedation with increased mortality in septic patients compared with dexmedetomidine sedation.[8]

OPIOIDS

Opioids are important analgesic sedatives employed in the critically ill to afford mechanical ventilation and patient comfort. The immunosuppressant effects of opioids were first demonstrated in 1898[66] with most subsequent research focusing on morphine use; little is known about the relative suppressing effects of other members of the opioid class of drugs. Therefore an opportunity exists to clarify the effects of different opioid receptor agonists on immune responses. However, present evidence suggests that the innate and adaptive immune systems are suppressed by opioid treatment.[67,68] Morphine has even been demonstrated to inhibit myeloid cell differentiation,[69] inhibiting immune responses at an early stage. The most heavily studied opioid, morphine, consistently demonstrates anti-inflammatory effects in vitro and increases mortality in vivo in animal models of infection.[70]

Macrophage

Morphine inhibits macrophage phagocytosis and activation,[71–74] chemotaxis,[75,76] nitric oxide (NO) production,[77–80] superoxide formation,[81,82] and cytokine expression[82] in vitro. The effects on phagocytosis and NO production seem to be dependent on μ opioid receptors as μ antagonists oppose morphine's effects; δ or κ antagonists had no effect.[71,77,78] Furthermore, μ opioid receptor gene deletion prevented morphine-mediated inhibition of phagocytosis.[83,84] Whereas several studies have reported an inhibition of respiratory burst activity,[77–80] others have reported an induction of superoxide and NO formation[82,85] with subsequent macrophage apoptosis. This result may be related to the opioid dose employed. Exogenous opioids inhibit respiratory bust activity at pharmacologic doses (10^8 M) whereas endogenous opioid peptides (β-endorphin and dynorphin) stimulate the production of superoxide at physiologic concentrations (10^{14}–10^{12} M).[68] Whether this purely represents a dose effect or

Table 2
Effects of sedatives in in vivo models of bacterial or lipopolysaccharide (LPS) infection

Drug	Pathogen	Brief Method	Results
Propofol[37,38]	Intravenous LPS	Baseline sedation with pentobarbital, ventilation, 100% O_2 in rats	LPS-induced mortality was 73%. Early treatment with propofol reduced mortality to 9%. Late treatment reduced mortality to 36%
Diazepam[46]	Intraperitoneal *Salmonella typhimurium*	Chronic intraperitoneal (infrasedative) diazepam (up to 60 days treatment)	Increased mortality with 30 days of pretreatment before infection
Diazepam[51]	Intraperitoneal *Klebsiella pneumoniae*	Intraperitoneal diazepam 3 days before infection	Diazepam reduced LD_{50} of *Klebsiella pneumoniae* by 72%
Morphine[52]	Intraperitoneal *Toxoplasma gondii*	Morphine treatment started 4.5 days before infection or on day of infection with continuous subcutaneous injections	85% mortality in animals treated with morphine 4.5 days before or on the day of infection (0% mortality in controls)
Morphine[53]	Oral *Salmonella typhimurium* infection	Simultaneous infection and opioid treatment	Morphine treatment precipitated 100% mortality at 40 days (median survival = 3.2 days); 46% mortality (median survival = 30 days) in controls
Morphine[54,55]	Intraperitoneal *Salmonella enterica*	Intraperitoneal morphine treatment started 24 h before infection and continued through infection	Morphine treatment precipitated 100% 8-day mortality; 0% control mortality
Morphine[56,57]	*Streptococcus pneumoniae* lung infection	Morphine administration (using pellet) started 24 h before infection	Morphine treatment precipitated 87% 7-day mortality; 20% mortality in controls

Morphine[58]	Intraperitoneal *Listeria monocytogenes* and *Salmonella enteridis*	Morphine treatment precipitated 100% mortality (0% in controls). No effect of morphine treatment of *Salmonella* or *Escherichia coli* infections
Morphine[59]	Single sublethal LPS injection	Morphine–LPS treatment precipitated 100% mortality. LPS controls had 0% mortality; morphine controls had 33% mortality
	24 h of opioid exposure followed by LPS challenge with ongoing opioid administration	
Morphine[60]	Repeated LPS injections	48 h mortality was 85% with morphine + LPS; 50% with LPS; 0% with morphine alone
	Simultaneous LPS injection and opioid treatment	
Dexmedetomidine[61,62]	Intravenous LPS	Mortality after LPS injection was 94% (0% in saline controls). Dexmedetomidine alone induced 10% mortality. Dexmedetomidine + LPS improved mortality to 44%
	Baseline sedation with pentobarbital, ventilation, 100% O_2 in rats	In follow-up experiments: Mortality was 81% (LPS group), 26% (LPS + low-dose Dex), 32% (LPS + medium dose Dex), and 20% (LPS + high-dose Dex) Mortality was 83% (LPS alone), 33% (early Dex treatment 1 h after LPS), and 58% (late Dex treatment 2 h after LPS)

other contributing factors (timing effect [acute vs long-term exposure] or variation in paradigms [eg, in vitro vs in vivo or species effect]) is currently unclear.

Morphine also exerts a dichotomous effect on inflammatory cytokine signaling. At low doses morphine exerts a proinflammatory effect acting through m opioid receptors.[68] At higher doses morphine exerts an anti-inflammatory effect reducing TNF-α, IL-1, and IL-6 production; this effect may involve μ and other receptors.[68]

Natural Killer Cells

Morphine suppresses NK cell activity rapidly after acute administration and after chronic administration.[68] It seems that this action is mediated from a central nervous system locus; N-methyl morphine (a quaternary morphine analogue that does not readily diffuse across the blood–brain barrier) fails to inhibit NK cell activity.[86] Similarly, morphine does not inhibit NK cell function when administered in vitro.[68]

Lymphocytes

Morphine treatment results in a shift in lymphocyte subsets, function, and apoptosis. For example, chronic morphine treatment reduced double-positive T cells (CD4+CD8+) by 80% whereas it increased the single-positive CD4+ group by 60% in mice. In contrast the CD8+ subset did not change.[87] However, in monkeys an opposite finding was observed: morphine administration decreased the circulating CD4+ cells by 10% but increased CD8+ T cells by 20%.[88]

Chronic morphine treatment reduces proliferation of thymocytes and T lymphocytes. Morphine and fentanyl treatment of lymphocytes results in impaired concanavalin A (Con A)-induced proliferation, IL-2 and IFN-γ production, and increased apoptosis.[89,90] Chronic morphine treatment also produces a shift from Th1 to Th2 CD4+ cells; naive CD4+ T cell differentiation is shifted toward Th2 through an adenylyl-cyclase–mediated mechanism.[91,92] Morphine inhibits the Th1 cytokines, IL-2 and IFN-γ, while increasing IL-4 and IL-5 (Th2 cytokines). Chronic morphine application leads to increased cyclic AMP (cAMP) levels, inducing IL-4 expression that contributes to the Th2 shift in lymphocytes.[92,93] Studies suggest that exogenous opioids activate lymphocytes, provoking the release of the immunosuppressant factor transforming growth factor-β (TGF-β) that inhibits respiratory burst activity in macrophages,[68] although direct effects on macrophages also contribute.[94]

Morphine also induces apoptosis in lymphocytes and macrophages[82,85,89,95,96] upregulating the cell death receptor Fas which, when activated, stimulates the extrinsic apoptotic cell death cascade.[95] Caspase-dependent cell death then ensues. As this apoptotic cell death of lymphocytes seems critical to septic pathogenesis, involving intrinsic and extrinsic apoptotic mechanisms[3] with subsequent caspase activation, sensitization to septic injury (through increased Fas and caspase activation) by morphine is a real possibility. Studies are urgently required to clarify the effects of opioids on sepsis-induced apoptosis.

Morphine also suppresses the transition of B cells to plasma cells, further inhibiting the adaptive immune response. Again this effect is dependent on μ opioid receptors. Morphine exposure also downregulates MHC class II expression, indicating a defect in antigen presentation.[97]

Systemic Immune Response

Morphine treatment increases mortality in multiple animal models of infection with diverse pathogens. Increased mortality with morphine treatment has been noted with *Streptococcus pneumoniae*,[56,57] *Salmonella typhimurium*,[53] *Salmonella enterica*,[54,55] *Toxoplasma gondii*,[52] and *Listeria monocytogenes* (see **Table 2**).[58] Increased mortality was not observed with *E coli* treatment.[58] In contrast to propofol[37,38] and dexmedetomidine,[61,62] morphine also increased mortality from LPS[59,60] although the experimental models were not identical. Furthermore, mice treated chronically with morphine developed spontaneous infections with enteric bacteria, suggesting that morphine treatment may contribute to the translocation of gram-negative bacteria in critically ill patients.[59] Morphine treatment shows a curious interaction with viral infection, showing a mild protective effect if given before the virus and a detrimental effect if given after,[98] although morphine does potentiate HIV-induced neuronal apoptosis.[99] Therefore there are significant data suggesting that morphine worsens outcome in the setting of infection.

Mechanism of Opioid Effect

Whereas extensive evidence shows that morphine-induced immune suppression is mediated by μ opioid receptors, their precise locus is unclear. Macrophages and lymphocytes express these receptors but accumulating data suggest evidence for another indirect mechanism of action stemming from the central nervous system by way of stimulation of the hypothalamic-pituitary axis (HPA) and the SNS, allowing morphine to produce immunosuppression.[67,68,70] It is of interest that the α_2-adrenoceptor agonist clonidine ameliorated the immune effects of morphine withdrawal.[100] Given the intrinsic involvement of μ opioid receptors in each of these effects, it is likely that any agonist of m opioid receptors will induce a similar response, thus it is likely that all opioids used in the critically ill will suffer these drawbacks. Certainly preliminary evidence suggests fentanyl and remifentanil have similarities to morphine in this regard.[90,101]

Opioids Summary

Morphine's effects on lymphocytes may have great clinical significance in critically ill patients because a shift to Th2 cytokine predominance is associated with increased infection by intracellular microbes.[3,7] This shift is also observed in the late phase of sepsis and has been suggested to contribute to secondary infections in the ICU; a contribution of opioids to this effect cannot be excluded. Similarly, apoptotic injury of lymphocytes and failure of the adaptive immune response is a critical step in the pathogenesis of sepsis. Opioid administration may therefore contribute to the immunosuppression observed in the critically ill.

α2-ADRENOCEPTOR AGONISTS

The SNS exerts an anti-inflammatory effect in the immune system by direct stimulation of α_1- and β-adrenoceptors on immune effectors. Stimulation of α_1- and β-adrenoceptors stimulates cAMP formation that in turn triggers signaling cascades, which reduce the expression of the proinflammatory cytokines and increase the expression of the anti-inflammatory cytokine IL-10[102,103]; this mimics the cytokine shift in sepsis. The SNS also contributes to activation-induced apoptotic cell death of lymphocytes[104,105] that also suppresses inflammation.[3] Indeed the detrimental effect of SNS stimulation on infection has been known for more than three decades with the demonstration that reserpine treatment prolonged survival from *S aureus* and *E coli* sepsis.[12] Thus control of SNS activity through appropriate sedation is likely to be an important mechanism of the management of critically ill patients. Parasympathetic nervous system activation also induces an anti-inflammatory effect. The relative immune effects or benefits of shifting autonomic activity between the two systems need further investigation.

Conversely, stimulation of local α_2-adrenoceptors provokes a proinflammatory response in vitro[106] and in some in vivo studies[107]; however, in most animal studies and all human studies in vivo their administration is anti-inflammatory (as assessed by plasma cytokine effects).[61,62,108–110] This curious, dichotomous response may stem from different peripheral and central nervous system (CNS) actions of these drugs. Peripherally, α_2-adrenoceptor agonists may stimulate innate immunity.[111–113] Centrally the sympatholytic actions may enhance the relative parasympathetic tone to control inflammation.[103,114] Thus, peripherally α_2-adrenoceptor stimulation may induce proinflammatory effects and central effects may shift towards an anti-inflammatory phenotype. Furthermore, inflammation itself may alter the coupled response of α_2-adrenoceptor stimulation from pro- to anti-inflammation.[115] Thus in the presence of inflammation, a sedative such as dexmedetomidine may act in an anti- rather than proinflammatory manner. Finally, effects on the adaptive immune system may act to control inflammation; further research is required to explore these possible different explanations for the observed responses.

Macrophage

In contrast to the hypnotic benzodiazepines[18–20] and propofol,[44] α_2-adrenoceptor stimulation provokes increased phagocytosis and nitric oxide dependent killing of *Mycobacterium avium* and *T gondii*[111–113] with the generation of increased free radicals, superoxide, nitric oxide, and proinflammatory cytokines in vitro.[111] These effects do not occur with stimulation of other adrenoceptors. A dose-dependent stimulation of TNF-α production is noted with α_2-adrenoceptor agonist stimulation in vitro.[106] α_2-Adrenoceptor agonists also stimulate IL-12 production by monocytes in vitro that may stimulate cell-mediated and Th1 immune responses.[116] Indeed this proinflammatory effect has been shown to have a role in acute lung injury in mice whereby α_2-adrenoceptor agonist treatment provoked an increased inflammatory response.[107] The phagocytes themselves were able to produce the catecholamines in question. However, in another study dexmedetomidine attenuated ventilator-induced lung injury correlating with reduced local inflammatory responses.[117] Whether the differences between these two latter studies relate to species differences (mice vs rats) or paradigm differences remains to be seen.

Neutrophil

At clinically relevant doses clonidine and dexmedetomidine did not affect chemotaxis, phagocytosis, and superoxide formation in human neutrophils.[118]

Lymphocyte

Few studies have explored the potential effects of α_2-adrenoceptor agonists on lymphocytes although α_2-adrenoceptor expression has been demonstrated by these cells.[119] Reduced lymphocyte proliferation in response Con A has been observed with clonidine treatment through the α_2-adrenoceptor,[119] although conflicting reports exist on this matter.[120] Coincident reduction in IFN-γ and IL-4 were noted. Similar to other sedatives and the opioids, in the setting of inflammation a shift toward predominance of Th2 in T cell subsets has been noted in humans and animals.[121] Thus in contrast to proinflammatory responses induced in macrophages in vitro, lymphocytic responses seem to shift to an anti-inflammatory phenotype in vivo. The effects of α_2-adrenoceptor agonists on the humoral response needs further evaluation, especially as SNS activity seems to promote this immune defense.[13]

Systemic Studies

Extensive studies with dexmedetomidine infusion in LPS-treated rats have demonstrated that the α_2-adrenoceptor agonist has potent anti-inflammatory properties, reducing TNF-α and IL-6 levels and improving mortality.[61,62] Indeed, similar reductions in inflammatory cytokine signaling have been noted in clinical studies of critically ill patients comparing dexmedetomidine and midazolam[108] and dexmedetomidine and propofol.[109] Preoperative clonidine also reduced TNF-α levels in plasma and cerebrospinal fluid in patients undergoing peripheral revascularization procedures.[110] The difference between the findings of proinflammatory effects on the innate immune system and systemic findings showing reduced levels of proinflammatory cytokines may be related to CNS or adaptive immune effects. As stated earlier, sympatholysis may reduce inflammation by way of relative stimulation of the parasympathetic nervous system.[114] Either way it is clear that α_2-adrenoceptor agonists interact with the immune system in a complex manner. Thus it is clear that preclinical research is required for information on the complex interaction of α_2-adrenoceptor agonists and the immune system.

α_2-Adrenoceptor Agonists Summary

Patients may benefit from α_2-adrenoceptor agonist sedation in many ways. Dexmedetomidine possesses (1) superior anti-inflammatory effects,[108–110] (2) improved macrophage function, (3) antiapoptotic activity,[11,122] and (4) a superior sedative profile compared with other sedatives.[10,11] It is also possible that the positive effects on delirium stem from the anti-inflammatory activity of these drugs.[8,9] Dexmedetomidine also prevents apoptotic cell death in neurons from various stimuli. Whether α_2-adrenoceptor agonists can prevent apoptotic death of lymphocytes (as occurs in sepsis) is currently under investigation.

SEDATION IN SEPSIS

The authors have recently performed a subgroup analysis of the MENDS study whereby they identified septic patients as likely to benefit from dexmedetomidine sedation, due to the benefits afforded by the α_2-adrenoceptor agonist or by the avoidance of the benzodiazepine lorazepam.[8] This a priori arranged subgroup analysis included 39 septic patients (19 in the dexmedetomidine group and 20 in the lorazepam group). Baseline demographics, ICU type, and admission diagnoses of the sepsis patients were well balanced between the groups. Dexmedetomidine-treated patients had more delirium- and mechanical ventilation-free days. In patients with sepsis the risk of dying at 28 days was reduced by 70% in dexmedetomidine patients as compared with lorazepam patients ($P = .04$).[8] This was a small secondary analysis and further studies are required to evaluate this remarkable finding, although it is possible that the immune effects of α_2-adrenoceptor agonists contribute significantly to this finding.

Nonetheless this intriguing result, which was based on a scientifically driven hypothesis, has revealed that choice of sedative may improve mortality in septic patients. A follow-up study has recently shown that compared with midazolam, patients sedated with dexmedetomidine incurred fewer secondary infections in the ICU.[123] This result would fit with a superior preservation of the innate immune response with dexmedetomidine sedation. Given the incredible burden of infection in the ICU and sepsis as a modality of death, randomized controlled trials of dexmedetomidine sedation to prevent infections and septic mortality are urgently required.

SUMMARY

As the armamentarium for sedation in the critically ill expands, opportunities will develop to modulate the immune responses of patients by way of the direct immune and neural-immune interactions of the sedatives. Control of autonomic activity through the use of appropriate sedation may be critical in this matter. Likewise analgesic-based sedation, with increased opioid dosage, may not prove beneficial in the setting of infection; whether avoidance of morphine in preference for a fentanyl derivative will help is unclear. However, as the immune effects seem dependent on the μ receptor, it is improbable that a significant difference would be uncovered. Similarly, the present evidence suggests benzodiazepines are deleterious in infection; further studies are required urgently to evaluate this evidence. As an alternative to benzodiazepine-based sedation, dexmedetomidine has shown a remarkable 70% mortality benefit in a small secondary analysis of septic patients from the MENDS trial. Further powered clinical studies should now be undertaken to investigate the potential benefit of the α_2-adrenoceptor agonist in this setting, with comparisons with propofol.

REFERENCES

1. Harrison DA, Welch CA, Eddleston JM. The epidemiology of severe sepsis in England, Wales and Northern Ireland, 1996 to 2004: secondary analysis of a high quality clinical database, the ICNARC Case Mix Programme Database. Crit Care 2006;10(2):R42.
2. Angus DC, Linde-Zwirble WT, Lidicker J, et al. Epidemiology of severe sepsis in the United States: analysis of incidence, outcome, and associated costs of care. Crit Care Med 2001;29:1303–10.
3. Hotchkiss RS, Nicholson DW. Apoptosis and caspases regulate death and inflammation in sepsis. Nat Rev Immunol 2006;6(11):813–22.
4. Matute-Bello G, Frevert CW, Martin TR. Animal models of acute lung injury. Am J Physiol Lung Cell Mol Physiol 2008;295(3):L379–99.
5. Wan L, Bagshaw SM, Langenberg C, et al. Pathophysiology of septic acute kidney injury: what do we really know? Crit Care Med 2008;36(4 Suppl): S198–203.
6. MacDonald A, Adamis D, Treloar A, et al. C-reactive protein levels predict the incidence of delirium and recovery from it. Age Ageing 2007;36:222–5.
7. Annane D, Bellisant E, Cavaillon JM. Septic shock. Lancet 2005;365:63–78.
8. Pandharipande PP, Sanders RD, Girard T, et al. Comparison of sedation with dexmedetomidine versus lorazepam in septic ICU patients. Critical Care 2008;12:P275.
9. Pandharipande PP, Pun BT, Herr DL, et al. Effect of sedation with dexmedetomidine vs lorazepam on acute brain dysfunction in mechanically ventilated patients. The MENDS randomized controlled trial. JAMA 2007;298:2644–53.
10. Nelson LE, Lu J, Guo T, et al. The alpha2-adrenoceptor agonist dexmedetomidine converges on an endogenous sleep-promoting pathway to exert its sedative effects. Anesthesiology 2003;98:428–36.
11. Sanders RD, Maze M. Alpha2-adrenoceptor agonists. Curr Opin Investig Drugs 2007;8:25–33.
12. Smith IM, Kennedy LR, Regné-Karlsson MH, et al. Adrenergic mechanisms in infection. III. Alpha- and beta-receptor blocking agents in treatment. Am J Clin Nutr 1977;30(8):1285–8.
13. Nance DM, Sanders VM. Autonomic innervation and regulation of the immune system (1987–2007). Brain Behav Immun 2007;21(6):736–45.

14. Heine J, Leuwer M, Scheinichen D, et al. Flow cytometry evaluation of the in vitro influence of four i.v. anaesthetics on respiratory burst of neutrophils. Br J Anaesth 1996;77:387–92.
15. Kelbel I, Weiss M. Anaesthetics and immune function. Curr Opin Anaesthesiol 2001;14(6):685–91.
16. Mikawa K, Akamatsu H, Nishina K, et al. Propofol inhibits human neutrophil functions. Anesth Analg 1998;87:695–700.
17. Corcoran TB, Engel A, Sakamoto H, et al. The effects of propofol on neutrophil function, lipid peroxidation and inflammatory response during elective coronary artery bypass grafting in patients with impaired ventricular function. Br J Anaesth 2006;97(6):825–31.
18. Heller A, Heller S, Blecken S, et al. Effects of intravenous anesthetics on bacterial elimination in human blood in vitro. Acta Anaesthesiol Scand 1998;42:518–26.
19. Krumholz W, Endrass J, Hempelmann G. Propofol inhibits phagocytosis and killing of *Staphylococcus aureus* and *Escherichia coli* by polymorphonuclear leukocytes in vitro. Can J Anaesth 1994;41:446–9.
20. Chen RM, Wu CH, Chang HC, et al. Propofol suppresses macrophage functions and modulates mitochondrial membrane potential and cellular adenosine triphosphate synthesis. Anesthesiology 2003;98:1178–85.
21. Chang H, Tsai SY, Chang Y, et al. Therapeutic concentration of propofol protects mouse macrophages from nitric oxide-induced cell death and apoptosis. Can J Anaesth 2002;49:477–80.
22. Chen RM, Wu GJ, Tai YT, et al. Propofol reduces nitric oxide biosynthesis in lipopolysaccharide-activated macrophages by downregulating the expression of inducible nitric oxide synthase. Arch Toxicol 2003;77:418–23.
23. Chen RM, Chen TG, Chen TL, et al. Anti-inflammatory and antioxidative effects of propofol on lipopolysaccharide-activated macrophages. Ann N Y Acad Sci 2005;1042:262–71.
24. Kotani N, Hashimoto H, Sessler DI, et al. Expression of genes for proinflammatory cytokines in alveolar macrophages during propofol and isoflurane anesthesia. Anesth Analg 1999;89(5):1250–6.
25. Ploppa A, Kiefer RT, Nohe B, et al. Dose-dependent influence of barbiturates but not of propofol on human leukocyte phagocytosis of viable *Staphylococcus aureus*. Crit Care Med 2006;34(2):478–83.
26. Huettemann E, Jung A, Vogelsang H, et al. Effects of propofol vs. methohexital on neutrophil function and immune status in critically ill patients. J Anesth 2006; 20(2):86–91.
27. Heine J, Jaeger K, Osthaus A, et al. Anaesthesia with propofol decreases FMLP-induced neutrophil respiratory burst but not phagocytosis compared with isoflurane. Br J Anaesth 2000;85:424–30.
28. Inada T, Taniuchi S, Shingu K, et al. Propofol depressed neutrophil hydrogen peroxide production more than midazolam, whereas adhesion molecule expression was minimally affected by both anesthetics in rats with abdominal sepsis. Anesth Analg 2001;92(2):437–41.
29. Galley HF, Dubbels AM, Webster NR. The effect of midazolam and propofol on interleukin-8 from human polymorphonuclear leukocytes. Anesth Analg 1998; 86(6):1289–93.
30. O'Donnell NG, McSharry CP, Wilkinson PC, et al. Comparison of the inhibitory effects of propofol, thiopentone and midazolam on neutrophil polarization in vitro in the presence or absence of human serum albumin. Br J Anaesth 1992;69:70–4.

31. Nagata T, Kansha M, Irita K, et al. Propofol inhibits FMLP-stimulated phosphorylation of p42 mitogen-activated protein kinase and chemotaxis in human neutrophils. Br J Anaesth 2001;86:853–8.
32. Inada T, Yamanouchi Y, Jomura S, et al. Effect of propofol and isoflurane anaesthesia on the immune response to surgery. Anaesthesia 2004;59:954–9.
33. Pirttikangas CO, Salo M, Mansikka M, et al. The influence of anaesthetic technique upon the immune response to hysterectomy. A comparison of propofol infusion and isoflurane. Anaesthesia 1995;50:1056–61.
34. Devlin EG, Clarke RS, Mirakhur RK, et al. Effect of four i.v. induction agents on T-lymphocyte proliferations to PHA in vitro. Br J Anaesth 1994;73(3):315–7.
35. Mozrzymas JW, Teisseyre A, Vittur F. Propofol blocks voltage-gated potassium channels in human T lymphocytes. Biochem Pharmacol 1996;52(6):843–9.
36. Song HK, Jeong DC. The effect of propofol on cytotoxicity and apoptosis of lipopolysaccharide-treated mononuclear cells and lymphocytes. Anesth Analg 2004;98:1724–8.
37. Taniguchi T, Yamamoto K, Ohmoto N, et al. Effects of propofol on hemodynamic and inflammatory responses to endotoxemia in rats. Crit Care Med 2000;28(4): 1101–6.
38. Taniguchi T, Kanakura H, Yamamoto K. Effects of posttreatment with propofol on mortality and cytokine responses to endotoxin-induced shock in rats. Crit Care Med 2002;30(4):904–7.
39. Takemoto Y. Dose effects of propofol on hemodynamic and cytokine responses to endotoxemia in rats. J Anesth 2005;19(1):40–4.
40. Hsu BG, Yang FL, Lee RP, et al. Effects of post-treatment with low-dose propofol on inflammatory responses to lipopolysaccharide-induced shock in conscious rats. Clin Exp Pharmacol Physiol 2005;32(1-2):24–9.
41. Kelbel I, Koch T, Weber A, et al. Alterations of bacterial clearance induced by propofol. Acta Anaesthesiol Scand 1999;43(1):71–6.
42. Helmy SA, Al-Attiyah RJ. The immunomodulatory effects of prolonged intravenous infusion of propofol versus midazolam in critically ill surgical patients. Anaesthesia 2001;56(1):4–8.
43. Kim SN, Son SC, Lee SM, et al. Midazolam inhibits proinflammatory mediators in the lipopolysaccharide-activated macrophage. Anesthesiology 2006;105(1): 105–10.
44. Massoco C, Palermo-Neto J. Effects of midazolam on equine innate immune response: a flow cytometric study. Vet Immunol Immunopathol 2003;95(1-2): 11–9.
45. Matsumoto T, Ogata M, Koga K, et al. Effect of peripheral benzodiazepine receptor ligands on lipopolysaccharide-induced tumor necrosis factor activity in thioglycolate-treated mice. Antimicrob Agents Chemother 1994;38(4):812–6.
46. Galdiero F, Bentivoglio C, Nuzzo I, et al. Effects of benzodiazepines on immunodeficiency and resistance in mice. Life Sci 1995;57(26):2413–23.
47. da Silva FR, Lazzarini R, de Sá-Rocha LC, et al. Effects of acute and long-term diazepam administrations on neutrophil activity: a flow cytometric study. Eur J Pharmacol 2003;478(2-3):97–104.
48. Mühling J, Sablotzki A, Fuchs M, et al. Effects of diazepam on neutrophil (PMN) free amino acid profiles and immune functions in vitro. Metabolical and immunological consequences of L-alanyl-L-glutamine supplementation. J Nutr Biochem 2001;12(1):46–54.
49. Weiss M, Mirow N, Birkhahn A, et al. Benzodiazepines and their solvents influence neutrophil granulocyte function. Br J Anaesth 1993;70(3):317–21.

50. Finnerty M, Marczynski TJ, Amirault HJ, et al. Benzodiazepines inhibit neutrophil chemotaxis and superoxide production in a stimulus dependent manner; PK-11195 antagonizes these effects. Immunopharmacology 1991;22(3):185–93.

51. Laschi A, Descotes J, Tachon P, et al. Adverse influence of diazepam upon resistance to *Klebsiella pneumoniae* infection in mice. Toxicol Lett 1983;16(3-4):281–4.

52. Chao CC, Sharp BM, Pomeroy C, et al. Lethality of morphine in mice infected with *Toxoplasma gondii*. J Pharmacol Exp Ther 1990;252:605–9.

53. MacFarlane AS, Peng X, Meissler JJ Jr, et al. Morphine increases susceptibility to oral *Salmonella typhimurium* infection. J Infect Dis 2000;181:1350–8.

54. Asakura H, Watarai M, Shirahata T, et al. Viable but nonculturable *Salmonella* species recovery and systemic infection in morphine-treated mice. J Infect Dis 2002;186:1526–9.

55. Feng P, Truant AL, Meissler JJ Jr, et al. Morphine withdrawal lowers host defense to enteric bacteria: spontaneous sepsis and increased sensitivity to oral *Salmonella enterica* serovar *Typhimurium* infection. Infect Immun 2006;74:5221–6.

56. Wang J, Barke RA, Charboneau R, et al. Morphine impairs host innate immune response and increases susceptibility to *Streptococcus pneumoniae* lung infection. J Immunol 2005;174:426–34.

57. Wang J, Barke RA, Charboneau R, et al. Morphine induces defects in early response of alveolar macrophages to *Streptococcus pneumoniae* by modulating TLR9-NF-kappa B signaling. J Immunol 2008;180(5):3594–600.

58. Asakura H, Kawamoto K, Igimi S, et al. Enhancement of mice susceptibility to infection with *Listeria monocytogenes* by the treatment of morphine. Microbiol Immunol 2006;50:543–7.

59. Hilburger ME, Adler MW, Truant AL, et al. Morphine induces sepsis in mice. J Infect Dis 1997;176:183–8.

60. Roy S, Cain KJ, Charboneau RG, et al. Morphine accelerates the progression of sepsis in an experimental sepsis model. Adv Exp Med Biol 1998;437:21–31.

61. Taniguchi T, Kidani Y, Kanakura H, et al. Effects of dexmedetomidine on mortality rate and inflammatory responses to endotoxin-induced shock in rats. Crit Care Med 2004;32:1322–6.

62. Taniguchi T, Kurita A, Kobayashi K, et al. Dose- and time-related effects of dexmedetomidine on mortality and inflammatory responses to endotoxin-induced shock in rats. J Anesth 2008;22(3):221–8.

63. Ugaz EM, Pinheiro SR, Guerra JL, et al. Effects of prenatal diazepam treatment on *Mycobacterium bovis*-induced infection in hamsters. Immunopharmacology 1999;41(3):209–17.

64. Hak E, Bont J, Hoes AW, et al. Prognostic factors for serious morbidity and mortality from community-acquired lower respiratory tract infections among the elderly in primary care. Fam Pract 2005;22(4):375–80.

65. Decaudin D. Peripheral benzodiazepine receptor and its clinical targeting. Anticancer Drugs 2004;15(8):737–45.

66. Cantacuzene J. Nouvelles recherches sur le monde de destruction des vibrions dans l'organisme. Ann Inst Pasteur 1898;12:273–300.

67. Vallejo R, de Leon-Casasola O, Benyamin R. Opioid therapy and immunosuppression: a review. Am J Ther 2004;11(5):354–65.

68. Roy S, Wang J, Kelschenbach J, et al. Modulation of immune function by morphine: implications for susceptibility to infection. J Neuroimmune Pharmacol 2006;1(1):77–89.

69. Tian M, Broxmeyer HE, Fan Y, et al. Altered hematopoiesis, behavior, and sexual function in mu opioid receptor-deficient mice. J Exp Med 1997;185(8):1517–22.

70. Weinert CR, Kethireddy S, Roy S. Opioids and infections in the intensive care unit should clinicians and patients be concerned? J Neuroimmune Pharmacol 2008;3(4):218–29.
71. Szabo I, Rojavin M, Bussiere JL, et al. Suppression of peritoneal macrophage phagocytosis of Candida albicans by opioids. J Pharmacol Exp Ther 1995;267: 703–6.
72. Tubaro E, Santiangeli C, Belogi L, et al. Methadone vs morphine: comparison of their effect on phagocytic functions. Int J Immunopharmacol 1987;9(1):79–88.
73. Tomei EZ, Renaud FL. Effect of morphine on Fc-mediated phagocytosis by murine macrophages in vitro. J Neuroimmunol 1997;74(1-2):111–6.
74. Tomassini N, Renaud F, Roy S, et al. Morphine inhibits Fc-mediated phagocytosis through μ and δ opioid receptors. J Neuroimmunol 2004;147(1-2):131–3.
75. Choi Y, Chuang LF, Lam KM, et al. Inhibition of chemokine-induced chemotaxis of monkey leukocytes by mu-opioid receptor agonist. In Vivo 1999;13: 389–96.
76. Miyagi T, Chuang LF, Lam KM, et al. Opioid suppress chemokine-mediated migration of monkey neutrophils and monocytes – an instant response. Immunopharmacology 2001;47:53–62.
77. Fecho K, Maslonek KA, Coussons-Read ME, et al. Macrophage-derived nitric oxide is involved in the depressed con A-responsiveness of splenic lymphocytes from rats administered morphine in vivo. J Immunol 1994;152:5845–52.
78. Pacifici R, Minetti M, Zuccaro P, et al. Morphine affects cytostatic activity of macrophages by the modulation of nitric oxide release. Int J Immunopharmacol 1995;17(9):771–7.
79. Stefano GB, Cadet P, Fimiani C, et al. Morphine stimulates iNOS expression via a rebound from inhibition in human macrophages: nitric oxide involvement. Int J Immunopathol Pharmacol 2001;14(3):129–38.
80. Wang J, Charboneau R, Balasubramanian S, et al. The immunosuppressive effects of chronic morphine treatment are partially dependent on corticosterone and mediated by the mu-opioid receptor. J Leukoc Biol 2002;71(5):782–90.
81. Sharp BM, Keane WF, Suh HJ, et al. Opioid peptides rapidly stimulate superoxide production by human polymorphonuclear leukocytes and macrophages. Endocrinology 1985;117(2):793–5.
82. Bhat RS, Bhaskaran M, Mongia A, et al. Morphine-induced macrophage apoptosis: oxidative stress and strategies for modulation. J Leukoc Biol 2004; 75(6):1131–8.
83. Roy S, Barke RA, Loh HH. Mu-receptor knockout mice: the role of mu-opioid receptor in immune functions. Brain Res Mol Brain Res 1998;61(1-2):190–4.
84. Roy S, Charboneau R, Barke RA, et al. Role of mu-opioid receptor in immune function. Adv Exp Med Biol 2001;493:117–26.
85. Singhal PC, Bhaskaran M, Patel J, et al. Role of p38 mitogen-activated protein kinase phosphorylation and Fas–Fas ligand interaction in morphine-induced macrophage apoptosis. J Immunol 2002;168(8):4025–33.
86. Lysle DT, Hoffman KE, Dykstra LA. Evidence for the involvement of the caudal region of the periaqueductal gray in a subset of morphine-induced alterations of immune status. J Pharmacol Exp Ther 1996;277:1533–40.
87. Roy S, Wang JH, Balasubramanian S, et al. Role of hypothalamic–pituitary axis in morphine-induced alteration in thymic cell distribution using mu-opioid receptor knockout mice. J Neuroimmunol 2001;116(2):147–55.
88. Carr DJ, France CP. Immune alterations in chronic morphine treated rhesus monkeys. Adv Exp Med Biol 1993;335:35–9.

89. Wang J, Charboneau R, Balasubramanian S, et al. Morphine modulates lymph node-derived T lymphocyte function: role of caspase-3, -8, and nitric oxide. J Leukoc Biol 2001;70(4):527–36.

90. Flores LR, Hernandez MC, Bayer BM. Acute immunosuppressive effects of morphine: lack of involvement of pituitary and adrenal factors. J Pharmacol Exp Ther 1994;268:1129–34.

91. Roy S, Wang JH, Sumandeep G, et al. Chronic morphine treatment differentiates T helper cells to Th2 effector cells by modulating transcription factors GATA 3 and T bet. J Neuroimmunol 2004;147:78–81.

92. Roy S, Wang JH, Charboneau RG, et al. Morphine induces CD4+ T cell IL-4 expression through an adenylyl cyclase mechanism independent of the protein kinase A pathway. J Immunol 2005;175(10):6361–7.

93. Avidor-Reiss T, Nevo I, Levy R, et al. Chronic opioid treatment induces adenylyl cyclase V superactivation: involvement of Gbg. J Biol Chem 1996;271(35):21309–15.

94. Singhal PC, Kapasi AA, Franki N, et al. Morphine-induced macrophage apoptosis: the role of transforming growth factor-beta. Immunology 2000;100(1):57–62.

95. Yin D, Mufson RA, Wang R, et al. Fas-mediated cell death promoted by opioids. Nature 1999;397(6716):218.

96. Singhal P, Kapasi A, Reddy K, et al. Opiates promote T cell apoptosis through JNK and caspase pathway. Adv Exp Med Biol 2001;493:127–35.

97. Bayer BM, Daussin S, Hernandez M, et al. Morphine inhibition of lymphocyte activity is mediated by an opioid dependent mechanism. Neuropharmacology 1990;29:369–74.

98. Veyries ML, Sinet M, Desforges B, et al. Effects of morphine on the pathogenesis of murine Friend retrovirus infection. J Pharmacol Exp Ther 1995;272:498–504.

99. Hu S, Sheng WS, Lokensgard JR, et al. Morphine potentiates HIV-1 gp120-induced neuronal apoptosis. J Infect Dis 2005;191:886–9.

100. West JP, Dykstra LA, Lysle DT. Immunomodulatory effects of morphine withdrawal in the rat are time dependent and reversible by clonidine. Psychopharmacology (Berl) 1999;146(3):320–7.

101. Sacerdote P, Gaspani L, Rossoni G, et al. Effect of the opioid remifentanil on cellular immune response in the rat. Int Immunopharmacol 2001;1(4):713–9.

102. Deng J, Muthu K, Gamelli R, et al. Adrenergic modulation of splenic macrophage cytokine release in polymicrobial sepsis. Am J Physiol Cell Physiol 2004;287(3):C730–6.

103. Sternberg EM. Neural regulation of innate immunity: a coordinated nonspecific host response to pathogens. Nat Rev Immunol 2006;6(4):318–28.

104. Oberbeck R, Schmitz D, Wilsenack K, et al. Adrenergic modulation of survival and cellular immune functions during polymicrobial sepsis. Neuroimmunomodulation 2004;11(4):214–23.

105. Stevenson JR, Westermann J, Liebmann PM, et al. Prolonged alpha-adrenergic stimulation causes changes in leukocyte distribution and lymphocyte apoptosis in the rat. J Neuroimmunol 2001;120(1-2):50–7.

106. Spengler RN, Allen RM, Remick DG, et al. Stimulation of alpha-adrenergic receptor augments the production of macrophage-derived tumor necrosis factor. J Immunol 1990;145(5):1430–4.

107. Flierl MA, Rittirsch D, Nadeau BA, et al. Phagocyte-derived catecholamines enhance acute inflammatory injury. Nature 2007;449(7163):721–5.

108. Memiş D, Hekimoğlu S, Vatan I, et al. Effects of midazolam and dexmedetomidine on inflammatory responses and gastric intramucosal pH to sepsis, in critically ill patients. Br J Anaesth 2007;98:550–2.

109. Venn RM, Bryant A, Hall GM, et al. Effects of dexmedetomidine on adrenocortical function, and the cardiovascular, endocrine and inflammatory responses in post-operative patients needing sedation in the intensive care unit. Br J Anaesth 2001;86:650–6.

110. Nader ND, Ignatowski TA, Kurek CJ, et al. Clonidine suppresses plasma and cerebrospinal fluid concentrations of TNF-alpha during the perioperative period. Anesth Analg 2001;93:363–9.

111. Weatherby KE, Zwilling BS, Lafuse WP. Resistance of macrophages to *Mycobacterium avium* is induced by alpha2-adrenergic stimulation. Infect Immun 2003;71:22–9.

112. Miles BA, Lafuse WP, Zwilling BS. Binding of -adrenergic receptors stimulates the anti-mycobacterial activity of murine peritoneal macrophages. J Neuroimmunol 1996;71:19–24.

113. Gets J, Monroy FP. Effects of alpha- and beta-adrenergic agonists on *Toxoplasma gondii* infection in murine macrophages. J Parasitol 2005;91(1):193–5.

114. Tracey KJ. Physiology and immunology of the cholinergic antiinflammatory pathway. J Clin Invest 2007;117(2):289–96.

115. Sud R, Spengler RN, Nader ND, et al. Antinociception occurs with a reversal in alpha 2-adrenoceptor regulation of TNF production by peripheral monocytes/macrophages from pro- to anti-inflammatory. Eur J Pharmacol 2008;588(2–3):217–31.

116. Kang BY, Lee SW, Kim TS. Stimulation of interleukin-12 production in mouse macrophages via activation of p38 mitogen-activated protein kinase by alpha2-adrenoceptor agonists. Eur J Pharmacol 2003;467(1–3):223–31.

117. Yang CL, Tsai PS, Huang CJ. Effects of dexmedetomidine on regulating pulmonary inflammation in a rat model of ventilator-induced lung injury. Acta Anaesthesiol Taiwan 2008;46(4):151–9.

118. Nishina K, Akamatsu H, Mikawa K, et al. The effects of clonidine and dexmedetomidine on human neutrophil functions. Anesth Analg 1999;88(2):452–8.

119. Bao JY, Huang Y, Wang F, et al. Expression of alpha-AR subtypes in T lymphocytes and role of the alpha-ARs in mediating modulation of T cell function. Neuroimmunomodulation 2007;14(6):344–53.

120. Cook-Mills JM, Cohen RL, Perlman RL, et al. Inhibition of lymphocyte activation by catecholamines: evidence for a non-classical mechanism of catecholamine action. Immunology 1995;85(4):544–9.

121. von Dossow V, Baehr N, Moshirzadeh M, et al. Clonidine attenuated early proinflammatory response in T-cell subsets after cardiac surgery. Anesth Analg 2006;103(4):809–14.

122. Ma D, Hossain M, Rajakumaraswamy N, et al. Dexmedetomidine produces its neuroprotective effect via the α_{2A}-adrenoceptor subtype. Eur J Pharmacol 2004;502:87–97.

123. Riker RR, Shehabi Y, Bokesch PM, et al. SEDCOM (Safety and Efficacy of Dexmedetomidine Compared With Midazolam) Study Group. Dexmedetomidine vs midazolam for sedation of critically ill patients: a randomized trial. JAMA 2009;301:489–99.

Pharmacoeconomics of Sedation in the ICU

Joseph F. Dasta, MSc[a,b,c,]*, Sandra Kane-Gill, PharmD, MSc[d]

KEYWORDS

- Economics • Pharmaceuticals • Costs and cost analysis
- Cost-effectiveness • Health resources • Length of stay
- Critical illness • Critical care • Intensive care units

The typical patient admitted to the ICU today is older, is sicker, and has more comorbid conditions than in the past. Their anxiety and resulting agitation is a manifestation of the frightening environment of the ICU in conjunction with multiple acute illnesses. Patients who are critically ill generate a financial burden to the institution. Examples of the cost of common acute illnesses in these patients include attributable costs of $12,000 (2003 dollars) for ventilator-associated pneumonia, doubling of the ICU costs in patients developing acute kidney injury following cardiac surgery compared with matched patients not developing renal dysfunction, and hospital costs averaging nearly $19,000 (2003 dollars) in patients admitted with acute heart failure.[1–3] At an academic medical center, the ICU drug expense was approximately one third of the total hospital drug expense.[4] The drug cost per day in 2002 averaged $312 for patients in the ICU versus $112 for patients not admitted in the ICU, and the percentage increase in ICU drug cost per year was double that of the non-ICU drug cost. An important way to keep hospital costs minimal is to optimize diagnosis and treatment to minimize the time spent in the ICU.

One recent study quantified the average cost per day for a patient in the ICU.[5] This large database of 51,000 patients revealed that the average daily cost of a day in the ICU ranged from $3000 to $4000 depending on the type of ICU. An additional finding was the incremental cost of mechanical ventilation that averaged $1522 per day. Excessive doses of sedatives that depress respiration can prolong the time a patient remains on mechanical ventilation. These data provide the basis for potentially beneficial economic impact of not only reducing the stay of a patient in the ICU but

A version of this article appeared in the 25:3 issue of *Critical Care Clinics*.

Conflicts of interest statement: Professor Dasta is a consultant to Baxter and Hospira and a member of the Academy for Continued Healthcare Learning speakers' bureau. Dr Kane-Gill is a consultant to Baxter and Hospira.

[a] The Ohio State University, College of Pharmacy, Columbus, OH, USA
[b] University of Texas, College of Pharmacy, Austin, TX, USA
[c] PO Box 967, Hutto, TX 78634-0967, USA
[d] University of Pittsburgh, School of Pharmacy, Pittsburgh, PA 15261, USA
* Corresponding author. PO Box 967, Hutto, TX 78634-0967.
E-mail address: jdasta@mail.utexas.edu

successfully weaning the patient from mechanical ventilation by optimizing the dose of sedatives, even if the patient remains in the ICU.

Treating agitation with sedatives, analgesics, and drugs for delirium marginally adds to the cost of care for these complex ICU patients since most of these drugs are available in generic form. However, inappropriately treating the symptoms of agitation without determining the cause of the altered mental status can delay diagnosis and prolong the stay in the ICU, increasing the costs of ICU care. Hence it is important to diagnose and treat conditions such as pain, sleep deprivation, drug and alcohol withdrawal, acute hypoxemia, hyponatremia, hypercapnea, and central nervous system toxicity from drugs such as anticholinergics, quinolones, lidocaine, and sodium nitroprusside (thiocyanate toxicity).[6] If the patient remains agitated, sedative therapy should be optimized.

Despite an increasingly large body of literature on pharmacotherapy and optimal use of sedatives in the ICU, the quantity and quality of pharmacoeconomic evaluations of sedation in the ICU is poor. Many studies only report drug acquisition cost and don't take into consideration the full scope of managing agitated patients in the ICU with sedatives. The purpose of this article is to discuss the various components that contribute to the cost of treating the agitated patient in the ICU and to critically review the articles published since 2000 that evaluated costs and cost-effectiveness of patients in the ICU receiving drugs for agitation and/or pain.

COST COMPONENTS OF ICU SEDATION

One of the most challenging tasks in health economics is establishing the actual cost of an intervention. It is easy to look up charges on the hospital bill of a patient Unified-Bill (UB) 92. Charge is the monitory amount a hospital bills a payor or patient for a product or service. Hospital financial departments use a cost-to-charge ratio to estimate costs associated with charges for various treatments or procedures. These are thought to be reasonable estimates of costs.[7] Cost-to-charge ratios may be inadequate because they include direct and indirect costs. It should be noted that cost data from ICU studies are not only sparse, but also fraught with inadequate or nonspecific cost estimates.[8] Despite these limitations, costs are used to determine the profit or loss from third-party reimbursements.

For drugs, the acquisition price by the hospital's buying group will reflect the cost per vial or ampule of an intravenous product. One can add the number of vials or ampules used during a patient's stay to determine the cost of that particular drug. However, drug cost is only one factor of the total cost of care; others include the degree of effectiveness and development of adverse drug events. A better method of evaluating the value of a pharmaceutical for an institution is a cost-effectiveness analysis. Examples of cost-effectiveness metrics include the cost per ventilator-free day, cost per delirium avoided, or cost per quality-adjusted life year. This type of information provides clinicians with better data to assist with formulary evaluation of new drugs and decisions to include particular drugs in sedation protocols.

To appreciate the total cost associated with treating the agitated patient in the ICU, an examination of the issues surrounding over- and undersedation, costs of monitoring, and additional issues such as pain, delirium, and long-term psychological effects is necessary. When costs associated with these topics are known, they will be listed; otherwise the topics will be described in a qualitative manner.

Costs of Undersedation

A patient who is inadequately sedated will exhibit tachycardia and increased myocardial oxygen consumption. In patients with ischemic heart disease, this may result in worsening ischemia leading to an acute myocardial infarction. Many of these patients progress to congestive heart failure. The 2009 statistics from the American Heart Association reveal that the annual direct hospital cost for coronary heart disease is $54.6 billion, and $20.1 billion for heart failure.[9] Patients who are undersedated are at risk for self-extubation, which can result in direct injury to the trachea and possibly aspiration, which may require prolonged ICU treatment. Patients who are agitated may also pull out their intravenous lines and catheters. One study reported 10 patients who removed 42 devices, 88% of which were gastrointestinal tubes and vascular catheters.[10] Significant agitation was recorded within 2 hours before 74% of the events. The estimated cost of this device removal in 1997 dollars for the 42-bed ICU was $181 per event, and over $250,000 annually.

It is more difficult to perform a thorough physical examination on a patient who is inadequately sedated. As such, delays in diagnosis may result in prolonged time in the ICU. A day in the ICU costs about $3,000–$4,000.[5] It is also difficult to assess the patient for pain during this period. This may result in either inadequate or excessive use of opioids. In patients with persistent agitation and anxiety, there may be a reflex shift toward oversedation. The trigger for this reaction is to prevent the patient from harming themselves or their caregivers. In some cases, these patients who are agitated may be administered paralytics. These agents require additional monitoring such as a peripheral nerve stimulator. The costs of patients who develop prolonged persistent effects of these drugs are three times higher than patients not exhibiting prolonged neuromuscular blockade.[11]

Inadequate sedation in patients after surgery may result in excessive movement by the patient producing wound dehiscence, and exposing patients to wound infection and related costs. A surgical site infection for ICU and non-ICU care was $12,149 per patient in 1998.[12] The economic consequences of undersedation may result in excessive time on the mechanical ventilator and hence increased costs of a longer ICU stay. Patients who are agitated require the nurse at the bedside to devote more time to manage agitation and less time to other critical needs; the financial implications of this are difficult to assess. Finally, considering costs from a societal perspective, undersedation may result in long-term psychological effects. Posttraumatic stress disorder is a complication that brings with it additional costs of psychotherapy and potential lost wages. These psychological effects and lost wages are also extended to the relatives of the critically ill.[13]

Costs of Oversedation

The most obvious economic impact of oversedation is prolonged time on the mechanical ventilator and in the ICU. The incremental cost of each day on the ventilator is $1522.[5] In the ICU there are additional clinical and economic consequences of prolonged mechanical ventilation caused by sedatives. Initially, the treatment of the excessively sedated patient may be inexpensive, ie, reduce dosage or discontinue sedatives and/or analgesics. If the patient remains unresponsive, clinicians may administer the opioid antagonist naloxone or the benzodiazepine antagonist romazecon. Adverse drug reactions of these agents include seizures and acute myocardial infarction. The patient who is unresponsive may also require additional diagnostic tests such as a computed tomography (CT) scan and a neurology consult. The inability to perform a thorough physical examination may also delay the diagnosis and appropriate therapy. These patients are unable to communicate with the nurse about their degree of pain. Physiologic parameters such as heart rate and sweating are used as a surrogate. The patient may receive excessive opioids if the cause of tachycardia, for example, is not pain. Opioid toxicity has clinical and economic effects. Excessive sedation resulting from high-dose intravenous lorazepam has additional considerations. Loraze-pam is associated with propylene glycol toxicity from the intravenous formulation, and the development of delirium from lorazepam occurs in a dose-dependent manner.[14,15] These complications generate additional costs. A comprehensive estimation of the costs associated with adverse drug reactions to sedatives has been previously published.[16]

The resulting immobility further predisposes the patient to develop deep venous thrombosis. The incremental cost of deep venous thrombosis is estimated to be $3000 in 2000 dollars.[17] Decubitus ulcers are another consequence of immobilization and the infections associated with this condition have additional costs. There are substantial costs associated with ventilator-associated pneumonia, and for the patient one of the main predisposing factors to this condition is the prolonged time on the ventilator.[1]

Additional Costs

In addition to the cost of prolonged mechanical ventilation from the respiratory depressive effects of opioids, these agents can reduce gastrointestinal transit time and may cause ileus. The resulting ileus, particularly postoperatively, can prolong stay in the ICU or hospital ward. The cost of postoperative ileus in one study was over $17,000 more than matched patients' not developing ileus postoperatively.[18]

It is estimated that 80% of patients on mechanical ventilation in the ICU develop delirium.[19] A subset of these patients display agitation and are often inadequately diagnosed and treated. Patients with delirium have longer ICU stay and prolonged mechanical ventilation. Patients with delirium have an incremental increase in ICU cost of $9000 per patient with an estimated annual increase in national health care costs of $6.5 to $20.4 billion.[20] Drug therapy that can prevent or treat patients with delirium in the ICU has the potential to significantly reduce hospital costs.

Optimal use of sedatives in the ICU requires constant monitoring for safety and efficacy as part of an institutionally approved protocol or guideline. Sedation scale results often dictate the dosage of sedatives. Sedation-assessment scale findings may be recorded once per hour, once per shift, or once daily. Although it is difficult to ascribe a cost to the nursing time required for documentation, it should be taken into consideration when determining the cost of sedating patients in the ICU. Some ICUs use objective sedation monitoring devices such as the bispectral index. There is the initial cost of the monitor followed by continual cost of the sensors. A recent review of the literature found no data that showed that using the bispectral index improved ICU outcome.[21]

Another important component of the cost of sedation is the cost associated with protocol development, implementation, and updating. Although not specific for sedation, one study determined the economic impact of a sepsis protocol.[22] It was found that the protocol reduced sepsis-related costs compared with the pre-protocol time. The cost of protocol development was estimated at $5000. This included nurse educator time for in-services, information technology services time for computer development, and pharmacist protocol development time. Sedation protocols have resulted in a reduction in ventilator-associated pneumonia, mechanical ventilation time, tracheostomies, and ICU and hospital stay.[23–25] Even with the recommendation to increase sedative use by pharmacists with the application of a sedation protocol a reduction in the duration of mechanical ventilation, ICU and hospital stay can be obtained.[26] However, a study on the cost of sedation protocols is needed.

REVIEW OF PHARMACOECONOMIC STUDIES OF SEDATION IN THE ICU SINCE 2000

There have been several reviews of economic evaluations of patients who were sedated in the ICU published in the past 10–15 years.[16,27] The authors have chosen to evaluate the more recent studies published since 2000 to provide a more contemporary analysis of the current state of the science. Compared with earlier studies, many of the recent studies evaluated the cost of care associated with sedation. A summary of these studies is shown in **Table 1**.

A multicenter, randomized, open-label economic evaluation of propofol compared with midazolam was conducted in 2002.[28] The first important observation from this study is that patients treated with propofol spent significantly more time adequately sedated as measured by a targeted Ramsay sedation score (60% vs 44%; $P = .01$). Also, patients receiving propofol were extubated an average of 5 hours sooner than patients receiving midazolam ($P = .001$). Despite these clinical differences financial benefit of total cost per patient was not shown. The median costs of propofol and midazolam were \$5,718 and \$5,950, respectively ($P = .94$). A plausible explanation for the lack of financial difference is the similarities in the length of ICU stay, even with faster extubation time for the propofol group. Clarity concerning the discharge process is needed to determine if logistics prevented ICU transfer or if patients receiving propofol needed additional care after extubation, thus hampering discharge.

A comparison of all practical sedative therapies would provide the most insight about cost-effective selection; however, this is difficult to perform. So, a hypothetical decision analysis model was used to estimate the costs of propofol, lorazepam, and midazolam, to provide short-, intermediate-, and long-term sedation in patients who are critically ill.[29] This analysis included cost of preparation and administration of medications and adverse drug events (hypotension, hypertriglyceridemia, ventilator-associated pneumonia, oversedation, and undersedation). Incidence and cost parameters were obtained from published literature. Costs were reported in 2002 US dollars. The least costly alternatives varied by duration of therapy, and included propofol (\$272), midazolam (\$587), and lorazepam (\$1604) for short-, intermediate-, and long-term sedations, respectively. Monte Carlo simulations were completed for each drug and duration of therapy showed consistent findings for >80% of cases. The most substantial cost driver for all 3 therapies was drug acquisition cost. Incorporating cost of delirium as an adverse event associated with sedative use may influence these results.[20]

An economic analysis was performed on a prospective, open-label study of 80 postoperative cardiac surgery patients randomized to remifentanil and propofol (if additional sedation was required) versus midazolam and fentanyl (simultaneously administered and titrated to effect) for ICU sedation of 12 to 72 hours.[30] The collected economic variables included the cost of drugs, personnel, and adverse events, based on 2003 data. Clinical findings included a similar sedation efficacy; however, time for extubation and discharge from the ICU were significantly shorter for the remifentanil/propofol group. Despite higher costs of study drugs in the remifentanil/propofol group, the total cost of care was not significantly different between the two study populations. It was noted that the remifentanil dosage was higher than what is used in routine clinical practice. When the mean dosage was reduced from 41.2 µg/kg/h to 9 µg/kg/h and the propofol dosage was increased from 1.2 mg/kg/h to 4 mg/kg/h, with an assumed equal clinical response, the drug costs were lesser by 56% and a net savings of €214 was observed in the remifentanil/propofol group. Although this study has limitations, it shows that more expensive drugs can have economic benefit if clinical effects such as less time in the ICU and on the mechanical ventilator occur.

Table 1
Summary of economic evaluations

Author/ Reference	Study Design	Sedatives Compared and Duration	Costs Considered	Result	Limitations	Interpretation
Anis et al[28]	Randomized, unblinded, multicenter pharmacoeconomic trial	Midazolam, propofol for short to intermediate therapy (21–30 hours)	ICU physician visits, nursing time, other professional contacts, diagnostic tests, medications	Clinical benefit but no economic benefit for total ICU cost associated with propofol use; in fact propofol acquisition costs were higher	Evaluating total ICU costs introduces costs other than those associated with sedative use, potentially influencing the results	Use of propofol may result in faster extubation times and more time spent on adequate sedation, but the logistics of ICU discharge need to be better delineated to determine the financial benefit
MacLaren and Sullivan[29]	Hypothetical decision analysis model	Lorazepam, midazolam, propofol for short-, intermediate-, and long-term therapy	Preparation and administration of sedatives, ADRs, therapeutic failures	Least costly sedative treatment varied by duration of therapy	Hypothetical model, so costs were obtained from various sources Costs of an ADR were obtained from literature outside the ICU Delirium was not included as an ADR, and associated costs were not considered	Selection of the least costly treatment may not be as easy as selecting one agent. An estimation of the patient's duration of therapy may assist with selecting a cost-effective therapy

Study	Design	Drugs	Costs measured	Results	Limitations	Conclusions
Muellejans et al[30]	Randomized, open-label, single-center cost consequence model of 80 cardiac surgery patients	Remifentanil + propofol, midazolam + fentanyl	Drug costs (including wastage), cost of materials for analogo-sedation, and personnel costs in 2003	Similar sedation efficacy, time to extubation and time to ICU discharge shorter, yet higher drug costs with remifentanil + propofol group. No difference in total cost of care	Open-label design, no data on concomitant therapy, data from one ICU	More expensive sedation therapy can have overall economic benefit
Dasta et al[31]	Retrospective economic evaluation of an administrative database of cardiac surgery patients from 250 hospitals	Midazolam + propofol in 9996 patients, midazolam + propofol + dexmedetomidine in 356 patients	Total and departmental charges	Dexmedetomidine cohort had lower hospital and ICU charges despite having higher pharmacy charges	Retrospective analysis, drug usage not causally related to outcome, sequence of drug administration not evaluated	Potential economic benefit of a more expensive drug, suggesting a formal pharmacoeconomic study be conducted
Dasta et al[32]	Piggyback cost minimization evaluation of a multicenter randomized clinical trial	Dexmedetomidine, median 3.5 days, midazolam median 4.1 days	Costs of ICU stay, mechanical ventilation, treatment of ADRs, and wholesale acquisition cost of study drugs	Dexmedetomidine group had total ICU costs lower by $9679 (95% CI $2314 to $17,045) despite higher acquisition cost of $1000	ICU costs were estimated from the literature; departmental costs and total hospital costs were not obtained	Although ICU stay was not significantly different, a more expensive drug results in lower total ICU costs

(continued on next page)

Table 1
(continued)

Author/ Reference	Study Design	Sedatives Compared and Duration	Costs Considered	Result	Limitations	Interpretation
Panharipande et al[33]	Randomized clinical trial with economic analysis	Dexmedetomidine, lorazepam until extubation	Total costs by procedure-based cost accounting	Median acquisition costs of dexmedetomidine \$4675 vs lorazepam \$2335 Although total hospital costs in dexmedetomidine group were \$22,000 higher, it was not significantly different, but most costs accrued before randomization	No formal cost-effectiveness evaluation	Higher acquisition costs of dexmedetomidine did not increase total hospital costs yet produced more days alive and without coma plus delirium
Cox et al[34]	Decision analysis model comparing value of sedatives from 2 randomized clinical trials, Monte Carlo simulation of 1000 scenarios	Propofol vs intermittent lorazepam and propofol vs midazolam	Study drug wholesale acquisition costs, ICU and hospital costs, and physician billing	Propofol was the most cost-effective compared with lorazepam and lowered hospital costs by \$6378. Propofol was the cost-effective choice in 91% of simulations. No difference in propofol vs midazolam	Used data from different studies, not able to evaluate drug-associated delirium	Propofol is cost-effective compared with intermittent lorazepam. Not able to detect an economic benefit over midazolam

| Al et al[35] | Micro-simulation Markov model of extrapolating data from the UltiSAFE trial | Conventional sedation compared to remifentanil-based sedation | Micro-costing of sedatives, diagnostics, consumables, hotel, nutrition, labor | There was approximately a $2000 increase in costs between the conventional group and the remifentanil group at 28-days including a 1 day shorter duration in ICU LOS and duration of mechanical ventilation | Data from the UltiSAFE trial was evaluated for short-term so the data in this evaluation was extrapolated to 28-days; confounders such as infections not evaluated | The cost savings associated with the remifentanil based analgosedation may exist but are still unclear at this time; but additional costs with this approach are not appearent |

Abbreviations: ADR, adverse drug reaction; ICU, intensive care unit; short-term therapy, 24 h; intermediate-term therapy, 24–72 h; long-term therapy, >72 h.

In 2006 a retrospective economic evaluation of dexmedetomidine, added to commonly used sedatives, was conducted.[31] An administrative claims database from 250 hospitals in the United States was analyzed and charge data were obtained from the UB 92 forms used for submitting claims. Patients with a cardiac vessel or valve procedure based on a corresponding primary International Classification of Disease, Ninth Revision, Clinical Modification (ICD-9-CM) procedure code and a charge for dexmedetomidine, midazolam or propofol were studied. The two most common drug regimens served as the basis for comparison of hospital and departmental charges. Two cohorts were midazolam plus propofol (n = 9996) versus dexmedetomidine plus midazolam and propofol (n = 356). Patient charge, not cost, was used in this study. Patients with dexmedetomidine added to their sedative regimen had fewer days in the ICU (1.4 vs 5.3) and a lower mortality rate (1% vs 3%). As expected, the average total hospital charges were lower ($86,678 vs $106,468). Significantly lower ICU and other departmental charges were seen despite higher pharmacy charges ($16,674 vs $12,676) in the dexmedetomidine cohort. This study is limited by the retrospective nature of the design and the inability to ascribe causality to the addition of dexmedetomidine to the midazolam and propofol regimen. This study also emphasizes the potential economic benefit of a more expensive drug and suggests a formal pharmacoeconomic evaluation be performed. As such, an economic evaluation of a randomized clinical trial[36] of dexmedetomidine versus midazolam in patients on mechanical ventilation with long-term sedative requirements was recently reported in abstract form.[32] Sedation equivalency was shown, as indicated by equivalent sedation scores. Patients randomized to dexmedetomidine experienced a shorter time to extubation, reduced incidence of delirium, and more delirium-free days. The stay in the ICU was numerically lesser in the dexmedetomidine group but not statistically different. Using a cost-minimization analysis, patients randomized to dexmedetomidine had significantly lesser ICU costs with an adjusted median cost savings of $9679 (95% CI $2314 to $17,045). Primary drivers of cost savings in patients in the dexmedetomidine group were reduced length of stay costs (median savings $6584) and reduced mechanical ventilation costs (median savings $2958), which accounts for 98% of the cost savings. This cost saving was seen despite higher study drug cost incurred by dexmedetomidine versus midazolam (median cost $1166 vs $60, respectively).

This study documents the reduction in ICU costs associated with dexmedetomidine usage in patients who are on long-term mechanical ventilation. It emphasizes that even if the ICU stay is not statistically lesser with a given therapy it can have an economic benefit and can be an important factor for reducing costs in the ICU. It also shows the clinical and economic benefit of a drug with a higher acquisition cost.

A recently published clinical trial of patients on mechanical ventilation in the ICU randomized to dexmedetomidine or lorazepam revealed that patients receiving dexmedetomidine had more time at their target sedation goal.[33] Patients who received dexmedetomidine experienced more days alive and without coma, and alive with a combination of coma plus delirium. Their cost analysis revealed that the cost of the study drug was $2340 higher for dexmedetomidine compared with lorazepam. The total costs were numerically more in the dexmedetomidine group for pharmacy, respiratory care, ICU, and hospital; however, these costs did not achieve statistical significance. It was reported that median total hospital costs were $22,500 more in patients randomized to dexmedetomidine, but most of this increase occurred before randomization to study drugs. This study therefore reveals equivalent hospital costs between the 2 groups, despite higher study drug costs with dexmedetomidine, with better sedation and a lower incidence of coma and the composite clinical finding of coma plus delirium.

Finally, a recent study used a decision analytic model to determine the cost-effectiveness of several sedatives.[34] The base-case analysis used the findings of a clinical trial of patients on mechanical ventilation randomized to receive intermittent lorazepam or propofol and daily awakening. Secondary analysis used the findings of the original study of daily awakening that evaluated propofol versus midazolam. Direct costs were used and included the wholesale acquisition cost for study drugs, daily ICU costs from the literature, and ward costs from the medical provider database. Efficacy was defined as mechanical ventilator-free days and mechanical ventilator-free survival, up to 28 days after intubation. Probabilistic analyses were performed using Monte Carlo simulation of 1000 scenarios.

In the base-case scenario, propofol was the most cost-effective regimen and was associated with lesser hospitalization costs of $6378, increases of 3.7 in mechanical ventilator–free days and 3.4 more mechanical ventilator–free survival days. Propofol dominance occurred in 91% of the simulations. Secondary analyses revealed no difference between propofol and midazolam in either costs or effectiveness. This study suggests propofol is cost-effective, despite higher acquisition price compared with lorazepam. It further questions the routine use of lorazepam as suggested by the 2002 Society of Critical Care Medicine guidelines.[37] The authors conclude that additional studies are needed to assess if midazolam has a comparable economic advantage.

Data are mounting on a paradigm shift from sedative-hypnotic based sedation to analgosedation, also referred to as A1 sedation.[6,38] One of the benefits is the reduction in the duration of mechanical and ICU length of stay.[39] The potential cost advantages of analgosedation using remifentanil compared to conventional therapy using morphine or fentanyl and propofol, midazolam or lorazepam was evaluated in a Markov Model indicating about a $2000 cost savings at 28-days with remifentanil.[35]

TEMPLATE FOR AN IDEAL PHARMACOECONOMIC STUDY

It is recommended that comparative effectiveness research methods be applied. An optimal cost-effectiveness analysis, otherwise known as a cost-utility analysis, should be conducted from a societal perspective, otherwise known as a cost utility analysis.[40] However, as the authors have indicated, it is difficult enough to obtain institutional costs without extending to a societal perspective.[40] Accurately capturing costs of lost wages and posttraumatic stress disorder for patients who are critically ill or itemizing the cost impact on relatives of patients who are critically ill would be extremely challenging. From an institutional perspective the authors propose an ideal pharmacoeconomic study for the use of sedatives in the ICU.

The components of a pharmacoeconomic study conducted under the premise of unlimited resources and time would include the following:

1. A multidisciplinary panel of experts would convene to develop an inclusive sedation pathway incorporating all aspects of oversedation, undersedation, and other potential adverse drug reactions. This will allow the important cost variables to be determined before data collection.
2. Each branch of the clinical pathway would be investigated for necessary cost components. For example a branch containing an adverse drug reaction such as hypotension would be evaluated for cost components of hypotension including dispensing, prescribing, administering, and monitoring time associated with its treatment. There is time associated with the nurse identifying an event, the physician's time for treating the event, the pharmacist's time for preparing the medication, and the team's time for monitoring the event. There may also be additional laboratory tests.

3. A homogeneous population would be selected for study so that sedation requirements would be similar.
4. The clinically relevant sedatives would be selected for comparison.
5. A multi-institutional, prospective, randomized trial would be initiated that is sufficiently powered to answer the primary objective.
6. All the data elements deemed appropriate by the expert panel in step one would be collected. These would include duration of mechanical ventilation, ICU and hospital stay, percentage time at target sedation, number of dosage adjustments, nursing satisfaction, patient's ability to communicate and cooperate with the nurse, incidence and duration of delirium, and adverse drug reactions.
7. Time-and-motion studies would be completed to determine health care professional time associated with providing sedation. Two separate analyses would be completed: (a) including time and (b) not including time, since cost shifting would be a factor.
8. If a nurse needs assistance from another nurse to manage extreme agitation, the possible consequences and complications of the patient for the nurse providing this assistance. For example, another patient may be in distress while the nurse is helping with the agitated patient.
9. Results would be presented as the incremental cost and a cost-effectiveness ratio. This could be presented as broadly as the cost of sedation per patient or more specifically as the cost per mechanical ventilator–free day, cost per delirium-free day, cost per patient cooperativeness, cost per adverse drug reaction avoided, cost per ICU day avoided, and cost per hour at targeted sedation score.

The ideal study contains a micro-costing approach to determine the absolute value of sedative therapy providing a more accurate measurement. One common micro-costing approach is activity based costing. Macro-costing using the total ICU stay introduces many confounding variables that influence this cost measurement.

In summary, the few pharmacoeconomic studies of sedatives performed to date have limitations. They do, however, provide some insight into the characteristics of a sedative that either reduce the cost of care or are cost-effective. These include a relatively short duration of action, lack of accumulation with long-term therapy, minimal effect on respiratory rate, no promotion of delirium, and ease of titration to achieve the target sedation goal. The ideal pharmacoeconomic study is recommended, although it would be resource intensive and expensive. These factors are a likely explanation for the existing data relying on cost estimations from clinical studies or from large administrative databases. As indicated in this review, some costs of sedative therapy are known, such as adverse drug events, mechanical ventilation, and delirium; however, many are unknown. It appears that clinicians have only begun to understand the cost of sedation. It is suggested that clinicians look beyond the acquisition cost of a sedative and include the effect of sedatives on the cost of care when selecting the most appropriate sedative.

REFERENCES

1. Warren DK, Shukla SJ, Olsen MA, et al. Outcome and attributable cost of ventilator-associated pneumonia among intensive care unit patients in a suburban medical center. Crit Care Med 2003;31(5):1312–7.
2. Dasta JF, Kane-Gill S, Durtschi AJ, et al. Costs and outcomes of acute kidney injury (AKI) following cardiac surgery. Nephrol Dial Transplant 2008;23(6): 1970–4.

3. Ng T, Dasta JF, Feldman DF, et al. Differences in patients with a primary vs secondary discharge diagnosis of heart failure from a database of 2.5 million admissions: implications for health care policy reform. Congest Heart Fail 2008; 14(4):202–10.

4. Weber RJ, Kane SL, Oriolo VA, et al. Impact of intensive care unit (ICU) drug use on hospital costs: a descriptive analysis, with recommendations for optimizing ICU pharmacotherapy. Crit Care Med 2003;31(Suppl 1): S17–24.

5. Dasta J, Kim SR, McLaughlin TP, et al. Incremental daily cost of mechanical ventilation in patients receiving treatment in an intensive care unit. Crit Care Med 2005; 33(6):1266–71.

6. Sessler CN, Varney K. Patient-focused sedation and analgesia in the ICU. Chest 2008;133(2):552–65.

7. Shartz M, Young DW, Siegrist R. The ratio of costs to charges: how good a basis for estimating costs? Inquiry 1995;32(4):476–81.

8. Glydmark M. A review of cost studies of intensive care units: problems with the cost concept. Crit Care Med 1995;23(8):964–72.

9. Lloyd-Jones D, Adams R, Carnethon M, et al. Heart disease and stroke statistics-2009 update. Circulation 2009;119(3):480–6.

10. Fraser G, Riker RR, Prato S, et al. The frequency and cost of patient-initiated device removal in the ICU. Pharmacotherapy 2001;21(1):1–6.

11. Rudis MI, Guslits BJ, Peterson EL, et al. Economic impact of prolonged motor weakness complicating neuromuscular blockade in the intensive care unit. Crit Care Med 1996;24(10):1749–56.

12. Jenney AW, Harrington GA, Russo PL, et al. Cost of surgical site infections following coronary artery bypass surgery. ANZ J Surg 2001;71(11):662–4.

13. Martin RA, Perez A, San Georgio MA. Psychological adaptation in relatives of critically injured patients admitted to an intensive care unit. Span J Psychol 2005; 8(1):36–44.

14. Nelson JL, Haas CE, Habtemariam B, et al. A prospective evaluation of propylene glycol clearance and accumulation during continuous-infusion lorazepam in critically ill patients. J Intensive Care Med 2008;23(3):184–94.

15. Pandharipande P, Shintani A, Peterson J, et al. Lorazepam is an independent risk factor for transitioning to delirium in intensive care unit patients. Anesthesiology 2006;104(1):21–6.

16. MacLaren R, Sullivan PW. Economic evaluation of sustained sedation/analgesia in the intensive care unit. Expert Opin Pharmacother 2006;7(15):2047–68.

17. Dasta JF, Durtschi AJ, Kane-Gill SL. Pharmacoeconomics, in critical care. In: Fink MP, Abraham E, Vincent JL, et al, editors. Textbook of critical care. Philadelphia: Elsevier Saunders; 2005. p. 1732–9.

18. Senagore AJ. Pathogenesis and clinical and economic consequences of postoperative ileus. Am J Health Syst Pharm 2007;64(Suppl 3):S3–7.

19. Pun BT, Ely EW. The importance of diagnosing and managing ICU delirium. Chest 2007;132(8):624–36.

20. Milbrandt EB, Seppen S, Harrison PL, et al. Costs associated with delirium in mechanically ventilated patients. Crit Care Med 2004;32(4):955–62.

21. LeBlanc J, Dasta JF, Kane-Gill SL. The role of bispectral index monitoring in the ICU. Ann Pharmacother 2006;40(3):490–500.

22. Shorr A, Micek ST, Jackson WL. Economic implications of an evidence-based sepsis protocol: can we improve outcomes and lower costs? Crit Care Med 2007;35(5):1257–62.

23. Quenot JP, Ladoire S, Devoucoux F, et al. Effect of a nurse-implemented sedation protocol on the incidence of ventilator-associated pneumonia. Crit Care Med 2007;35(9):2031–6.
24. Brook AD, Ahrens TS, Schaiff R, et al. Effect of a nursing-implemented sedation protocol on the duration of mechanical ventilation. Crit Care Med 1999;27(12):2609–15.
25. Devlin JW, Nasraway SA. Reversing oversedation in the intensive care unit: the role of pharmacists in energizing guideline efforts and overcoming protocol fatigue. Crit Care Med 2008;36(2):626–8.
26. Marshalll J, Finn CA, Theodore AC. Impact of a clinical pharmacist-enforced intensive care unit sedation protocol on duration of mechanical ventilation and hospital stay. Crit Care Med 2008;36:427–33.
27. Wittbrodt ET. Analysis of pharmacoeconomics of sedation and analgesia. Crit Care Clin 2001;17(4):1003–13.
28. Anis AH, Wang XH, Leon H, et al. Economic evaluation of propofol for sedation of patients admitted to intensive care units. Anesthesiology 2002;96(1):196–201.
29. MacLaren R, Sullivan PW. Pharmacoeconomic modeling of lorazepam, midazolam, and propofol for continuous sedation in critically ill patients. Pharmacotherapy 2005;25(10):1319–28.
30. Muellejans B, Matthey T, Scholpp J, et al. Sedation in the intensive care unit with remifentanil/propofol versus midazolam/fentanyl: a randomized, open-label, pharmacoeconomic trial. Crit Care 2006;10:R91.
31. Dasta JF, Jacobi J, Sesti A, et al. Addition of dexmedetomidine to standard sedation regimens after cardiac surgery: an outcomes analysis. Pharmacotherapy 2006;26(6):798–805.
32. Dasta JF, Kane-Gill SL, Pencina M, et al. A cost-minimization analysis of dexmedetomidine compared with midazolam for long-term sedation in the intensive care unit. Crit Care Med 2010;38:497–503.
33. Panharipande PP, Pun BT, Herr D, et al. Effect of sedation with dexmedetomidine vs lorazepam on acute brain dysfunction in mechanically ventilated patients. JAMA 2007;298(22):2644–53.
34. Cox CE, Reed SD, Govert JA, et al. Economic evaluation of propofol and lorazepam for critically ill patients undergoing mechanical ventilation. Crit Care Med 2008;36(3):706–14.
35. Al MJ, Hakkaart L, Tan SS, et al. Cost-consequence analysis of remifentanil-based analog-sedation vs conventional analgesia and sedation for patients on mechanical ventilation in the Netherlands. Crit Care 2010;14:R195.
36. Riker RR, Shehabi Y, Bokesch PM, et al. Dexmedetomidine vs. midazolam for sedation of critically ill patients: a randomized trial. JAMA 2009;305(5):489–99.
37. Jacobi J, Fraser GL, Coursin DB, et al. Clinical practice guidelines for the sustained use of sedatives and analgesics in the critically ill adult. Crit Care Med 2002;30(1):119–41.
38. Egerod I. Cultural changes in ICU sedation management. Qual Health Res 2009; 19:687–96.
39. Rozendaal FW, Spronk PE, Snellen FF, et al. Remifentanil-propofol analog-sedation shortens duration of ventilation and length of ICU stay compared to a conventional regimen: a centre randomised, cross-over, open-label study in the Netherlands. Intens Care Med 2009;35:291–8.
40. American Thoracic Society. Understanding costs and cost-effectiveness in critical care. Am J Respir Crit Care Med 2002;165(2):540–50.

Delirium Prevention and Treatment

Yoanna Skrobik, MD, FRCP(C)[a,b]

KEYWORDS

- Delirum • Critical care • Prevention • Pharmacology
- Non-pharmacologic management

Delirium is characterized by an acute change or fluctuation in mental status, inattention, and either disorganized thinking or an alteration in level of consciousness. It occurs in 35% to 80% of critically ill hospitalized patients. The variability in delirium rates described in the surgical or medical critically ill depends partly on the severity of illness and partly on the type of instrument used to screen for delirium.

Brain dysfunction (delirium and coma) in nonneurologic intensive care unit (ICU) patients has been the subject of increased study in recent years; coma and delirium appear to be independent predictors of longer hospital stay, higher hospital costs, and higher mortality.[1–3] Delirium may be associated with prolonged cognitive impairment, impaired activities of daily living, and decreased quality of life in survivors of critical illness.

DEFINITIONS AND CATEGORIES OF DELIRIUM

Delirium can be diagnosed in ICU settings by psychiatrists and trained nonpsychiatric personnel. It can be detected in mechanically ventilated and other nonverbal patients using validated instruments such as the Confusion Assessment Method for the ICU[4] and the Intensive Care Delirium Screening Checklist (ICDSC).[5] Verbal communication limits descriptions of specific symptoms in intubated patients. Agitation and slowing occur frequently (in more than 90% of patients), and specific symptoms may be markers of prognosis.[6]

SUBSYNDROMAL DELIRIUM

Subsyndromal delirium occurs when patients have one or more delirium symptoms but do not meet criteria for full-blown clinical delirium.[7] This clinical syndrome is well described in the geriatric literature. In the ICU, its identification is possible with the ICDSC, a graded scale at the patient's bedside, with clinical criteria rated from zero to eight.[7] Delirious patients have four clinical abnormalities or more. Patients

A version of this article appeared in the 25:3 issue of *Critical Care Clinics*.
[a] Department of Medicine (Critical Care), Université de Montréal, Montréal, Québec, Canada
[b] Intensive Care Unit, Hôpital Maisonneuve Rosemont, Montréal, Québec, Canada
E-mail address: skrobik@sympatico.ca

Anesthesiology Clin 29 (2011) 721–727
doi:10.1016/j.anclin.2011.09.010   anesthesiology.theclinics.com
1932-2275/11/$ – see front matter © 2011 Elsevier Inc. All rights reserved.

with no abnormalities (ie, an ICDSC of 0) are considered cognitively normal. Those with ICDSC ratings of one to three items are labeled as having "subsyndromal delirium."[7] Subsyndromal delirium affects roughly one-third of the critically ill, as reported in the only paper published to date on the subject. This incidence, when combined with the number of patients considered delirious with the ICDSC, adds to a combined 70% incidence of delirium-like cognitive abnormalities. It is possible that the discrepancies in incidence descriptions for delirium (35% by some and 80% by others) are related to separate identification or confounding of these two syndromes. Whether subsyndromal delirium constitutes a graded step in the spectrum of brain dysfunction severity (from normal to subsyndromal delirium to delirium) or not is unclear. Although subsyndromal delirium resembles delirium in that it is associated with longer hospital stay and a higher probability of dependent living upon hospital discharge, it does not have the same risk factors and is probably preventable.

PREVENTION

Delirium has untoward consequences, on the one hand, and potentially preventable associated factors, on the other. Studies addressing delirium prevention and prophylaxis can be separated into those evaluating nonpharmacologic, pharmacologic, and combined (pharmacologic and nonpharmacologic) approaches.

Nonpharmacologic Delirium Prevention

Controversy exists as to whether factors associated with delirium are causative. Nonpharmacologic intervention aims to prevent or reverse these potential contributors. Although no studies have been published to date on nonpharmacologic delirium prevention in the ICU, two prevention strategy studies in non-ICU patients deserve mention. The first[8] to successfully demonstrate the effectiveness of nonpharmacologic intervention targeted specific aspects of care in a high-risk medical geriatric population. Treated patients underwent systematic orientation; therapeutic activities designed to lessen cognitive impairment; early mobilization; nonpharmacologic minimization of psychoactive drug use; prevention of sleep deprivation; enhancement of communication, including provision of eyeglasses and hearing aids; and early intervention for volume depletion.[8] The incidence of delirium was 9.9% with this intervention compared with 15.0% in the group receiving usual care (odds ratio [OR], 0.60; 95% confidence interval [CI], 0.39, 0.92).[8] In those patients who did develop delirium, exposure to "preventive" measures did not change the severity or the duration of delirium or any of the complications associated with it.[8]

The second nonpharmacologic intervention study,[9] the first randomized clinical trial, allocated hip fracture patients to "standard care" versus care in which treating physicians requested a routine geriatric consultation. The consultation incorporated standardized recommendations targeting 10 domains: systemic oxygenation monitoring, as a surrogate for oxygen delivery to the brain; fluid and electrolyte balance; pain management; minimization of psychoactive drug use; optimal bowel and bladder function; nutrition; early mobilization; prevention of postoperative complications; appropriate environmental stimuli; and treatment of delirium symptoms.[9] A 77% adherence to the geriatric consultant's recommendations was achieved in this study, and the total cumulative incidence of delirium during hospitalization was 32% in the proactive geriatric-consultation group versus 50% in the "usual care" group (OR, 0.48 [95% CI, 0.23, 0.98]; relative risk [RR], 0.64 [95% CI, 0.37, 0.98]).[9]

One study documented the incidence of delirium in 49 patients randomized to early physiotherapy and occupational therapy versus 55 patients randomized to routine care.[10] There were fewer days of delirium in the ICU [2.0 (0.0, 6.0) vs 4.0 (2.0, 7.0); P = .034] and in the hospital [2.0 (0.0, 6.0) vs 4.0 (2.0, 8.0); P = .017] in the early mobilization group.[10] Likewise, there were a lower percentage of ICU days with delirium [33.0% (0.0%, 58.0%) vs 57.0% (33.0%, 69.0%); P = .015] and percentage of hospital days with delirium [25.0% (0.0%, 43.0%) vs 39.0% (22.0%, 62.0%); P = .009] in the early mobilization group.[10] Risk factors for delirium between groups were similar.

The features that link these studies are careful and systematic assessments of non–life-threatening patient characteristics, medications, and needs. Most of the interventions focus on dimensions that are not part of the culture of most ICUs. Some interventions, for instance prevention of sleep deprivation, may be challenging to implement in an ICU where sleep is abnormal in the majority of patients.[11] Further, it is a secondary consideration in the context of caring for acute emergencies. Other interventions, such as early mobilization, have been shown to be of benefit but are nonetheless not yet part of routine practice.

Until ICU-based delirium prevention studies are available, it seems reasonable to implement patient-focused care, and to broaden this perspective to include reorientation, communication, mobilization, and minimization of pharmacologic exposure. At the very least, it is difficult to see how such approaches, when administered by well-educated health care professionals, could place the patient at risk.

Pharmacologic Delirium Prevention

Aizawa and colleagues[12] hypothesized that sleep disturbances are critical factors in the etiology of postoperative delirium. In this study, patients were admitted to the ICU after abdominal surgery and were then randomized to pharmacologic sleep-wake cycle adjustment or to conventional care. The "Delirium Free Protocol" involved nightly routine administration of intramuscular diazepam at 20:00 hours and intravenous 8-hour long infusions of flunitrazepam and meperidine. The incidence of delirium in the 7 days after surgery was significantly lower in the intervention group (5% vs the controls' 35%) (OR, 0.10 [95% CI, 0.01, 0.89]; RR, 0.14 [95% CI, 0.02, 1.06]).[12] However, the protocol caused some sedation upon waking, and this may have interfered with delirium assessment.

There are no trials evaluating antipsychotic drugs or anticholinesterase inhibitors for delirium prevention in the ICU. Outside the ICU, a trial evaluating prophylactic haloperidol was not effective in preventing delirium but did reduce its severity and duration.[13] A second study that compared donepezil with placebo reported an incidence of delirium of 18.8% after surgery in treatment and placebo groups (RR, 1.2 [95% CI, 0.48, 3.00]).[14]

Dexmedetomidine has been compared with midazolam in the sedation of critically ill patients.[15] The prevalence of delirium during sedative treatment was strikingly lower in dexmedetomidine-treated patients: 54% (n = 132/244) versus 76.6% (n = 93/122) in midazolam-treated patients ([95% CI, 14%–33%]; P<.001).[15] Dexmedetomidine-treated patients were more likely to develop bradycardia (42.2% [103/244] vs 18.9% [23/122]; P<.001).[15] It can be speculated that dexmedetomidine, a potent central alpha-2-receptor antagonist, which is described for the treatment of alcohol withdrawal, has a potential role to play in delirium prevention or treatment. Conversely, the benzodiazepines used in the nondexmedetomidine group may have contributed to the increased incidence of delirium.[16]

Combined Pharmacologic and Nonpharmacologic Prevention

The use of sedatives[16,17] and analgesics[18] has been linked to delirium, particularly in the context of excessive sedation. The author's group implemented and compared, in a PRE-POST fashion, a symptom-driven protocol in a single tertiary ICU.[19] They routinely distinguished among the clinical features of pain, agitation, and delirium and provided protocolized pharmacologic and nonpharmacologic approaches that were individualized to specific symptoms. After the institution of this protocol (POST), more patients remained cognitively intact (32.5% PRE vs 41.2% POST; $P = .004$). The rate of delirium was similar (34.7% PRE vs 34.2% POST; $P = .9$), but the number of patients manifesting subsyndromal (ie, subclinical) delirium was significantly less in POST. There was no difference in antipsychotic use between the PRE and POST groups.

Combined pharmacologic and nonpharmacologic prevention strategies are challenging and onerous to implement in any inpatient unit. Problems with adherence to protocols have been described, and they likely limit the effectiveness. Further studies are needed but, of necessity, are likely to be limited in scope and in number. Risk stratification may aid in identifying patients most likely to benefit from multimodal interventions. Strategies to improve intervention implementation and adherence, such as shared "ownership" and interactive education, may also serve to improve interdisciplinary protocols. Such combined approaches are likely to be an integral part of any delirium intervention package.

ALCOHOLIC PATIENTS

Alcoholic patients deserve special mention. About 1 in 10 North Americans purportedly consumes excess alcohol and is therefore at risk for alcohol withdrawal. In addition, alcoholism contributes to as many as 21% of admissions to ICU.[20,21] Validated questionnaires (eg, CAGE questionnaires or Clinical Institute Withdrawal Assessment for Alcohol Scales) are not routinely administered in the critical care setting. Alcoholism doubles the incidence of delirium without necessarily developing into alcohol withdrawal syndrome.[22,23] Screening for alcohol consumption should be part of every ICU admission case history, whenever feasible.

DELIRIUM TREATMENT
Nonpharmacologic

Addressing delirium management in the ICU requires routine screening for its presence. Validated pedagogic interventions targeting nurses are useful in establishing reliable delirium screening.[24] Early delirium recognition and management in the medical and surgical ICU setting may aid in delirium resolution and shorten the length of stay. Although interventions focused on increasing exposure to daylight, avoiding use of restraints, and boosting family contact are endorsed by intensivists and other caregivers, none of these interventions have been rigorously evaluated.[25]

Pharmacologic

Delirium is distressing for patients, families, and caregivers. Pharmacologic sedation of the agitated or frightened patient is therefore broadly perceived as desirable. Although no double-blind, randomized, placebo-controlled trial has ever established the efficacy or safety of any antipsychotic medication in the management of delirium, administration of antipsychotics is endorsed by guideline recommendations, and it is part of routine clinical practice for the majority of intensive care specialists.[26,27]

Any discussion of antipsychotic medication as a category is complicated by the variety and the differences in the receptor-adherence profiles characteristic to each.[28,29] All conventional and atypical antipsychotics appear to be equally efficacious in the treatment of psychosis, and at present there is no evidence of differential effects on delirium. Two studies evaluating antipsychotic use in the ICU have been published. In the first,[30] delirious patients able to tolerate enteral nutrition were randomized to receive enteral olanzapine or intravenous haloperidol. Both groups of patients improved with time in their delirium severity score. Benzodiazepine requirements, which reflected the need for sedation, decreased equally in both groups.[30] Patients in the olanzapine arm had less extrapyramidal side effects than those receiving haloperidol.[30] In the second study,[31] 30 delirious patients able to tolerate enteral nutrition were randomized to receive quetiapine (50 mg every 12 h) or placebo in addition to as-needed intravenous haloperidol. Patients receiving quetiapine achieved a "nondelirium" score (ie, Intensive Care Delirium Checklist score <4) faster, had a shorter ICU stay (54 vs 138 hours, $P = .007$), spent less time agitated (6 vs 36 hours, $P = .03$), and required a shorter treatment duration. It is not clear whether these findings are generalizable, as the studies are limited by their inclusion of patients able to tolerate enteral drugs, thereby limiting the generalizability of the findings.

There are no intravenous second-generation antipsychotics available for ICU use. The use of other sedatives, such as benzodiazepines, has generated much scientific and academic interest over the last 10 years; however, the focus has been the titration of sedation and the disadvantages of its excess rather than optimal therapy for agitation. Well-established sedation scales, such as the Richmond Agitation and Sedation Scale,[32] are better validated for sedation than for agitation. Optimal pharmacologic treatment of delirium in the ICU thus remains to be established.

THE SPECIFIC CASE OF DELIRIUM AND ALCOHOL WITHDRAWAL

Pharmacologic interventions shown to be beneficial in the prevention of alcohol withdrawal have been best described with the administration of sedatives.[33] Although providing alcohol to patients stratified to be at high risk for alcohol withdrawal seems effective, the heterogeneity in the design of the studies and the potential risks of alcohol administration preclude the recommendation of this practice.[21,34] Benzodiazepines, major tranquilizers, and central alpha-blockers, alone or in combination, are the cornerstone of conventional alcohol withdrawal symptom management. The addition of phenobarbital and propofol, in addition to titrated benzodiazepines, not only benefits patients but also reduces the necessity for intubation in patients admitted to the ICU with alcohol withdrawal syndrome (AWS).[35] Titrating sedative drugs to patient need benefits the critically ill.[36,37] For alcoholic patients, this is particularly true; however, screening for patients at risk and use of an appropriate alcohol withdrawal scale (AWS or Clinical Institute Withdrawal Assessment) is essential. In the context of careful titration, administering additional sedation early in the course of alcohol withdrawal symptoms in ICU patients yields a better outcome.[21]

SUMMARY

Little is known of nonpharmacologic and pharmacologic delirium prevention and treatment in the critical care setting. Trials emphasizing early mobilization suggest that this nonpharmacologic approach is associated with an improvement in delirium incidence. Titration and reduction of opiate analgesics and sedatives may improve subsyndromal delirium rates. All critical care caregivers should rigorously screen for alcohol abuse, apply alcohol withdrawal scales in alcoholic patients, and titrate sedative drugs accordingly. No nonpharmacologic approach or drug has been shown to be beneficial once delirium is established. Considering the importance and the consequences of delirium in the critical care setting, studies to further address prevention and rigorous trials addressing pharmacologic intervention are urgently needed.

REFERENCES

1. Ely EW, Shintani A, Truman B, et al. Delirium as a predictor of mortality in mechanically ventilated patients in the intensive care unit. JAMA 2004;291:1753–62.
2. Ouimet S, Kavanagh BP, Gottfried SB, et al. Incidence, risk factors and consequences of ICU delirium. Intensive Care Med 2007;33:66–73.
3. Thomason JW, Shintani A, Peterson JF, et al. Intensive care unit delirium is an independent predictor of longer hospital stay: a prospective analysis of 261 non-ventilated patients. Crit Care 2005;9:R375–81.
4. Ely EW, Inouye SK, Bernard GR, et al. Delirium in mechanically ventilated patients: validity and reliability of the confusion assessment method for the intensive care unit (CAM-ICU). JAMA 2001;286:2703–10.
5. Bergeron N, Dubois MJ, Dumont M, et al. Intensive care delirium screening checklist: evaluation of a new screening tool. Intensive Care Med 2001;27:859–64.
6. Marquis F, Ouimet S, Riker R, et al. Individual delirium symptoms: do they matter? Crit Care Med 2007;35:2533–7.
7. Ouimet S, Riker R, Bergeon N, et al. Subsyndromal delirium in the ICU: evidence for a disease spectrum. Intensive Care Med 2007;33:1007–13.
8. Inouye SK, Bogardus ST Jr, Charpentier PA, et al. A multicomponent intervention to prevent delirium in hospitalized older patients. N Engl J Med 1999;340:669–76.
9. Marcantonio ER, Flacker JM, Wright RJ, et al. Reducing delirium after hip fracture: a randomized trial. J Am Geriatr Soc 2001;49:516–22.
10. Schweickert WD, Pohlman MC, Pawlik A, et al. The impact of early mobilization on ICU delirium in mechanically ventilated (MV) patients. Lancet 2009;373:1874–82.
11. Cooper AB, Thornley KS, Young GB, et al. Sleep in critically ill patients requiring mechanical ventilation. Chest 2000;117:809–18.
12. Aizawa K, Kanai T, Saikawa Y, et al. A novel approach to the prevention of postoperative delirium in the elderly after gastrointestinal surgery. Surg Today 2002; 32:310–4.
13. Kalisvaart KJ, de Jonghe JF, Bogaards MJ, et al. Haloperidol prophylaxis for elderly hip-surgery patients at risk for delirium: a randomized placebo-controlled study. J Am Geriatr Soc 2005;53:1658–66.
14. Liptzin B, Laki A, Garb JL, et al. Donepezil in the prevention and treatment of post-surgical delirium. Am J Geriatr Psychiatry 2005;13:1100–6.
15. Riker RR, Shehabi Y, Bokesch PM, et al. Dexmedetomidine vs midazolam for sedation of critically ill patients: a randomized trial. JAMA 2009;301:489–99.
16. Pandharipande P, Shintani A, Peterson J, et al. Lorazepam is an independent risk factor for transitioning to delirium in intensive care unit patients. Anesthesiology 2006;104:21–6.
17. Pandharipande P, Cotton B, Shintani A, et al. Prevalence and risk factors for development of delirium in surgical and trauma intensive care unit patients. J Trauma 2008;65:34–41.
18. Marcantonio ER, Juarez G, Goldman L, et al. The relationship of postoperative delirium with psychoactive medications. JAMA 1994;272:1518–22.
19. Ouimet, et al. Delirium prevention strategies: targeting and improving outcomes. ICM 2006;32(Suppl 1):S141.
20. de Wit M, Wan SY, Gill S, et al. Prevalence and impact of alcohol and other drug use disorders on sedation and mechanical ventilation: a retrospective study. BMC Anesthesiol 2007;7:3.
21. Moss M, Burnham EL. Alcohol abuse in the critically ill patient. Lancet 2006;368: 2231–42.

22. Blondell RD, Powell GE, Dodds HN, et al. Admission characteristics of trauma patients in whom delirium develops. Am J Surg 2004;187:332–7.
23. Marcantonio ER, Goldman L, Mangione CM, et al. A clinical prediction rule for delirium after elective noncardiac surgery. JAMA 1994;271:134–9.
24. Devlin JW, Marquis F, Riker RR, et al. Combined didactic and scenario-based education improves the ability of intensive care unit staff to recognize delirium at the bedside. Crit Care 2008;12:R19.
25. Cheung CZ, Alibhai SM, Robinson M, et al. Recognition and labeling of delirium symptoms by intensivists: does it matter? Intensive Care Med 2008;34:437–46.
26. Jacobi J, Fraser GL, Coursin DB, et al. Clinical practice guidelines for the sustained use of sedatives and analgesics in the critically ill adult. Crit Care Med 2002;30:119–41.
27. Seitz DP, Gill SS, van Zyl LT. Antipsychotics in the treatment of delirium: a systematic review. J Clin Psychiatry 2007;68:11–21.
28. Kapur S, Seeman P. Antipsychotic agents differ in how fast they come off the dopamine D2 receptors. Implications for atypical antipsychotic action. J Psychiatry Neurosci 2000;25:161–6.
29. Nordstrom AL, Farde L, Wiesel FA, et al. Central D2-dopamine receptor occupancy in relation to antipsychotic drug effects: a double-blind PET study of schizophrenic patients. Biol Psychiatry 1993;33:227–35.
30. Skrobik YK, Bergeron N, Dumont M, et al. Olanzapine vs haloperidol: treating delirium in a critical care setting. Intensive Care Med 2004;30:444–9.
31. Devlin, et al. Crit Care Med 2008;36(12):A17.
32. Ely EW, Truman B, Shintani A, et al. Monitoring sedation status over time in ICU patients: reliability and validity of the Richmond Agitation-Sedation Scale (RASS). JAMA 2003;289:2983–91.
33. Spies CD, Otter HE, Huske B, et al. Alcohol withdrawal severity is decreased by symptom-orientated adjusted bolus therapy in the ICU. Intensive Care Med 2003; 29:2230–8.
34. Hodges B, Mazur JE. Intravenous ethanol for the treatment of alcohol withdrawal syndrome in critically ill patients. Pharmacotherapy 2004;24:1578–85.
35. Gold JA, Rimal B, Nolan A, et al. A strategy of escalating doses of benzodiazepines and phenobarbital administration reduces the need for mechanical ventilation in delirium tremens. Crit Care Med 2007;35:724–30.
36. Kress JP, Vinayak AG, Levitt J, et al. Daily sedative interruption in mechanically ventilated patients at risk for coronary artery disease. Crit Care Med 2007;35: 365–71.
37. Girard TD, Kress JP, Fuchs BD, et al. Efficacy and safety of a paired sedation and ventilator weaning protocol for mechanically ventilated patients in intensive care (awakening and breathing controlled trial): a randomised controlled trial. Lancet 2008;371:126–34.

Delirium: An Emerging Frontier in the Management of Critically Ill Children

Heidi A.B. Smith, MD, MSCI[a,*], D. Catherine Fuchs, MD[b],
Pratik P. Pandharipande, MD, MSCI[c], Frederick E. Barr, MD, MSCI[d],
E. Wesley Ely, MD, MPH[e]

KEYWORDS

- Brain dysfunction • Confusion • Delirium • Encephalopathy
- Pediatric • Critical care • Psychosis

Acute brain dysfunction is a common and significant complication associated with critical illness. The development of delirium, or acute brain dysfunction, is largely considered an expected and trivial component of critical disease.[1–3] With the advent of well-validated and reliable diagnostic instruments for delirium in critically ill adults, there has been rapid and significant progress in the body of knowledge on this topic.[4] Furthermore, better understanding of delirium has prompted new recommendations for delirium monitoring to be a component of daily usual care for all intensive care unit (ICU) patients.[5] Delirium remains essentially unrecognized in the pediatric critical care setting because of the inability of prompt diagnosis and uncertainty of clinical significance. Therefore, the pediatric knowledge base regarding delirium occurring during critical illness drastically lags behind adult literature. There are ongoing studies in Europe and the United States to develop and implement pediatric instruments to

---

A version of this article appeared in the 25:3 issue of *Critical Care Clinics.*

This work was supported by National Institutes of Health (AG001023); Veterans Affairs Clinical Science Research and Development Service (VA Merit Review Award and Career Development Award), and the Veterans Affairs Tennessee Valley Geriatric Research, Education, and Clinical Center (GRECC).

[a] Department of Anesthesiology, Vanderbilt University School of Medicine, Nashville, TN 37232, USA

[b] Department of Psychiatry, Vanderbilt University School of Medicine, Nashville, TN 37232, USA

[c] Division of Critical Care, Department of Anesthesiology, Vanderbilt University School of Medicine, Nashville, TN 37232, USA

[d] Department Chair of Pediatrics, University of Mississippi Medical Center, Jackson, MS 39216, USA

[e] Veterans Affairs Geriatric Research Education Clinical Center (VA-GRECC), Center for Health Services Research, Division of Allergy/Pulmonary/Critical Care Medicine, Vanderbilt University School of Medicine, Nashville, TN 37232, USA

* Corresponding author.

E-mail address: heidi.smith@vanderbilt.edu

Anesthesiology Clin 29 (2011) 729–750

doi:10.1016/j.anclin.2011.09.011

anesthesiology.theclinics.com

diagnose and monitor delirium in critically ill children. This article provides an overview of the diagnosis, clinical significance, pathophysiology, and treatment of delirium, based on adult studies, and it highlights the emerging and exciting areas of pediatric delirium research.

DEFINITION

Delirium is a disturbance of consciousness and cognition that develops acutely with a fluctuating course of inattention and an impaired ability to receive, process, store, or recall information.[6,7] Historically, *delirium* was used to describe an agitated and confused person, whereas *lethargus* was used to depict a quietly confused person.[1] ICU literature traditionally describes delirium as "ICU psychosis, ICU syndrome, acute confusional state, encephalopathy, and acute brain failure."[1,8,9] The remarkable variation in terminology for delirium (acute brain dysfunction) has greatly limited successful collaboration within the medical community.[4] To this end, the American Psychiatric Association recommended that "delirium" be consistently used to describe the "acute state of brain dysfunction" in critical care literature.[6]

Clinical Presentation and Subtypes

Delirium presents with a wide range of symptoms and a continuum of psychomotor behavior.[10,11] Hypoactive delirium is characterized by apathy, decreased responsiveness, and withdrawal,[10] historically a condition referred to by neurologists as "encephalopathy."[4] Patients with hypoactive delirium are often assumed erroneously to be thinking clearly. Hypoactive delirium does not commonly arouse concern by the medical team, which leads to minimal monitoring or treatment, despite these patients being at substantial risk for poor outcomes.[2,12,13] Hyperactive delirium is characterized by restlessness, agitation, and emotional liability,[10] classically referred to as "delirium" by physicians across a wide range of disciplines.[4] Combative patients with hyperactive delirium are perceived to be at greatest risk for self-extubation and self-inflicted harm and, therefore, are closely monitored and administered substantial doses of sedatives and narcotics to diminish their symptoms.[14] However, the administration of standard sedatives to mask symptoms of delirium may actually contribute to worse clinical outcomes in these patients.

A study of subtype prevalence in a large cohort of adult medical ICU patients demonstrated that hypoactive delirium was considerably more common than hyperactive delirium (43.5% vs 1.6%), whereas a combined clinical picture referred to as "mixed delirium" was the most frequently observed (54.1%).[11] The high prevalence of hypoactive delirium in critically ill patients may contribute to its underrecognition, particularly in critically ill children.[6,15] When the brain does not have the capacity to function normally, the imbalance of neurotransmitter release and cellular damage, as currently understood, is expressed clinically in various ways. Transition from one clinical expression of delirium to another does not describe a "new condition," but rather a fluctuation in brain function. Psychiatrists and intensivists increasingly use "delirium" to appropriately refer to all motoric subtypes (hypoactive, hyperactive, and mixed) of acute brain dysfunction because patients often fluctuate between these clinical states with time.[4]

Though the prevalence of all motoric subtypes of delirium has not been adequately described in the pediatric population, Turkel and colleagues[15] suggest that symptomatology may be very similar between children and adults. Manifestations of delirium, most commonly reported in adults and children, include impaired alertness, inattention, fluctuation in mental status, confusion, and disturbances in sleep-wake cycles.[15]

However, there is concern that pediatric delirium may be extremely subtle and may be complicated by the developmental variability in clinical presentations. Pediatric delirium may also be associated with other neuropsychiatric symptoms, such as purposeless actions, inconsolability, and signs of autonomic dysregulation.[16] Recognition of differences in delirium presentation between children and adults highlights the need for a pediatric-focused diagnostic approach to delirium in the pediatric ICU (PICU).[15,17,18]

DIAGNOSIS

Intensivists are experts in identifying and treating multiorgan failure. Modern technology provides the ability to monitor organ function decisively—pulmonary dysfunction by compliance curves, pulse oximetry, and blood gases; cardiac dysfunction by blood pressure, electrocardiography, and indices of oxygen delivery; and renal dysfunction by urine output and serum creatinine.[1] However, the systematic monitoring of the central nervous system has been inadequate in the identification of disturbances of consciousness and content, otherwise *delirium*. Consciousness consists of two distinct components: (1) *arousal*, or the appearance of wakefulness, and (2) *the content of consciousness*, or the sum of mental function.[19] Although arousal is routinely monitored using the Glasgow Coma Scale[20] and/or various sedation scales, such as the Modified Motor Activity Sedation Scale[21] or the Richmond Agitation Sedation Scale (RASS),[22] the assessment of the content of consciousness has been extremely limited. See **Box 1** for commonly used terms in the assessment of delirium.[1,23]

Historically, psychiatric consultation using the Diagnostic and Statistical Manual of Mental Disorders (DSM-IV) criteria, family and nurse interviews, and patient examination has been required to assess content of consciousness and ultimately diagnose delirium.[24] Delirium is diagnosed based on four major DSM-IV criteria: (1) an acute onset or fluctuating course of impaired cognition; (2) disturbance of consciousness which leads to the inability to focus, shift, or maintain attention; (3) an altered level of cognition, which may present with disorientation, language disturbance, memory deficit, or perceptual disturbances; (4) a general medical condition that directly triggers delirium.[7,16] Many clinicians assume that agitation or hallucinations must be present for diagnosis of delirium. Although these features may be present, they are not required.[25] A complete psychiatric evaluation is time consuming and limited by available personnel and patient needs, and frankly unrealistic in the ICU setting. Furthermore, delirium is a syndrome that represents brain dysfunction as assessed by specialists in both psychiatry and neurology. It is a clinical expression of brain dysfunction caused either from primary disease of the brain or secondary from a variety of complications associated with critical illness. Therefore, tools that can be used at the bedside for rapid diagnosis and ongoing monitoring of delirium in critically ill patients are vital to exploring this new frontier of pediatric critical care medicine.

Adult ICU Diagnostic Tools

In the adult population, several delirium-screening tools have been created and validated against formal psychiatric assessments as the reference standard. The Delirium Rating Scale,[26] Confusion Assessment Method for the ICU (CAM-ICU),[27,28] and the Intensive Care Delirium Screening Checklist (ICDSC)[29] are reliable screening tools for delirium in adult critically ill patients. Of these, the CAM-ICU[27,28] and the ICDSC[29] are validated for use by nonpsychiatrically trained medical professionals in the ICU setting. The CAM-ICU is the most commonly used diagnostic tool for delirium of

> **Box 1**
> **Terms used in the diagnosis of delirium**
>
> **Alertness**: A level of consciousness where a person is spontaneously and fully aware of their environment with appropriate interactions.
>
> **Mental status**: The current state of mind, which can be evaluated using domains of appearance, attitude, behavior, mood and affect, speech, thought process, thought content, perception, cognition, insight, and judgment.
>
> **Comatose**: Lacking consciousness. A comatose patient is unarouseable and unaware of the surroundings. A comatose patient may have acute brain dysfunction or delirium.
>
> **Consciousness**: A type of mental state, and a way of perceiving, particularly the perception of a relationship between self and other. In practical terms, it denotes being awake and responsive to the environment, in contrast to being asleep or in a coma.
>
> **Confusion**: A symptom of a pathologic condition such as delirium or acute brain dysfunction, which is characterized by a deficit in orientation (ability to place oneself correctly in the world by time, location, and personal identity), memory (ability to correctly recall previous events or learn new material), and executive functions.
>
> **Delirium**: A disturbance of consciousness characterized by an acute onset and a fluctuating course of impaired cognition. Delirium develops acutely, is usually reversible, and is caused by a general medical condition, substance intoxication or withdrawal, medication, or toxin exposure.
>
> **Lethargy**: A level of consciousness where a person is drowsy but easily arouseable. Though this patient is unaware of certain elements within their environment, they become fully aware and can interact appropriately with minimal provocation.
>
> **Psychosis**: A major mental disorder characterized by the inability to distinguish reality from fantasy, the presence of hallucinations or delusions, and the inability to maintain interpersonal relations, which compromises daily functioning. A psychotic individual may be able to perform actions that require a high level of intellectual effort in clear consciousness, whereas a delirious individual has impaired memory and cognitive function.
>
> **Stupor**: A level of consciousness where a person is difficult to arouse and is unaware of certain elements within their environment. A stuporous patient may become incompletely aware and interactive when provoked significantly.
>
> *Adapted from* Ely EW, Siegel MD, Inouye SK. Delirium in the intensive care unit: an under-recognized syndrome of organ dysfunction. Sem Resp Crit Care Med 2001;22(2):115–26; with permission. See also reference.[23]

critical illness, also validated for use in patients who require mechanical ventilation and are therefore nonverbal. With the ability for prompt diagnosis of delirium in critically ill adults,[25,30–32] there has been an explosion of literature on prevalence, associated outcomes, risks, and treatment of this disease state.

Pediatric ICU Diagnostic Tools

The adult tools previously described, in their present form, cannot be applied to the pediatric population because of differences in developmental expression of cognition between these diverse populations. The lack of age-appropriate diagnostic tools in children results in a knowledge deficit regarding the incidence, clinical presentation, response to treatment, and consequence of pediatric delirium in the ICU.[15,17,18]

The Pediatric Anesthesia Emergence Delirium (PAED) scale screens children as young as 2 years for emergence delirium (ED) after anesthesia during the postoperative period.[33] ED is defined as a disturbance in mentation after general anesthesia, which is associated with hallucinations, delusions, or confusion, manifested by frequently observed symptoms such as restlessness, involuntary physical activity, and extreme agitation.[34] What has been referred to as ED by anesthesiologists would in large part be considered hyperactive delirium. The PAED scale is made up of five items, which are scored 0 to 4, with a final summation, and the degree of ED increases directly with the total score (**Box 2**).[33] Two salient features of delirium are represented in this scale: (1) disturbance of consciousness (items A and C) and (2) changes in cognition (item B).[7] The limitations of the scale are easily recognized because of its subjective nature and lack of validation against DSM-IV criteria for diagnosis of delirium. The purpose of the scale is to identify hyperactive delirium, which is the least common form of delirium described in the critically ill. This scale may provide a foundation for the creation of tools to diagnose all subtypes of delirium, particularly that occurring in children aged less than 5 years.

The Pediatric Confusion Assessment Method for the ICU (pCAM-ICU) is the first delirium diagnostic tool to be validated in critically ill children at least 5 years of age, both ventilated and nonventilated, developed by the Vanderbilt Pediatric Delirium Group (**Fig. 1**).[35] This tool is an adaptation of the adult CAM-ICU. The pCAM-ICU demonstrated a sensitivity of 83% and a specificity of 99%, in addition to high inter-rater reliability. A rapid diagnosis of delirium by clinicians could guide critical therapeutic decisions, such as maneuvers to improve cerebral oxygen delivery, choice of sedative and analgesic medications, and influencing the timing of extubation. The pCAM-ICU is reliable when used by non-psychiatric trained healthcare providers, which provides an opportunity of bedside monitoring for delirium.

The pCAM-ICU mirrors diagnosis of delirium by the CAM-ICU with a two-step approach: (1) assessment of *level of consciousness* using a standardized sedation scale and (2) assessment of *content of consciousness* using the pCAM-ICU. The level of consciousness for both tools is evaluated by the Richmond Agitation Sedation Scale,[36,37] which ranges from −5 (comatose) to +4 (combative), with 0 describing an alert and calm patient (**Table 1**). By design, the pCAM-ICU requires an interactive patient to assess content of consciousness. Therefore, patients with a RASS score of −4 or −5, those who require physical stimulation for arousal, or those who do not arouse are defined as being in a comatose state and cannot be assessed for delirium. This does not mean that the patient does not have brain dysfunction; it simply means that the patient cannot be adequately assessed for content of consciousness by the pCAM-ICU. If patients have a level of consciousness other than comatose, they are then evaluated on *4 key features of delirium diagnosis* based on DSM-IV criteria to

---

Box 2
The Pediatric Anesthesia Emergence Delirium scale

Item A: The child makes eye contact with the caregiver.

Item B: The child's actions are purposeful.

Item C: The child is aware of his/her surroundings.

Item D: The child is restless.

Item E: The child is inconsolable.

Items A, B, and C are scored as follows: **4**, not at all; **3**, just a little; **2**, quite a bit; **1**, very much; **0**, extremely. Items D and E are scored as follows: **0**, not at all; **1**, just a little; **2**, quite a bit; **3**, very much; **4**, extremely. The scores of all items are summed to obtain a total PAED scale score. The degree of ED increases directly with the total score.
Adapted from Sikich N, Lerman J. Development and psychometric evaluation of the pediatric anesthesia emergence delirium scale. Anesthesiology 2004;100(5):1138–45.

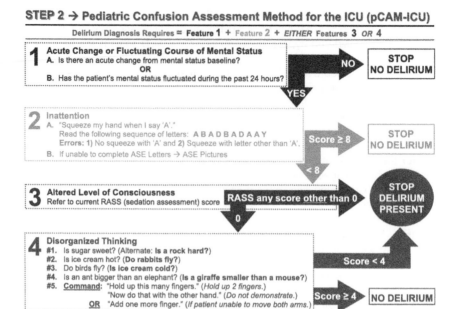

Fig. 1. The pCAM-ICU shown above can be used by bedside nurses to monitor for delirium following assessment of arousal using a sedation scale of choice. The pCAM-ICU is a valid and highly reliable tool for diagnosis of delirium in children at least 5 years of age. (Copyright © 2008, Heidi A.B. Smith, MD, MSCI and Monroe Carell Jr, Children's Hospital at Vanderbilt, all rights reserved.)

include (1) acute onset of mental status changes or a fluctuating course *and* (2) inattention, with *either* (3) altered level of consciousness *or* (4) disorganized thinking.

The pCAM-ICU diverges from the traditional CAM-ICU in features 2 and 4, where "inattention" and "disorganized thinking" are evaluated. Because of limitations in developmental expression of cognition, the assessments for both "inattention" and "disorganized thinking" required adaptation to differentiate children with and without delirium. In particular, the Attention Screening Examination (ASE) pictures used in feature 2 were replaced with bold-colored nonthreatening figures that children could easily recognize (**Fig. 2**). In addition, the questions used for evaluation of "disorganized thinking" were substituted with those of age-appropriate content. The pCAM-ICU may emerge as a beneficial tool because of its foundation on DSM-IV criteria of delirium diagnosis; and it may have the ability to diagnose and screen for all subtypes of delirium, including the most prevalent and most subtle subtype, hypoactive delirium. The limitation of this tool is the inability to use it in children aged younger than 5 years. It is recognized that the evaluation of the content of consciousness is a challenge in young children and infants. Refinement of the pCAM-ICU for this age group is currently underway at Vanderbilt referred to as the preschool CAM-ICU (psCAM-ICU).

PREVALENCE AND PROGNOSTIC SIGNIFICANCE
Delirium in Critically Ill Adults

Brain dysfunction is very common in adults with critical illness. Delirium has been observed in 60% to 80% of ventilated adult ICU patients and 40% to 60% of nonventilated adult ICU patients.[29,31,38–41] The high incidence of delirium during critical illness

Table 1
Richmond agitation-sedation scale[36,37a]

Scale	Label	Description
+4	Combative	Combative, violent, immediate danger to staff
+3	Very agitated	Pulls to remove tubes or catheters: aggressive
+2	Agitated	Frequent nonpurposeful movement, fights ventilator
+1	Restless	Anxious, apprehensive, movements not aggressive or violent
+0	Alert and calm	—
−1	Drowsy	Not fully alert, but has sustained awakening to voice (eye opening and contact >10 sec)
−2	Light sedation	Briefly awakens to voice (eye opening and contact <10 sec)
−3	Moderate sedation	Movement or eye opening to voice (but no eye contact)
−4	Deep sedation	No response to voice Movement or eye opening to physical stimulation
−5	Unarouseable	No response to voice or physical stimulation

[a] Patients are assessed for delirium with the pCAM-ICU if their level of consciousness is such that it requires only the caregivers voice to stimulate them to some degree of arousal. The RASS was used by Smith and colleagues due to its objectivity in patient assessment. Patients with a RASS of (−)3 or higher can be assessed for delirium using the pCAM-ICU, while patients who are comatose or have a RASS score of −4 or −5 are reassessed at a later time.

makes its association with morbidities and adverse outcomes in survivors extremely important. Critically ill patients with delirium have more failed and self-extubations,[30,42] prolonged requirement of mechanical ventilation,[30,31] inadvertent removal of catheters,[30] prolonged hospital stay,[30,41] higher health care costs,[43] and increased mortality.[31,44,45] Delirium is associated with a threefold increase in risk for death in adults after controlling for presence of coma, severity of illness, and preexisting comorbidities.[31]

The development of delirium during hospitalization has been implicated in the development of complications in survivors, such as long-term cognitive impairment (LTCI) and posttraumatic stress disorder (PTSD).[32,46,47] Critical illness alone leads to neuropathologic changes, ultimately associated with neurologic dysfunction.[48] Evidence from 11 studies, totaling ~500 adult patients, suggests that 25% to 78% of patients develop LTCI following critical illness.[49–57] There is mounting evidence that the causal link between critical illness and the development of LTCI is delirium,[58] with many studies demonstrating delirium as one of the strongest predictors for LTCI in survivors.[25,31,32,59,60]

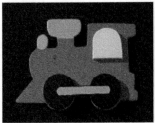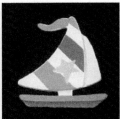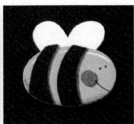

Fig. 2. ASE pictures used for assessment of "Feature 2: Inattention" for the pCAM-ICU are adapted for pediatrics with use of bold colors and child-friendly images. (*Courtesy of* Heidi A.B. Smith, MD, and Jenny Boyd, MD, Nashville, TN.)

The physiologic and psychiatric consequences of critical illness have just begun to be recognized.[61,62] Experts almost uniformly acknowledge that experiencing life-threatening illnesses often leads to acute stress disorder and PTSD.[61–64] A review of 20 studies involving adults demonstrates that the reported rates of PTSD symptoms in adult ICU survivors may be more than 40%, and they may easily eclipse the rates occurring in other medical populations.[61,62,65] There is an association between critical illness and PTSD, and an important risk factor for its development may be delirium.[66]

Delirium in Critically Ill Children

Pediatric delirium in the critically ill population remains in its infancy regarding diagnosis, treatment, and associations of risk. Literature available on pediatric delirium is biased toward general medical populations that exhibit hyperactive symptoms that have triggered consultation by psychiatric services. In one of the largest pediatric retrospective studies on delirium, Turkel and colleagues[24] reported that of 1027 consecutive patients evaluated by the child psychiatric service, 84 patients (9%) carried a diagnosis of delirium. Schieveld and colleagues[16] reported that of 877 critical care patients prospectively referred to the child psychiatry service, 40 patients (4.5%) were diagnosed with delirium. Both studies describe patient cohorts that were identified through clinical symptoms associated with hyperactive delirium, which is reported as the least common manifestation of delirium in the critically ill.[11] Therefore, the true prevalence of pediatric delirium in critical care populations remains unknown.

The actual prognostic significance of pediatric delirium during critical illness is also limited by a scarcity of prospective studies, none of which include patients on mechanical ventilation. In a large retrospective study, Turkel and colleagues[24] revealed increased morbidity and a 20% mortality rate in children diagnosed with delirium. In the critically ill pediatric population, mortality alone may not be a realistic outcome measure for the significance of delirium and potential treatment effects because mortality is a rare event with rates of 3% to 15% nationally. As the diagnosis of pediatric delirium increases, the use of functional outcome measures in addition to monitoring mortality will be important to truly describe the effects of brain dysfunction.[67]

Critical illness causes acute and chronic organ dysfunction, which may include progression to long-term neurologic sequelae in the pediatric patient.[68] Research is limited in the area of LTCI in pediatrics; however, recent investigations using validated rating scales suggest that a significant percentage of pediatric patients develop unfavorable neurocognitive and functional morbidity after critical illness.[69] Alievi and colleagues[70] assessed outcomes of 443 PICU survivors using validated functional outcome scales and found that PICU treatment and critical illness contributed to considerable declines in neurocognitive and functional performance in a significant proportion of this study cohort. Fiser and colleagues[71] also used functional outcome scales to prospectively assess a cohort of 11,106 patients following critical illness. They found that patients with mild to moderate disability at the time of discharge from the PICU subsequently had neurocognitive and functional impairments that affected school performance. With early pediatric research showing evidence of LTCI after critical illness, it is imperative to evaluate the relationship between the development of delirium and LTCI.

PTSD is prevalent among children with chronic illnesses such as cancer,[72] although little is known about the prevalence and adverse consequences of PTSD in pediatric survivors of critical illness.[63,73] Children may rely on coping resources more easily disrupted by the ICU environment compared with their adult counterparts, and they may have a less sophisticated ability to effectively process psychologically complex issues associated with life-threatening events.[63] Specifically, children's resilience to trauma may heavily rely on the maintenance of routine and presence of parents, both of which are disturbed in the PICU. When they are in a state of delirium, both children and adults commonly experience psychotic symptoms and delusions of a profoundly disturbing nature. Memories of these thought distortions, in turn, can trigger the dysregulation of the hypothalamic-pituitary-adrenal axis, presenting clinically with the symptoms of avoidance, anxiety, and hypervigilance, characteristic of PTSD. Existing literature on patients with chronic mental illness suggests that memories of psychotic episodes frequently form the basis for PTSD.[74] A similar dynamic appears to be at work in critically ill pediatric patients, with a 2008 article suggesting a link between delusional (as opposed to factual) memories and symptoms of PTSD.[75] These reports highlight the necessity for prompt delirium diagnosis and the subsequent ability to look at associations with brain dysfunction during critical illness and the long-term effects it initiates.

ETIOLOGY

Delirium is a neurobehavioral manifestation of imbalances in the synthesis, release, and inactivation of neurotransmitters that normally control cognitive function, behavior, and mood.[76] Many different global pathways are involved in the development of brain dysfunction. What begins as the stimulation of numerous diverse pathways may converge onto a few specific neural pathways that ultimately affect both arousal and the content of consciousness and cause delirium. Understanding the cellular response to critical illness, including neurotransmitter activity and neuroreceptor expression, may lead to innovative diagnostic and treatment modalities. Neurotransmitter imbalance, impaired oxidative metabolism, and inflammation are all implicated in the development of delirium.[25,76–79]

Three specific neurotransmitter systems are involved in the development of delirium, which include the glutamatergic, dopaminergic, and cholinergic pathways.[80–82] The cerebral cortex, striatum, substantia nigra, and thalamus are critical neuroanatomic areas that are most sensitive to alterations in neurotransmitter balances.[83] The thalamus, in particular, operates as a filter for information flowing to the cerebral cortex. When neurotransmitter balance becomes altered through disease or psychoactive medication administration, thalamic dysfunction may lead to sensory overload and hyperarousal (hyperactive delirium).[83,84]

Dopamine is a key neurotransmitter thought to be responsible for modulation of behavior, mood, and cognitive function.[85] The effect of dopamine on cortical function appears to fluctuate, following an inverted U-shaped curve based on concentration and specific receptor mediation.[86,87] In general, dopamine deficiency leads to extrapyramidal symptoms, whereas dopamine excess is associated with a range of psychotic disorders.[88] A balance in dopamine appears to be crucial, and a deficiency or excess of dopamine in the setting of delirium may be associated with hypoactive or hyperactive subtypes respectively.

Gamma aminobutyric acid (GABA) is the primary inhibitory neurotransmitter in the central nervous system (CNS).[79] Global and persistent inhibition of CNS arousal through GABAergic stimulation may cause disruption in cerebral functional connectivity and lead to unpredictable neurotransmission causing a constellation of acute brain dysfunction and LTCI.[25,89,90] Many common sedatives used in the ICU setting, like benzodiazepines and propofol, have high affinity for the GABAergic receptors and contribute to delirium through interference in sleep patterns and production of a central-mediated acetylcholine deficient state.[79,83,85]

Scarcity of acetylcholine has been linked to the development of delirium in critical illness.[91] Hyperactive delirium or psychosis associated with anticholinergic excess provides insight into the dysfunctional state of acetylcholine deficiency.[79] Numerous studies have demonstrated that the development of delirium and an increase in symptom severity of delirium is directly increased with the use of commonly used ICU drugs with significant anticholinergic properties.[92–94]

Both adults and pediatric patients present with similar types of critical illness, such as trauma, septic shock, myocardial insufficiency, and respiratory failure. There are numerous mechanisms, including hypoperfusion and inflammation, by which critical illness may lead to organ dysfunction. Hypoperfusion of tissues is recognized as 1 of the leading causes of organ dysfunction, and it may contribute to the development of delirium.[83] Whether due to decreased oxygen delivery or increased oxygen demands, neural ischemia leads to the inability to (1) maintain ionic gradients causing cortical depression,[95,96] (2) balance neurotransmitter synthesis, release, and metabolism,[97–101] and (3) eliminate neurotoxic byproducts from normal metabolic processes or disease states.[97,98,100]

Inflammation is another common and significant contributor of multiorgan dysfunction in the critically ill.[102] Inflammation initiates a cascade of activity that results in endothelial damage, thrombin formation, and ultimately microvascular compromise.[103] Animal studies have demonstrated that inflammatory mediators cross the blood-brain barrier,[104] increase vascular permeability in the brain,[105] and result in electroencephalographic (EEG) alterations consistent with those seen in septic patients diagnosed with delirium.[106] The diffuse slowing on EEG is thought to represent a reduction in cerebral oxidative metabolism or "cerebral insufficiency."[107,108] Girard and colleagues[109] demonstrated that a significant increase in key biomarkers of coagulation and inflammation were associated with the development of delirium among adult critical care patients.

RISK FACTORS

The cause of delirium in the critically ill is multifactorial and associated with numerous risk factors.[83] These risk factors can be categorized into three main groups: (1) predisposing factors or host factors, (2) precipitating factors including the severity and type of presenting illness, and (3) iatrogenic or environmental factors occurring in the ICU.[2,6,110–115] In critically ill adults, the most common risk factors are older age, pre-existing cognitive impairment, severity of illness in the ICU, and exposure to sedatives (Table 2).[6,39,45,116,117] There remains a dearth of literature on risk factors specific for the development of pediatric delirium in the critically ill.

Predisposing risk factors for pediatric delirium may be similar to those observed in adults, including age, genetic predisposition, chronic neurologic illnesses, or psychiatric disease. Genetic risk factors may impact pediatric and adult patients alike. Polymorphisms of apolipoprotein E4, previously linked to the development of Alzheimer disease[118] and poor patient outcomes in the setting of closed head injury and intracranial hemorrhage,[119,120] have been linked with delirium. Ely and colleagues[121] demonstrated a significant association between the Apo E4 polymorphism and duration of delirium in adult critical care patients. Leung and colleagues[122] also demonstrated that an Apo E4 carrier status was associated with a higher risk for development of delirium in patients postoperative from noncardiac surgery. Similar studies into genetic risk factors and other predisposing risk factors for the development of pediatric delirium need to be performed.

Iatrogenic Factors

Iatrogenic risk factors in the ICU, which significantly contribute to the development of delirium, include sleep deprivation and administration of sedatives and

Table 2
Risk factors for delirium[a]

| Predisposing Factors Host | Precipitating Factors | |
	Factors of Critical Illness	Iatrogenic Factors
Age	Acidosis	Few social interactions
Apolipoprotein E4 polymorphism	Anemia	Frequent nursing care
Cognitive impairment	CNS pathology	Immobilization
Depression	Electrolyte disturbances	Medications
Epilepsy	Endocrine derangement	Oversedation
Stroke history	Fever	Poorly controlled pain
Vision/hearing impairment	Hepatic failure	Sleep disturbances
	High severity of illness	Vascular access lines
	Hypoperfusion	
	Hypotension	
	Hypothermia	
	Hypoxia/anoxia	
	Intracranial hemorrhage	
	Infection/sepsis	
	Malnutrition	
	Metabolic disturbances	
	Myocardial failure	
	Poisoning	
	Respiratory failure	
	Shock	
	Trauma	

[a] See Refs.[2,6,38,44,82,109–124]

analgesics.[6,115,117,123] ICU patients sleep on average for 2 hours per day,[124] and less than 6% of that sleep is random eye movement sleep. Sleep deficiency may detrimentally affect protein synthesis, cellular and humoral immunity, energy expenditure, and ultimately organ function.[124] Excessive noise, diagnostic procedures, pain, fear, and frequency of patient-care activities are some recognized sources of sleep deprivation within the ICU.[83,125] However, exposure to sedatives and analgesics, mechanical ventilation, and other disease-associated complications may have even greater roles in affecting sleep patterns in the critically ill.[125]

Sedative Administration

Patients who require mechanical ventilation routinely receive sedative and analgesic medications to reduce pain and anxiety, per guidelines of the Society of Critical Care Medicine (SCCM).[5] Although the use of sedation and analgesia may facilitate patient care and safety,[126,127] their use may also depress spontaneous ventilation and prolong the requirement of mechanical ventilation, leading to greater costs and complications.[128–131] Patients on mechanical ventilation are often sedated to the point of stupor or coma to improve oxygenation, alleviate agitation, and to prevent them from removing support devices. When patients emerge from the effects of sedation, they may do so peacefully or in a combative manner, thereby experiencing the hypoactive or hyperactive form of delirium, respectively.[1]

Multiple studies on adults have shown significant associations between the administration of sedatives and the development of delirium,[45] of which benzodiazepines are the most commonly implicated.[114,117] Psychoactive medications represent a significant iatrogenic cause of delirium,[13,115,132] with a relative risk for delirium of 3 to 11 times.[13,114] The temporal relationship between sedative administration and ICU delirium was examined by Pandharipande and colleagues,[117] where lorazepam was found to be an independent risk factor for the daily transition to delirium (odds ratio, 1.2; 95% confidence interval, 1.2–1.4). Although administration of midazolam and lorazepam has been consistently shown to be associated with the development of delirium, studies have been less consistent on the relationship between delirium and opioids.[6]

Greater than 90% of infants and children supported on mechanical ventilation receive psychoactive medications, most commonly combinations of opioids and benzodiazepines.[133,134] Colville and colleagues[75] reported that, of 102 consecutive children aged between 7 and 17 years admitted to the PICU, 1 of 3 reported having delusional memories following discharge. Delusional memories were significantly associated with a longer duration of psychoactive medication administration during PICU stay.[75] This association of sedative exposure and the delusional memories highlights the likelihood that pediatric patients may have a significant risk of delirium during critical illness.

TREATMENT STRATEGIES

The clinical approach to prevent or treat delirium may vary and be driven by different goals: (1) prevention through controlling precipitating risk factors, (2) management of delirium symptoms (psychosis or agitation), and/or (3) treatment of delirium through resolution of its underlying cause or modulation of the neurochemical cascade.[83] Multidisciplinary approaches to the prevention and overall management of delirium in critically ill adults and children have yet to be adequately studied. However, well-studied treatment protocols for delirium in noncritically ill patients may provide some insight into delirium management in ICU populations.[6] In general, the treatment of delirium in the ICU setting requires (1) an accurate delirium diagnosis, (2) means of consistent monitoring and reevaluation, (3) therapeutic intervention for hyperactive manifestations that may cause patient harm, (4) avoidance of risk factors to include certain ICU medications that may exacerbate delirium severity, and (5) diagnosis and treatment of the underlying etiology if possible.[83]

Nonpharmacologic Management

Iatrogenic risk factors for delirium in the ICU setting are numerous and fundamentally avoidable. Inouye and colleagues[135] conducted a study of a multicomponent delirium intervention protocol in critically ill adults, consisting of (1) cognitive stimulation and patient reorientation, (2) consistent nonpharmacologic sleep, (3) exercise and early mobilization, (4) use of hearing aids or glasses, and (5) timely removal of indwelling catheters. The protocol reduced delirium incidence significantly from 15% in the usual-care group to 9.9% in the intervention group. Other adult randomized controlled trials of similar multicomponent therapies have also shown similar improvements in the occurrence of delirium.[136,137] Schieveld and coworkers[16] instituted an intervention strategy for critically ill children with delirium to include parental presence, pictures of familiar people and objects, familiar music, and involvement of a child psychiatrist. All surviving patients demonstrated reduction of the assessed severity of delirium.

The goal of any multicomponent approach to delirium treatment and prevention will be based on minimizing risk factors. Some of the most common risk factors are infection, electrolyte abnormalities, sleep deprivation, and medication exposure.[6]

Maintaining as normal an environment as possible within the ICU setting allows for consistent patient orientation and, ultimately, reassurance. As part of this approach, promoting normal circadian light rhythm with light and noise control is likely to be paramount. Family involvement, adherence to patient routines, and removal of restraints when appropriate may specifically impact pediatric ICU patients. A mainstay of both prevention and treatment focuses on appropriate use and even avoidance of certain GABAergic agents, such as benzodiazepines and propofol.[138] Sedatives and analgesics are clearly intended to provide patient comfort through pain control and anxiety relief, which in many instances may decrease the risk of developing delirium.[139] However, oversedation must also be avoided because its association with transition to delirium is well documented, and the usefulness of validated sedation scales and daily interruption of sedatives are shown to significantly improve outcomes.[128,130,140]

Pharmacologic Management

Pharmacologic therapy for delirium in the ICU may be a helpful adjunct to the needed multicomponent approach to patient care. Once risk factors for delirium have been minimized, along with the alleviation of complications from critical disease, such as hypoxia, hypoglycemia, or shock, pharmacologic therapy can be considered.[6] Although medications used for delirium may improve cognition, there are many psychoactive effects that may worsen a patient's sensorium and lead to prolonged cognitive impairment.[25] Until prospective, randomized, double-blinded studies demonstrate clear treatment benefit of antipsychotic drugs, great caution must be exercised and only minimal doses required for potential benefit must be administered.

Haloperidol (Haldol) is a conventional antipsychotic most frequently used for the treatment of delirium.[141] Haloperidol antagonizes the D2 receptor in numerous higher cortical pathways, leading to restoration of hippocampal function.[25,83] With inhibition of the dopamine-2 receptor, the effects of dopamine excess are controlled, and symptoms such as unstructured thought patterns and hallucinations can be alleviated.[25] However in hypoactive delirium that is associated with dopamine scarcity versus excess, treatment with haloperidol may exacerbate the severity of delirium and prolong psychomotor retardation or even promote catatonic features.[83] SCCM guidelines recommend that adult patients with hyperactive delirium be treated with haloperidol, although the optimal dosing regimen has yet to be defined in clinical trials.[6] Successful treatment of hyperactive delirium in PICU patients with haloperidol was reported by Schieveld and colleagues[16] using a loading dose of 0.15 to 0.25 mg intravenous followed by 0.05 to 0.5 mg/kg every day for maintenance. In patients who could tolerate oral medication, an atypical antipsychotic, risperidone (Risperdal), was provided as a loading dose of 0.1 to 0.2 mg followed by 0.2 to 2.0 mg every day as maintenance. Schieveld and colleagues reported that the majority of treated patients had beneficial effects most noted immediately following the loading dose.

Atypical antipsychotics, such as risperidone, olanzapine (Zyprexa), and ziprasidone (Geodon) are considered alternatives to haloperidol for delirium treatment. The clinical benefit of this class of drugs is the global impact on not just dopamine receptors but also effects on serotonin, acetylcholine, and norepinephrine neurotransmission.[142] Patients with hypoactive delirium may benefit from the global effect on neurotransmitter equilibrium versus traditional focus on dopamine suppression. Skrobik and colleagues[142] completed a nonrandomized trial comparing haloperidol to olanzapine in 73 adult ICU patients. Although resolution of delirium was similar in both groups, the side effects were greatly decreased in those patients receiving olanzapine.

All antipsychotics have potentially serious side effects. The most concerning adverse effects include torsades de pointes, malignant hyperthermia, extrapyramidal movement disorders, hypotension, glucose and lipid dysregulation, laryngeal spasm, and anticholinergic effects, such as constipation, urinary retention, and dry mouth.[25] Any patient with prolonged QT or with significant cardiac arrhythmias should avoid treatment with antipsychotics. Schieveld and colleagues[16] demonstrated that, of 40 pediatric critical care patients treated for delirium with typical and atypical antipsychotics, only two patients developed acute dystonias that required further intervention. Although atypical antipsychotics are associated with fewer side effects, there remains a lack of well-designed, randomized, placebo-controlled trials studying the efficacy of either typical or atypical antipsychotics for the treatment or prevention of delirium in adult or pediatric critically ill patients.[6]

The use of sedatives, such as benzodiazepines, is a mainstay of treatment for agitation and withdrawal syndromes in the PICU. However, administration of lorazepam (Ativan) is now recognized to be a significant risk factor for the development of delirium in the ICU.[114,117] A novel α2-receptor agonist, dexmedetomidine (Precedex), has been used in the ICU setting for sedation and was not shown to have an association with the development of delirium. Maldonado and colleagues[138] were able to demonstrate that, of patients sedated after sternal closure, only 8% of those receiving dexmedetomidine developed delirium compared with 50% of patients treated with either propofol (Diprivan) or midazolam (Versed). Pandharipande and colleagues[143] completed a double-blinded randomized controlled trial, in which ICU patients treated with dexmedetomidine compared with lorazepam spent fewer days in coma and had more neurologically appropriate days. Pediatric studies of dexmedetomidine have been limited to patients treated for ED following anesthesia. These studies demonstrate less analgesic withdrawal complications with the use of dexmetetomidine.[6,144]

SUMMARY

Delirium is a syndrome of acute brain dysfunction that commonly occurs in critically ill adults and most certainly is prevalent in critically ill children all over the world. The dearth of information about the incidence, prevalence, and severity of pediatric delirium stems from the simple fact that there have not been well-validated instruments for routine delirium diagnosis at the bedside. This article reviewed the emerging solutions to this problem, including description of a new pediatric tool called the pCAM-ICU. In adults, delirium is responsible for significant increases in both morbidity and mortality in critically ill patients. The advent of new tools for use in critically ill children will allow the epidemiology of this form of acute brain dysfunction to be studied adequately, will allow clinical management algorithms to be developed and implemented following testing, and will present the necessary incorporation of delirium as an outcome measure for future clinical trials in pediatric critical care medicine.

REFERENCES

1. Ely EW, Siegel MD, Inouye SK. Delirium in the intensive care unit: an under-recognized syndrome of organ dysfunction. Semin Respir Crit Care Med 2001;22(2):115–26.
2. Francis J, Martin D, Kapoor WN. A prospective study of delirium in hospitalized elderly. JAMA 1990;263(8):1097–101.
3. Inouye SK. The dilemma of delirium: clinical and research controversies regarding diagnosis and evaluation of delirium in hospitalized elderly medical patients. Am J Med 1994;97(3):278–88.

4. Morandi A, Pandharipande P, Trabucchi M, et al. Understanding international differences in terminology for delirium and other types of acute brain dysfunction in critically ill patients. Intensive Care Med 2008;34:1907–15.
5. Jacobi J, Fraser GL, Coursin DB, et al. Clinical practice guidelines for the sustained use of sedatives and analgesics in the critically ill adult. Crit Care Med 2002;30(1):119–41.
6. Pandharipande P, Ely EW. Scoring and managing delirium in the PICU. In: Shanley TP, Zimmerman JJ, editors. Current concepts in pediatric critical care - society of critical care medicine. Mount Prospect (IL): Society of Critical Care Medicine; 2008. p. 69–77.
7. American Psychiatric Association Diagnostic and statistical manual of mental disorders. Fourth edition, text revision. Washington, DC: American Psychiatric Association; 2000.
8. Justic M. Does "ICU psychosis" really exist? Crit Care Nurse 2000;20(3):28–37.
9. McGuire BE, Basten CJ, Ryan CJ, et al. Intensive care unit syndrome: a dangerous misnomer. Arch Intern Med 2000;160(7):906–9.
10. Meagher DJ, Trzepacz PT. Motoric subtypes of delirium. Semin Clin Neuropsychiatry 2000;5(2):75–85.
11. Peterson JF, Pun BT, Dittus RS, et al. Delirium and its motoric subtypes: a study of 614 critically ill patients. J Am Geriatr Soc 2006;54(3):479–84.
12. O'Keefe ST, Chonchubhair AN. Postoperative delirium in the elderly. Br J Anaesth 1994;73:673–87.
13. Inouye SK, Schlesinger MJ, Lydon TJ. Delirium: a symptom of how hospital care is failing older persons and a window to improve quality of hospital care. Am J Med 1999;106(5):565–73.
14. Ely EW, Truman B, May L, et al. Validation of the CAM-ICU for delirium assessment in mechanically ventilated patients [abstract]. J Am Geriatr Soc 2001;49:S2.
15. Turkel SB, Trzepacz PT, Tavare CJ. Comparing symptoms of delirium in adults and children. Psychosomatics 2006;47(4):320–4.
16. Schieveld JN, Leroy PL, van OS J, et al. Pediatric delirium in critical illness: phenomenology, clinical correlates and treatment response in 40 cases in the pediatric intensive care unit. Intensive Care Med 2007;33:1033–40.
17. Martini DR. Commentary: the diagnosis of delirium in pediatric patients. J Am Acad Child Adolesc Psychiatry 2005;44(4):395–8.
18. Schieveld JN, Leentjens AF. Delirium in severely ill young children in the pediatric intensive care unit (PICU). J Am Acad Child Adolesc Psychiatry 2005;44(4):392–4.
19. Plum F, Posner J. The diagnosis of stupor and coma. Philadelphia: FA Davis Co; 1980.
20. Teasdale G, Jennett B. Assessment of coma and impaired consciousness: a practical scale. Lancet 1974;2:81–4.
21. Devlin JW, Boleski G, Mlynarek M, et al. Motor Activity Assessment Scale: a valid and reliable sedation scale for use with mechanically ventilated patients in an adult surgical intensive care unit. Crit Care Med 1999;27(7):1271–5.
22. Ramsay MA, Keenan SP. Measuring level of sedation in the intensive care unit. JAMA 2000;284:441–2.
23. Trzepacz PT, Baker RW. The psychiatric mental status examination. Oxford (UK): Oxford University Press; 1993. p. 202.
24. Turkel SB, Tavare CJ. Delirium in children and adolescents. J Neuropsychiatry Clin Neurosci 2003;15:431–5.
25. Pandharipande P, Jackson J, Ely EW. Delirium: acute cognitive dysfunction in the critically ill. Curr Opin Crit Care 2005;11(4):360–8.

26. Trzepacz PT, Mittal D, Torres R, et al. Validation of Delirium Rating Scale Revised-98: comparison to the delirium rating scale and cognitive test for delirium. J Neuropsychiatry Clin Neurosci 2001;13:229–42.
27. Ely EW, Margolin R, Francis J, et al. Evaluation of delirium in critically ill patients: validation of the Confusion Assessment Method for the Intensive Care Unit (CAM-ICU). Crit Care Med 2001;29(7):1370–9.
28. Ely EW, Inouye SK, Bernard GR, et al. Delirium in mechanically ventilated patients: validity and reliability of the confusion assessment method for the intensive care unit (CAM-ICU). JAMA 2001;286(21):2703–10.
29. Bergeron N, Dubois MJ, Dumont M, et al. Intensive Care Delirium Screening Checklist: evaluation of a new screening tool. Intensive Care Med 2001;27(5):859–64.
30. Ely EW, Gautam S, Margolin R, et al. The impact of delirium in the intensive care unit on hospital length of stay. Intensive Care Med 2001;27(12):1892–900.
31. Ely EW, Shintani A, Truman B, et al. Delirium as a predictor of mortality in mechanically ventilated patients in the intensive care unit. JAMA 2004;291(14):1753–62.
32. Jackson JC, Gordon SM, Hart RP, et al. The association between delirium and cognitive decline: a review of the empirical literature. Neuropsychol Rev 2004;14(2):87–98.
33. Sikich N, Lerman J. Development and psychometric evaluation of the pediatric anesthesia emergence delirium scale. Anesthesiology 2004;100(5):1138–45.
34. Wilson TA, Graves SA. Pediatric considerations in a general postanesthesia care unit. J Post Anesth Nurs 1990;5(1):16–24.
35. Smith HA, Boyd J, Fuchs DC, et al. Diagnosing delirium in critically ill children: validity and reliability of the Pediatric Confusion Assessment Method for the Intensive Care Unit. Crit Care Med 2011;39:150–7.
36. Sessler CN, Gosnell MS, Grap MJ, et al. The Richmond Agitation-Sedation Scale: validity and reliability in adult intensive care unit patients. Am J Respir Crit Care Med 2002;166(10):1338–44.
37. Ely EW, Truman B, Shintani A, et al. Monitoring sedation status over time in ICU patients: reliability and validity of the Richmond Agitation-Sedation Scale (RASS). JAMA 2003;289(22):2983–91.
38. Dubois MJ, Bergeron N, Dumont M, et al. Delirium in an intensive care unit: a study of risk factors. Intensive Care Med 2001;27(8):1297–304.
39. McNicoll L, Pisani MA, Zhang Y, et al. Delirium in the intensive care unit: occurrence and clinical course in older patients. J Am Geriatr Soc 2003;51(5):591–8.
40. Pandharipande P, Costabile S, Cotton B, et al. Prevalence of delirium in surgical ICU patients [abstract]. Crit Care Med 2005;33(12 Suppl):A45.
41. Thomason JW, Shintani A, Peterson JF, et al. Intensive care unit delirium is an independent predictor of longer hospital stay: a prospective analysis of 261 non-ventilated patients. Crit Care 2005;9(4):R375–81.
42. Salam A, Tilluckdharry L, Amoateng-Adjepong Y, et al. Neurologic status, cough, secretions and extubation outcomes. Intensive Care Med 2004;30:1334–9.
43. Milbrandt EB, Deppen S, Harrison PL, et al. Costs associated with delirium in mechanically ventilated patients. Crit Care Med 2004;32(4):955–62.
44. Lin SM, Liu CY, Wang CH, et al. The impact of delirium on the survival of mechanically ventilated patients. Crit Care Med 2004;32(11):2254–9.
45. Ouimet S, Kavanagh BP, Gottfried SB, et al. Incidence, risk factors and consequences of ICU delirium. Intensive Care Med 2007;33(1):66–73.

46. Jackson JC, Gordon SM, Girard TD, et al. Delirium as a risk factor for long term cognitive impairment in mechanically ventilated ICU survivors (under review) [abstract]. Am J Respir Crit Care Med 2007;175:A22.

47. Hopkins RO, Jackson JC. Long-term neurocognitive function after critical illness. Chest 2006;130(3):869–78.

48. Insel K, Morrow D, Brewer B, et al. Executive function, working memory, and medication adherence among older adults. J Gerontol B Psychol Sci Soc Sci 2006;61(2):102–7.

49. Heaton RK, Marcotte TD, Mindt MR, et al. The impact of HIV-associated neuropsychological impairment on everyday functioning. J Int Neuropsychol Soc 2004;10:317–31.

50. Hinkin CH, Castellon SA, Durvasula RS, et al. Medication adherence among HIV+ adults. Neurology 2002;59:1944–50.

51. Stewart JT, Gonzalez-Perez E, Zhu Y, et al. Cognitive predictors of restiveness in dementia patients. Am J Geriatr Psychiatry 1999;7:259–63.

52. Allen SC, Jain M, Ragab S, et al. Acquisition and short-term retention of inhaler techniques require intact executive function in elderly subjects. Age Ageing 2003;32(3):299–302.

53. Kalhan R, Mikkelsen M, Dedhiya P, et al. Underuse of lung protective ventilation: analysis of potential factors to explain physician behavior. Crit Care Med 2006; 34(2):300–6.

54. Biederman J, Petty C, Fried R, et al. Impact of psychometrically defined deficits of executive functioning in adults with attention deficit hyperactivity disorder. Am J Psychiatry 2006;163:1730–8.

55. Evans JD, Bond GR, PS Meyer, et al. Cognitive and clinical predictors of success in vocational rehabilitation in schizophrenia. Schizophr Res 2004;70:331–42.

56. McGurk SR, Mueser KT. Cognitive and clinical predictors of work outcomes in clients with schizophrenia receiving supported employment services: 4 year follow-up. Adm Policy Ment Health 2006;33:598–606.

57. Washburn AM, Sands LP. Social cognition in nursing home residents with and without cognitive impairment. J Gerontol B Psychol Sci Soc Sci 2006;61:P174–9.

58. Gunther ML, Jackson JC, Ely EW. The cognitive consequences of critical illness: practical recommendations for screening and assessment. Crit Care Clin 2007; 23(3):491–506.

59. Jackson JC, Hart RP, Gordon SM, et al. Six-month neuropsychological outcome of medical intensive care unit patients. Crit Care Med 2003;31(4):1226–34.

60. Hopkins RO, Weaver LK, Pope D, et al. Neuropsychological sequelae and impaired health status in survivors of severe acute respiratory distress syndrome. Am J Respir Crit Care Med 1999;160(1):50–6.

61. Tedstone JE, Tarrier N. Posttraumatic stress disorder following medical illness and treatment. Clin Psychol Rev 2003;23:409–48.

62. Jackson JC, Hart RP, Gordon SM, et al. Post-traumatic stress disorder and post-traumatic stress symptoms following critical illness in medical intensive care unit patients: assessing the magnitude of the problem. Crit Care 2007;11(1):R27.

63. Ward-Begnoche W. Posttraumatic stress symptoms in the pediatric intensive care unit. J Spec Pediatr Nurs 2007;12(2):84–92.

64. Kangas M, Henry JL, Bryant RA. Posttraumatic stress disorder following cancer: A conceptual and empirical review. Clin Psychol Rev 2002;22:499–524.

65. Davydow DS, Gifford JM, Desai SV, et al. Posttraumatic stress disorder in general intensive care unit survivors: a systematic review. Gen Hosp Psychiatry 2008;30(5):421–34.

66. Girard TD, Shintani AK, Jackson JC, et al. Risk factors for posttraumatic stress disorder symptoms following critical illness requiring mechanical ventilation: a prospective cohort study. Crit Care 2007;11(1):R28.

67. Fiser DH, Tilford JM, Roberson PK. Relationship of illness severity and length of stay to functional outcomes in the pediatric intensive care unit: a multi-institutional study. Crit Care Med 2000;28(4):1173–9.

68. Van Vielingen TE, Tuokko HA, Cramer K, et al. Awareness of financial skills in dementia. Aging Ment Health 2004;8:374–80.

69. Hopkins RO. Does critical illness and intensive care unit treatment contribute to neurocognitive and functional morbidity in pediatric patients? J Pediatr (Rio J) 2007;83(6):488–90.

70. Alievi PT, Carvalho PR, Trotta EA, et al. The impact of admission to a pediatric intensive care unit assessed by means of global and cognitive performance scales. J Pediatr (Rio J) 2007;83(6):505–11.

71. Fiser DH, Long N, Roberson PK, et al. Relationship of pediatric overall performance category and pediatric cerebral performance category scores at pediatric intensive care unit discharge with outcome measures collected at hospital discharge and 1- and 6-month follow-up assessments. Crit Care Med 2000;28(7):2616–20.

72. Geffen DB, Blaustein A, Amir MC, et al. Post-traumatic stress disorder and quality of life in long-term survivors of Hodgkin's disease and non-Hodgkin's lymphoma in Israel. Leuk Lymphoma 2003;44(11):1925–9.

73. Rees G, Gledhill J, Garralda ME, et al. Psychiatric outcome following paediatric intensive care unit (PICU) admission: a cohort study. Intensive Care Med 2004; 30(8):1607–14.

74. Jones C, Griffiths RD, Humphris G, et al. Memory, delusions, and the development of acute posttraumatic stress disorder-related symptoms after intensive care. Crit Care Med 2001;29(3):573–80.

75. Colville G, Kerry S, Pierce C. Children's factual and delusional memories of intensive care. Am J Respir Crit Care Med 2008;177(9):976–82.

76. Trzepacz PT. Update on the neuropathogenesis of delirium. Dement Geriatr Cogn Disord 1999;10:330–4.

77. Trzepacz PT, Delirium. Advances in diagnosis, pathophysiology, and treatment. Psychiatr Clin North Am 1996;19(3):429–48.

78. Meagher DJ, Moran M, Raju B, et al. Phenomenology of delirium. Assessment of 100 adult cases using standardized measures. Br J Psychiatry 2007;190:135–41.

79. Gunther ML, Morandi A, Ely EW. Pathophysiology of delirium in the intensive care unit. Crit Care Clin 2008;24(1):45–65.

80. Pavlov VA, Wang H, Czura CJ, et al. The cholinergic anti-inflammatory pathway: a missing link in neuroimmunomodulation. Mol Med 2003;9:125–34.

81. Webb JM, Carlton EF, Geeham DM. Delirium in the intensive care unit: are we helping the patient? Crit Care Nurs Q 2000;22(4):47–60.

82. Crippen D. Treatment of agitation and its comorbidities in the intensive care unit. In: Hill NS, Levy MM, editors. Ventilator Management Strategies for Critical Care(Lung Biology in Health and Disease). New York: Marcel Dekker, Inc; 2001. p. 243–84.

83. Maldonado JR. Delirium in the acute care setting: characteristics, diagnosis and treatment. Crit Care Clin 2008;24(4):657–722.

84. Gaudreau JD, Gagnon P, Roy MA, et al. Association between psychoactive medications and delirium in hospitalized patients: a critical review. Psychosomatics 2005;46(4):302–16.

85. Bloom FE, Kupfer DJ, Bunney BS, et al. Amines. Psychopharmacology: the fourth generation of progress. New York: Raven Press; 1995. p. 1287–359.

86. Meyer-Lindenberg A, Kohn PD, Kolachana B, et al. Midbrain dopamine and prefrontal function in humans: interaction and modulation by COMT genotype. Nat Neurosci 2005;8(5):594–6.

87. Meyer-Lindenberg A, Nichols T, Callicott JH, et al. Impact of complex genetic variation in COMT on human brain function. Mol Psychiatry 2006;11(9): 867–77, 797.

88. Bloom FE, Kupfer DJ, Bunney BS, et al. Schizophrenia. Psychopharmacology: the fourth generation of progress. New York: Raven Press; 1995. 1171–286.

89. Gunther ML, Jackson JC, Wesley EE. Loss of IQ in the ICU brain injury without the insult. Med Hypotheses 2007;69:1179–82.

90. Hopkins RO, Jackson JC. Assessing neurocognitive outcomes after critical illness: are delirium and long-term cognitive impairments related? Curr Opin Crit Care 2006;12:388–94.

91. Flacker JM, Cummings V, Mach JR Jr, et al. The association of serum anticholinergic activity with delirium in elderly medical patients. Am J Geriatr Psychiatry 1998;6(1):31–41.

92. Tune LE, Egeli S. Acetylcholine and delirium. Dement Geriatr Cogn Disord 1999; 10:342–4.

93. Tune LE, Strauss ME, Lew MF, et al. Serum levels of anticholinergic drugs and impaired recent memory in chronic schizophrenic patients. Am J Psychiatry 1982;139(11):1460–2.

94. Han L, McCusker J, Cole M, et al. Use of medications with anticholinergic effect predicts clinical severity of delirium symptoms in older medical inpatients. Arch Intern Med 2001;161(8):1099–105.

95. Basarsky TA, Feighan D, MacVicar BA. Glutamate release through volume-activated channels during spreading depression. J Neurosci 1999;19(15): 6439–45.

96. Somjen GG, Aitken PG, Balestrino M, et al. Extracellular ions, hypoxic irreversible loss of function and delayed post ischemic neuron degeneration studied in vitro. Acta Physiol Scand Suppl 1989;58:258.

97. Busto R, Globus MY, Dietrich WD, et al. Effect of mild hypothermia on ischemia-induced release of neurotransmitters and free fatty acids in rat brain. Stroke 1989;20(7):904–10.

98. Globus MY, Alonso O, Dietrich WD, et al. Glutamate release and free radical production following brain injury: effects of posttraumatic hypothermia. J Neurochem 1995;65(4):1704–11.

99. Globus MY, Busto R, Dietrich WD, et al. Effect of ischemia on the in vivo release of striatal dopamine, glutamate, and gamma-aminobutyric acid studied by intracerebral microdialysis. J Neurochem 1988;51(5):1455–64.

100. Globus MY, Busto R, Martinez E, et al. Ischemia induces release of glutamate in regions spared from histopathologic damage in the rat. Stroke 1990;21(11 Suppl):III43–6.

101. Takagi K, Ginsberg MD, Globus MY, et al. Effect of hyperthermia on glutamate release in ischemic penumbra after middle cerebral artery occlusion in rats. Am J Phys 1994;267(5 Pt 2):H1770–6.

102. Marshall JC. Inflammation, coagulopathy, and the pathogenesis of multiple organ dysfunction syndrome. Crit Care Med 2001;29(7 Suppl):S99–106.

103. Wheeler AP, Bernard GR. Treating patients with severe sepsis. N Engl J Med 1999;340(3):207–14.

104. Papadopoulos MC, Lamb FJ, Moss RF, et al. Faecal peritonitis causes oedema and neuronal injury in pig cerebral cortex. Clin Sci (Lond) 1999;96(5):461–6.

105. Huynh HK, Dorovini-Zis K. Effects of interferon-gamma on primary cultures of human brain microvessel endothelial cells. Am J Pathol 1993;142(4):1265–78.

106. Krueger JM, Walter J, Dinarello CA, et al. Sleep-promoting effects of endogenous pyrogen (interleukin-1). Am J Phys 1984;246(6 Pt 2):R994–9.

107. Engel GL, Romano J. Delirium, a syndrome of cerebral insufficiency. J Chronic Dis 1959;9(3):260–77.

108. Fink MP, Evans TW. Mechanisms of organ dysfunction in critical illness: report from a Round Table Conference held in Brussels. Intensive Care Med 2002; 28(3):369–75.

109. Girard TD, Shintani A, Thompson JL, et al. Biomarkers of inflammation and coagulopathy predict the duration of acute brain dysfunction in critically ill patients [abstract]. Crit Care Med 2006;34(12 Suppl):A19.

110. Wilson LM. Intensive care delirium. The effect of outside deprivation in a windowless unit. Arch Intern Med 1972;130(2):225–6.

111. Levkoff SE, Evans DA, Liptzin B, et al. Delirium. The occurrence and persistence of symptoms among elderly hospitalized patients. Arch Intern Med 1992;152(2): 334–40.

112. Francis J, Kapoor WN. Delirium in hospitalized elderly. J Gen Intern Med 1990;5: 65–79.

113. Williams-Russo P, Urquhart BL, Sharrock NE, et al. Post-operative delirium: predictors and prognosis in elderly orthopedic patients. J Am Geriatr Soc 1992;40(8):759–67.

114. Marcantonio ER, Juarez G, Goldman L, et al. The relationship of postoperative delirium with psychoactive medications. JAMA 1994;272(19):1518–22.

115. Inouye SK, Charpentier PA. Precipitating factors for delirium in hospitalized elderly persons. Predictive model and interrelationship with baseline vulnerability. JAMA 1996;275(11):852–7.

116. Aldemir M, Ozen S, Kara IH, et al. Predisposing factors for delirium in the surgical intensive care unit. Crit Care 2001;5(5):265–70.

117. Pandharipande P, Shintani A, Peterson J, et al. Lorazepam is an independent risk factor for transitioning to delirium in intensive care unit patients. Anesthesiology 2006;104(1):21–6.

118. Corder EH, Saunders AM, Strittmatter WJ, et al. Gene dose of apolipoprotein E type 4 allele and the risk of Alzheimer's disease in late onset families. Science 1993;261(5123):921–3.

119. Laskowitz DT, Sheng H, Bart RD, et al. Apolipoprotein E-deficient mice have increased susceptibility to focal cerebral ischemia. J Cereb Blood Flow Metab 1997;17(7):753–8.

120. Lynch JR, Pineda JA, Morgan D, et al. Apolipoprotein E affects the central nervous system response to injury and the development of cerebral edema. Ann Neurol 2002;51(1):113–7.

121. Ely EW, Girard TD, Shintani AK, et al. Apolipoprotein E4 polymorphism as a genetic predisposition to delirium in critically ill patients. Crit Care Med 2007;35(1):112–7.

122. Leung JM, Sands LP, Wang Y, et al. Apolipoprotein E e4 allele increases the risk of early postoperative delirium in older patients undergoing noncardiac surgery. Anesthesiology 2007;107(3):406–11.

123. Schor JD, Levkoff SE, Lipsitz LA, et al. Risk factors for delirium in hospitalized elderly. JAMA 1992;267(6):827–31.

124. Aurell J, Elmqvist D. Sleep in the surgical intensive care unit: continuous polygraphic recording of sleep in nine patients receiving postoperative care. Br Med J (Clin Res Ed) 1985;290(6474):1029–32.

125. Gabor JY, Cooper AB, Crombach SA, et al. Contribution of the intensive care unit environment to sleep disruption in mechanically ventilated patients and healthy subjects. Am J Respir Crit Care Med 2003;167(5):708–15.

126. Chevron V, Menard J, Richard J, et al. Unplanned extubation: risk factors of development and predictive criteria for reintubation. Crit Care Med 1998;26: 1049–53.

127. Marx CM, Smith PG, Lowrie LH, et al. Optimal sedation of mechanically ventilated pediatric critical care patients. Crit Care Med 1994;22:163–70.

128. Brook AD, Ahrens TS, Schaiff R, et al. Effect of a nursing-implemented sedation protocol on the duration of mechanical ventilation. Crit Care Med 1999;27(12): 2609–15.

129. Kollef M, Pittet D, Sanchez GM, et al. A Randomized Double-Blind Trial of Iseganan in Prevention of Ventilator-associated Pneumonia. Am J Respir Crit Care Med 2006;173(1):91–7.

130. Kress JP, Pohlman AS, O'Connor MF, et al. Daily interruption of sedative infusions in critically ill patients undergoing mechanical ventilation. N Engl J Med 2000;342(20):1471–7.

131. Randolph AG, Wypij D, Venkataraman ST, et al. Effect of mechanical ventilator weaning protocols on respiratory outcomes in infants and children: a randomized controlled trial. JAMA 2002;288(20):2561–8.

132. Francis J. Drug-induced delirium: diagnosis and treatment. CNS Drugs 1996;5: 103–14.

133. Twite MD, Rashid A, Zuk J, et al. Sedation, analgesia, and neuromuscular blockade in the pediatric intensive care unit: survey of fellowship training programs. Pediatr Crit Care Med 2004;5(6):521–32.

134. Rhoney DH, Parker D. Use of sedative and analgesic agents in neurotrauma patients: effects on cerebral physiology [abstract]. Neurol Res 2001;2-3:237–59.

135. Inouye SK, Bogardus ST Jr, Charpentier PA, et al. A multicomponent intervention to prevent delirium in hospitalized older patients. N Engl J Med 1999;340(9): 669–76.

136. Marcantonio ER, Flacker JM, Wright RJ, et al. Reducing delirium after hip fracture: a randomized trial. J Am Geriatr Soc 2001;49(5):516–22.

137. Lundstrom M, Edlund A, Karlsson S, et al. A multifactorial intervention program reduces the duration of delirium, length of hospitalization, and mortality in delirious patients. J Am Geriatr Soc 2005;53(4):622–8.

138. Maldonado JR, van der Starre PJ, Wysong A. Post-operative sedation and the incidence of ICU delirium in cardiac surgery patients [abstract]. Anesthesiology 2003;99:A465.

139. Morrison RS, Magaziner J, Gilbert M, et al. Relationship between pain and opioid analgesics on the development of delirium following hip fracture. J Gerontol A Biol Sci Med Sci 2003;58(1):76–81.

140. Kollef MH, Levy NT, Ahrens TS, et al. The use of continuous i.v. sedation is associated with prolongation of mechanical ventilation. Chest 1998;114(2):541–8.

141. Ely EW, Stephens RK, Jackson JC, et al. Current opinions regarding the importance, diagnosis, and management of delirium in the intensive care unit: a survey of 912 healthcare professionals. Crit Care Med 2004;32(1):106–12.

142. Skrobik YK, Bergeron N, Dumont M, et al. Olanzapine vs haloperidol: treating delirium in a critical care setting. Intensive Care Med 2004;30(3):444–9.

143. Pandharipande PP, Pun BT, Herr DL, et al. Effect of sedation with dexmedetomidine vs lorazepam on acute brain dysfunction in mechanically ventilated patients: the MENDS randomized controlled trial. JAMA 2007;298(22):2644–53.
144. Ibacache ME, Munoz HR, Brandes V, et al. Single-dose dexmedetomidine reduces agitation after sevoflurane anesthesia in children. Anesth Analg 2004; 98(1):60–3.

Cognitive Functioning, Mental Health, and Quality of Life in ICU Survivors: An Overview

James C. Jackson, PsyD[a],*, Nathaniel Mitchell[a],
Ramona O. Hopkins, PhD[b,c,d]

KEYWORDS

- Cognitive impairments • Critical illness • Critical care outcomes
- Psychiatric disorders • Quality of life

There has been increasing awareness of the fact that diseases, treatments, and events (such as surgery or the experience of critical care) often have significant and persistent consequences for cognitive and psychological functioning.[1] Progress in critical care has led to decreased mortality rates among individuals admitted to intensive care units (ICUs). However, for many survivors of critical illness, ICU hospitalization can lead to a life of significant limitations and obstacles, especially with regard to cognitive functioning. Although neurologic dysfunction is not as well studied in the critical care literature as it ought to be, current data suggest a high prevalence of neurologic disturbances in patients with critical illness admitted to medical/surgical (non-neurologic) ICUs.[2-4] Such disturbances can be severe and include encephalopathy and cognitive and psychiatric impairments. Important neurologic disturbances that are common during and after critical care are delirium and long-term cognitive impairments. Emerging research indicates that although these disorders are distinct, they are inextricably linked in critical care. **Fig. 1** shows possible relationships between premorbid state, critical illness, and outcomes. Recent investigations show that delirium is widely prevalent during critical illness and places patients at greater risk for development of cognitive impairment.[5] Further, long-term cognitive impairments may occur in more than half of all ICU survivors and are associated with poor functional outcomes.

A version of this article appeared in the 25:3 issue of *Critical Care Clinics*.
[a] Center for Health Services Research, Vanderbilt University Medical Center, Vanderbilt University School of Medicine, 6th Floor MCE Suite 6100, Nashville, TN 37232, USA
[b] Department of Psychology, Brigham Young University, Provo, UT 84602, USA
[c] Neuroscience Center, Brigham Young University, Provo, UT 84602, USA
[d] Department of Medicine, Pulmonary and Critical Care Division, Intermountain Medical Center, Murray, UT, USA
* Corresponding author.
E-mail address: james.c.jackson@vanderbilt.edu

Anesthesiology Clin 29 (2011) 751–764
doi:10.1016/j.anclin.2011.09.012
1932-2275/11/$ – see front matter © 2011 Elsevier Inc. All rights reserved.

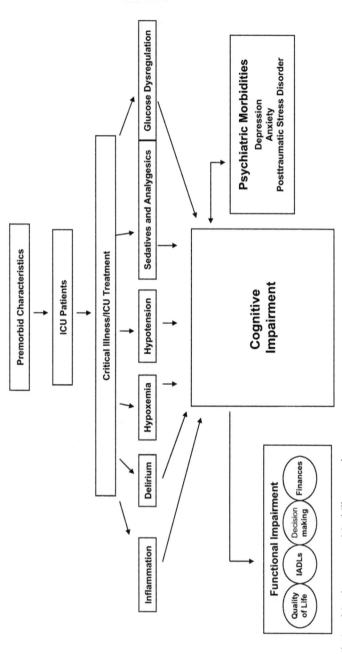

Fig. 1. Relationships between critical illness and outcomes.

DELIRIUM OR ACUTE COGNITIVE OUTCOMES IN ICU PATIENTS

Delirium is a neurobehavioral condition that occurs in a wide variety of health care settings, is associated with adverse outcomes, including death, and is the most common manifestation of acute brain dysfunction during critical illness.[6–8] It is a potentially toxic neuropsychiatric syndrome, characterized by a fluctuating course and pronounced inattention. It is highly prevalent among the hospitalized elderly, affecting between 15% and 20% of hospitalized medical patients,[9] 25% to 65% of surgical patients,[10,11] and as many as 80% of patients in ICU settings.[12] Although delirium was once considered benign, recent evidence has linked it with a variety of adverse outcomes, including prolonged hospitalization, poor surgical recovery, and increased morbidity and mortality.[13–16] Some researchers speculate that delirium may be a marker of subclinical dementia or cognitive impairment that might not otherwise develop for years or decades; indeed, data suggest that common pathogenic mechanisms might underlie development of cognitive impairments in delirium and dementia.[17]

Delirium is linked to poor cognitive outcomes in a variety of patient populations. A review by Maclullich and colleagues,[18] which looked at nine studies published after 2004 on the association between delirium and cognitive decline, documented a strong relationship between these two conditions. Their conclusions echoed those of Jackson and colleagues[19] in the 2004 review on the same topic, which focused on another nine investigations conducted since 2004. Together, these reviews represented a total of 18 investigations—most of them prospective cohort studies—from 1989 to 2008, with a combined total of nearly 4000 patients. These investigations almost uniformly demonstrated, with varying degrees of rigor and sophistication, that the emergence of delirium was a harbinger for greater, more severe, and more persistent neuropsychological decline. Although relevant research to date has focused on the link between delirium and global cognitive impairment, there is emerging evidence to suggest that delirium may be characterized by distinct anatomic patterns and processes.[20] Recent investigations employing sophisticated neuroimaging technologies have demonstrated that delirium results in significant cerebral hypoperfusion in several brain regions, including frontal, temporal, and subcortical regions.[21] Subcortical structures, which appear to mediate key elements of executive functioning, are particularly susceptible to even slight alterations in blood flow because of the small perforating vessels feeding these structures.[22] Evidence from clinical investigations suggests that executive dysfunction commonly develops secondary to reduced blood flow to vulnerable subcortical structures implicated in frontal-subcortical circuitry, even in the absence of frank ischemic injury.[23]

A variety of central nervous system insults, such as stroke and traumatic brain injury, can cause delirium and cognitive impairments, suggesting that widely distributed central nervous system abnormalities likely occur.[24] Neuroimaging data are lacking in critically ill patients with delirium or long-term cognitive impairments. One study found that neuropathologic abnormalities, including significant ventricular enlargement and generalized atrophy, occurred in elderly delirious patients compared with controls.[25] Focal lesions (infarcts and hemorrhage) were observed in frontal and parietal regions in these delirious patients.[25] A study of critically ill patients who underwent CT brain imaging for diminished level of consciousness, confusion, altered mental status, or prolonged delirium found that 61% had abnormalities on brain imaging, including generalized brain atrophy, ventricular enlargement, white matter lesions/hyperintensities, and cortical and subcortical lesions.[26] Although data are limited, future studies using increasingly sophisticated, hypothesis-driven brain imaging techniques will help advance the understanding of the neurologic effects of delirium, its relationship to cognitive impairments after critical illness, and its treatment, while potentially elucidating neuroscientific mechanisms that are now unknown.

PREVALENCE OF COGNITIVE IMPAIRMENT IN ICU SURVIVORS

The terms *cognitive dysfunction* and *cognitive impairment* are often used synonymously, although *impairment* implies a greater degree of permanence in contrast to *dysfunction*, which refers to an acute condition that may change or improve. Recognizing this distinction, it is perhaps most appropriate to discuss ICU survivors in the context of cognitive impairment, because the neuropsychological deficits that characterize these individuals may improve with time, but tend to be permanent in most cases.[27] Among mechanically ventilated general medical ICU survivors, approximately a third or more demonstrate moderate to severe cognitive impairment 6 months after discharge.[28] Among cohorts composed of both medical and surgical ICU survivors, including those with specific conditions such as sepsis and acute respiratory distress syndrome (ARDS), rates of impairment vary widely in part because of assessment timing and methods.[2,4] Among specific populations, notably patients with ARDS, the prevalence of cognitive impairments is particularly high and persistent, with 46% of patients at 1 year[29] and 25% of patients at 6 years reporting ongoing difficulties.[30] Although highly prevalent, cognitive impairment demonstrated by ICU survivors is also often quite severe. For example, the aforementioned ARDS patients with cognitive sequelae all fell below the sixth percentile of the normal distribution of cognitive functioning, displaying marked neuropsychological deficits in wide-ranging areas, including on tasks requiring memory, executive functioning, and mental processing abilities. Impairment does not impact all domains equally, and deficits in some areas rebound more completely than others.

Significant questions exist related to the relationship between premorbid cognitive functioning and the development of subsequent cognitive impairment among ICU survivors.[27] Although many individuals are cognitively normal before the onset of hospitalization, others, particularly those with multiple medical comorbidities that may impact cognition, such as vascular disease, diabetes, chronic obstructive pulmonary disease, and HIV, may have preexisting cognitive impairments.[31,32] They may be particularly vulnerable to the neurologic effects of critical illness. One of the most provocative issues in this regard is whether individuals with preexisting forms of cognitive impairment, particularly conditions such as mild cognitive impairment (MCI) or Alzheimer disease, which are characterized by a natural history of decline, may worsen more rapidly than they otherwise would after neurologic insults such as those occurring during the ICU stay. Conditions such as Alzheimer disease and its common precursor, MCI, affect large numbers of elderly patients—individuals who increasingly undergo and survive intensive care treatment and major surgery and who may be at particular risk to experience potentially toxic syndromes such as delirium.

PERSISTENCE OF COGNITIVE IMPAIRMENTS

It seems that many ICU survivors experience some or marked improvement in cognitive functioning in the year after hospital discharge (those already in the process of cognitive decline at the time of their critical illness may improve relative to their levels of cognitive functioning at hospital discharge, only to return to a pattern of gradual or accelerated deterioration).[4] However, despite demonstrating a clear trajectory of improvement, many individuals continue to have persistent cognitive impairment with time, infrequently returning to their pre-ICU baseline levels. For example 70%

of ARDS survivors had cognitive impairments at hospital discharge, but 45% had cognitive impairments at 1 year. There was no improvement in the cognitive impairment rate from 1 to 2 years.[33] A retrospective cohort study of 46 ARDS survivors found 25% had cognitive impairments 6 years after ICU treatment; only 21 patients returned to full-time employment, and all patients with cognitive impairments were disabled.[30] A second study in 30 ARDS survivors had impaired memory, attention, concentration, executive dysfunction, and motor impairments when assessed from 1 to more than 6 years post-hospital discharge (mean 6.2 years).[34] These studies suggest that the cognitive impairments in ARDS survivors are persistent, affect employment, and for a subset of the ICU population are resistant to significant improvement.

It may be that the effects of ARDS on cognitive functioning are accelerated among patients with specific sorts of vulnerabilities, such as frail elderly, although this proposition has largely been unstudied among critically ill patients. Nevertheless, the idea that the effects of ARDS on cognitive function may be magnified among some individuals, such as geriatric patients with preexisting MCI or dementia, is compelling. Although data are lacking, it may be that some ICU survivors suffer from a clinically distinct condition that is referred to as "ICU accelerated dementia." The phenomenon in which the rate of cognitive impairment increases after medical illness has been observed among other populations, including most notably in the well-known neuro-epidemiologic investigation, the Cache County study, which studied progression of dementia in medically ill patients with early Alzheimer disease.[35]

MECHANISMS OF COGNITIVE IMPAIRMENTS

It has been widely recognized that the brain is an immunologically active organ and therefore is vulnerable to systemic inflammatory reactions such as those resulting from sepsis or septic shock, similar to the findings in severe systemic illness. The inflammatory responses are mediated by cytokines, nonantibody proteins that penetrate the blood-brain barrier directly or indirectly to modulate and influence brain activity and potentially alter neurotransmitter release. Studies have shown that increased levels of biologic markers of inflammation, including IL-6 and TNF-α, predict the development of cognitive impairments among older patients without acute illness.[36,37] However, as is true with most cognitive impairments, including the family of dementias, there is probably not a single uniform cause; instead, a number of more or less significant factors interact dynamically with premorbid and genetic variables, resulting in adverse outcomes. Mechanisms of cognitive impairment implicated in the development of brain injury among ICU survivors include hypoxemia,[29] hyperglycemia,[38] delirium duration,[5] and hypotension.[39]

The use of sedatives or analgesics is associated with poor cognitive outcomes in other populations,[40,41] although their role in the development of cognitive impairment after critical illness has been largely unstudied. However, they may be powerfully implicated in the relationship that has been demonstrated between delirium and the emergence of subsequent neuropsychological deficits.[5] That is, sedatives and analgesics, particularly benzodiazepines, contribute to the development of delirium, which in turn is associated with an increased risk for cognitive impairment. Although the specific nature of the relationship between sedatives or analgesics has yet to be fully studied in ICU cohorts and is yet to be elucidated, there are reasons to believe that certain medications or medication classes could contribute to adverse cognitive outcomes, particularly in vulnerable populations. For example, in a recent investigation by Pomara and colleagues,[42] healthy elderly subjects with the *APOE4* allele, a well-known genetic risk factor for Alzheimer disease, experienced more pronounced cognitive impairment and were slower to recover after acute oral challenge with lorazepam. The cognitive impairment experienced by these subjects was not the result of pharmacokinetic factors, raising the possibility that factors unique to the effects of *APOE4* may have resulted in pronounced vulnerability to drug-related cognitive toxicity. Although the idea that certain genetic alleles may mediate and amplify the effects of specific drugs on the development of cognitive impairment is controversial and not unanimously supported by the literature, it highlights yet another possible mechanism through which neuropsychological deficits in ICU survivors might develop.

DEPRESSION AND ANXIETY IN ICU SURVIVORS

Psychological morbidity, such as depression and anxiety, occurs frequently after critical illness.[43,44] Depression occurs in 25%[33] to more than 50% of survivors of critical illness.[45] Angus and colleagues[45] reported that 50% of ARDS survivors had depression 1 year after treatment, whereas Cheung and colleagues[46] reported a 58% incidence of depression 2 years after ICU discharge. A study of 13 ICUs in four hospitals found that 26% of patients had symptoms of depression 6 months after acute lung injury.[47] Similar rates of depression are reported in 22% to 33% of medical inpatients[48] and in 25% to 28% of patients with cardiac and pulmonary disorders.[49,50] Psychiatric disorders after critical illness may be because of a psychological reaction to the emotional and physiologic stress, sequelae of brain injury sustained as a result of critical illness and its treatment, or both. Medications, physiologic changes, pain, altered sensory inputs, and an unfamiliar environment are all potential contributors in the development of psychological sequelae.[51]

There is little data available about risk factors for depression in survivors of critical illness. Depression is positively associated with longer ICU lengths of stay, longer duration of mechanical ventilation, and greater number of days on sedatives.[52] Two additional studies support the relationship between longer ICU lengths of stay and depression.[43] No information is available regarding factors related to longer ICU lengths of stay that lead to the development of depression. That is, it is not known if it is the time or the longer exposure to other factors such as sedatives or glucose dysregulation that results in depression. For example, a recent study found that hypoglycemia during ICU treatment was associated with greater symptoms of depression 3 months after acute lung injury.[47] Other factors related to depression are higher body mass index, premorbid depression or anxiety, and mean ICU benzodiazepine dose.[47] A study in 13 ICUs from four hospitals found depression at 6 months was related to surgical but not medical or trauma ICU admission, maximum organ failure score, and mean benzodiazepine dose.[53]

Although the above studies are starting to assess relationships between critical illness and ICU treatment with development of depression, research is in its infancy; additional studies are needed to determine risk factors, mechanisms, and potential treatments. Daily sedative interruption did not reduce the prevalence of depression at hospital discharge, but did reduce the rate of depression at 1 year.[54] A study that assessed prevalence of antidepressant treatment found that 37% of ARDS patients were taking antidepressant medications 2 months after ICU discharge.[44] Little is known regarding whether treatment of depression with antidepressant medications improves outcomes.

There is limited information on generalized or nonspecific anxiety in critically ill populations. The prevalence of nonspecific anxiety is less frequently reported than depression, but the rate of anxiety ranges from 23% to 41%.[43,54] The rates of anxiety in ICU survivors is higher than that observed in medical inpatients (5%–20%),[55] but similar to the reported rates of 10% to 40% observed in patients with pulmonary disorders.[56] Potential mechanisms of depression and anxiety in ICU survivors include organ dysfunction, medications, pain,[52] sleep deprivation, ICU treatment, elevated cytokines,[57] stress-related activation of the hypothalamic-pituitary axis, hypoxemia, and neurotransmitter dysfunction due to brain injury. The most frequently identified anxiety disorder is posttraumatic stress disorder (post traumatic stress disorder [PTSD], see discussion in the next section). The prevalence of psychological morbidity is high and research is in its early stages. Future investigations should assess mechanisms, risk factors, and possible interventions.

POST TRAUMATIC STRESS DISORDER IN ICU SURVIVORS

PTSD was once believed to result primarily from experiences such as combat, assault, and exposure to a natural disaster. Experts have recognized that a somewhat broader array of events may indeed be traumatic to individuals, including life-threatening illnesses and surgical procedures. A significant literature has emerged in this regard, particularly as it relates to the development of PTSD after the diagnosis of cancer. Researchers and clinicians are focusing on another experience believed to contribute to PTSD and PTSD symptoms—critical illness and the events associated with ICU hospitalization—although a debate on the prevalence and severity of PTSD in ICU survivors is ongoing.[58]

Of particular interest for ICU clinicians and research is the role of memory in mediating the development of PTSD, because a key impetus for employing strategies to keep critically ill patients heavily sedated has been the concern that memories of their ICU experience could facilitate the development of PTSD.[59] The importance of specific *explicit memories* (memories pertaining to facts and events, which are accessible to consciousness)[24,25] in the generation and maintenance of PTSD is difficult to estimate because they are the basis for nightmares, flashbacks, and intrusive thoughts, and they contribute to avoidant and reexperiencing symptoms. Although a detailed treatment of these issues is beyond the scope of this review, the authors briefly discuss several key findings from the literature as they relate to ICU populations. The preponderance of evidence suggests that the absence of episodic memory for a traumatic event is protective against the development of PTSD; most studies have shown that the risk of PTSD is markedly lower in individuals unable to recall a traumatic event than in those with explicit memory for the event(s).[26,60–63] The literature is not unanimous and is quite narrow in scope, with virtually all relevant studies having been conducted on victims of motor vehicle accidents or other traumas with concomitant traumatic brain injury.[64] Theories of information processing suggest that traumatic memories can be encoded *implicitly* during periods of impaired consciousness and may provide the basis for the generation of PTSD symptoms even if patients are not consciously aware of the memories.[65–68] Also, during periods of impaired consciousness, the encoding of emotional experiences such as panic or severe pain appears to be sufficient for the generation of PTSD symptoms.[69]

Many ICU patients report little, if any, conscious awareness of their critical illness, although as Jones and colleagues[70] have reported, delusional memories, often having violent and paranoid themes, are pervasive among these individuals. Among patients with delirium, particularly hyperactive delirium, psychotic symptoms including visual hallucinations are particularly common.[71,72] These hallucinations and delusions can be extremely gripping and are often characterized by paranoid and traumatic themes involving physical or sexual assault or torture. As is frequently the case, these hallucinations are integrated by patients into a narrative that sometimes involves benign actual events and, as such, tend to be entrenched. Even after hallucinations dissipate, their effects may persist in the form of delusional memories, particularly for those patients who remain convinced that the aversive experiences they remember actually happened. Importantly, sedative medications may be one factor that mediates the development of delusional memories.[73] Delusional memories may exist in the absence of factual memories, and factual memories provide markers of reality and may serve to orient the patient. For example, in one study, daily sedative interruption was associated with fewer symptoms of PTSD,[54] suggesting that even limited factual memories from brief awakening may reduce PTSD. In addition, delusional memories tend to be stable with time and are significantly more persistent than factual memories.[74] Delusional memories may be more refractory to the normal cognitive processes of habituation and reappraisal because they are not well integrated into the long-term memory. Although research is limited, the presence of delusional memories of the ICU is associated with increased levels of anxiety and PTSD.[75,76]

QUALITY OF LIFE IN ICU SURVIVORS

Health-related quality of life has emerged as an important measure of outcome in a variety of disease states and may be particularly important after ICU treatment, where interventions can maintain life but may lead to significant morbidity. Although definitions differ slightly across disciplines, health-related quality of life is defined as a set of causally linked dimensions of health, with biologic/physiologic, mental, physical, social function, cognitive, and health perceptions.[44] Critically ill patients with severe sepsis[77] and prolonged mechanical ventilation[78] have significantly lower quality of life. The quality-of-life scores for ARDS survivors are very low at extubation and then increase substantially at 3 months, with only slight additional improvement by 1 year.[44] The reduced quality of life occurs primarily in physical domains (eg, physical functioning, bodily pain, and role physical)[44] and is associated with pulmonary symptoms,[44] abnormal pulmonary function,[79] and persistent muscle wasting and weakness.[80] The perturbations in quality of life appear to be profound as Rothenhäusler and colleagues[30] state: "...the success of intensive care management of severe diseases such as ARDS is no longer judged solely by its effects on survival but by its influence on patients' psychosocial well-being."

Dowdy and colleagues,[81] in a recent meta-analysis of health-related quality of life in ARDS survivors, found that ARDS survivors consistently had lower quality-of-life scores compared with matched, normative controls at all time points after ICU discharge (from hospital discharge up to 66 months later). The magnitude of the quality-of-life differences between critically ill patients and healthy controls represent a moderate decline in physical domains and mild-to-moderate decline in emotional domains, particularly early after ICU discharge. Improvements in quality of life are uneven and are time- and domain-specific.[33] The greatest gains occur in physical functioning, social functioning, and role physical in the first 6 months, with only modest additional improvements thereafter. Role physical is the singular domain where improvement continues throughout the first several years.[33] Although quality-of-life scores improve with time in most longitudinal studies, these improvements do not necessarily reflect clinical meaningful changes in function. As Herridge and colleagues[80] state, health-related quality of life "will be profoundly influenced by the patient's prior health status and her expectations for a return to premorbid functional status."

The timing of quality-of-life assessment may influence the findings either by exaggerating or by underestimating patient perception of their quality of life relative to their critical illness and ICU treatment. Survivors may have shifting perceptions of their illness and recovery, leading to different responses with time, without a similar objective change in their actual capabilities. Conversely, report improvements in quality of life might be more relevant than objective changes in capabilities in predicting willingness and ability to contribute to society. The influence of the "ICU experience," such as invasive procedures and the amount and quality of caregiver support, on health-related quality of life scores has not been assessed. Given the importance of quality of life as a measure of global outcome in survivors of critical illness, it is imperative that clinicians understand that brain function, musculoskeletal function, and other components of medical care that influence quality of life should also be assessed.

Neurocognitive impairments are a major determinant of the ability to return to work, work productivity, life satisfaction, and reduced quality of life.[82] Two studies found that ARDS patients with cognitive impairment had lower quality of life compared with patients without cognitive impairment.[82] Rothenhäusler and colleagues[30] found that ARDS patients with and without neurocognitive impairments had lower quality of life compared with age- and gender-matched healthy controls. Alternatively, decreased quality of life was not associated with neurocognitive impairments in ARDS survivors or with executive dysfunction in a critically ill medical population.[83] Depression and anxiety are also associated with decreased quality of life for all domains, except physical functioning.[39] A study in patients with acute lung injury found that depression and psychosocial symptoms were associated with lower life satisfaction, but not with physical problems or limitations.[44] Depression correlated with poor functional status and decreased ability to perform activities of daily living in patients with chronic obstructive pulmonary disease.[84] Decreased quality of life on the psychosocial domains (eg, role emotional, mental health, and vitality) is associated with PTSD in ARDS patients.[43] Greater PTSD symptoms are associated with reduced quality-of-life scores.[85] Psychiatric disorders and their relationships with decreased quality of life are undoubtedly multifactorial. Data to date indicate that cognitive and emotional functions are associated with lower quality of life after critical illness. The effects of critical illness and ICU therapies extend well beyond hospital discharge and often lead to significant neurocognitive and psychiatric morbidities and reduced quality of life in survivors.[33,80] The observed morbidities and their adverse impact on quality of life raise questions regarding possible interventions to improve outcomes in these patients.

SUMMARY

The significant and sometimes permanent effects of critical illness on wide-ranging aspects of functioning are increasingly recognized. Among the areas affected are acute and long-term cognitive functioning, depression, anxiety, PTSD, and quality of life. These and other areas are increasingly being studied and indeed are increasingly the focus of clinical attention and investigations. These conditions have been a focus of attention for more than a dozen years, with much improvement occurring in the ability to characterize these phenomena. For instance, in intervening years, it has been learned that cognitive impairment is highly prevalent and functionally disruptive and that it occurs in wide-ranging domains. Key questions remain unanswered with regard to vital questions such as determining causes, risk factors, and mechanisms as well as the degree to which brain injuries associated with critical illness are amenable to rehabilitation. Little remains known about the effects of critical illness on elderly ICU cohorts and on the neurologic functioning of individuals with preexisting impairment versus those who are normal. Few data exist regarding the development of strategies designed to prevent the emergence of neuropsychological deficits after critical illness. Although great progress has been made and is ongoing, a pressing need exists for additional investigation of cognitive impairment and other conditions, such as PTSD and quality of life after critical illness, that will seek to untangle the many pertinent questions related to this condition and that will ultimately offer help and hope to the thousands of survivors affected by this condition.

REFERENCES

1. Angus DC, Carlet J. Surviving intensive care: a report from the 2002 Brussels Roundtable. Intensive Care Med 2003;29:368–77.
2. Hopkins RO, Brett S. Chronic neurocognitive effects of critical illness. Curr Opin Crit Care 2005;11(4):369–75.
3. Hopkins RO, Jackson JC. Assessing neurocognitive outcomes after critical illness: are delirium and long-term cognitive impairments related? Curr Opin Crit Care 2006;12:388–94.
4. Hopkins RO, Jackson JC. Long-term neurocognitive function after critical illness. Chest 2006;130(3):869–78.
5. Girard TD, Shintani AK, Jackson JC, et al. Duration of delirium in patients with severe sepsis predicts long-term cognitive impairment. 2006:A739.
6. Pandharipande P, Cotton BA, Shintani A, et al. Prevalence and risk factors for development of delirium in surgical and trauma intensive care unit patients. J Trauma 2008;65(1):34–41.
7. Pandharipande P, Jackson J, Ely EW. Delirium: acute cognitive dysfunction in the critically ill. Curr Opin Crit Care 2005;11(4):360–8.
8. Meagher DJ. Delirium: optimising management. Br Med J 2001;322(7279):144–9.
9. Lipowski ZJ. Delirium in the elderly patient. N Engl J Med 1989;320(9):578–82.
10. Galanakis P, Bickel H, Gradinger R, et al. Acute confusional state in the elderly following hip surgery: incidence, risk factors and complications. Int J Geriatr Psychiatry 2001;16(4):349–55.
11. O'Keefe ST, Chonchubhair AN. Postoperative delirium in the elderly. Br J Anaesth 1994;73:673–87.
12. Ely EW, Inouye SK, Bernard GR, et al. Delirium in mechanically ventilated patients: validity and reliability of the confusion assessment method for the intensive care unit (CAM-ICU). JAMA 2001;286(21):2703–10.
13. Inouye SK, Rushing JT, Foreman MD, et al. Does delirium contribute to poor hospital outcomes? A three-site epidemiologic study. J Gen Intern Med 1998; 13:234–42.
14. Ely EW, Shintani A, Truman B, et al. Delirium as a predictor of mortality in mechanically ventilated patients in the intensive care unit. JAMA 2004;291(14):1753–62.
15. ISIS-2. Randomised trial of intravenous streptokinase, oral aspirin, both, or neither among 17187 cases of suspected acute myocardial infarction: ISIS-2. Lancet 1988;2:349–60.
16. Uldall KK, Ryan R, Berghuis JP, et al. Association between delirium and death in AIDS patients. AIDS Patient Care 2000;14:95–100.
17. Eikelenboom P, Hoogendijk WJG. Do delirium and Alzheimer's dementia share specific pathogenetic mechanisms? Dement Geriatr Cogn Disord 1999;10(5): 319–24.
18. Maclullich AM, Beaglehole A, Hall RJ, et al. Delirium and long-term cognitive impairment. Int Rev Psychiatry 2009;21(1):30–42.

19. Jackson JC, Gordon SM, Hart RP, et al. The association between delirium and cognitive decline: a review of the empirical literature. Neuropsychol Rev 2004; 14(2):87–98.
20. Trzepacz PT. Is there a final common neural pathway in delirium? Focus on acetylcholine and dopamine. Semin Clin Neuropsychiatry 2000;5:132–48.
21. Fong TG, Bogardus ST, Daftary A, et al. Cerebral perfusion changes in older delirious patients using 99mTc HMPAO SPECT. J Gerontol A Biol Sci Med Sci 2007; 61A:1294–9.
22. Moody DM, Bell MA, Challa VR. Features of the cerebral vascular pattern that predict vulnerability to perfusion or oxygenation deficiency: an anatomic study. Am J Neuroradiol 2007;11:431.
23. Alexander GE, DeLong MR, Strick PL. Parallel organization of functionally segregated circuits linking basal ganglia and cortex. Annu Rev Neurosci 1986;9: 357–81.
24. Squire L. Declarative and non-declarative memory: multiple brain systems supporting learning and memory. J Cogn Neurosci 1992;4:232–43.
25. Parkin A. Human memory. Curr Biol 1999;9:582–5.
26. Sbordone R, Seyraniniana GD, Ruff RM. Are the subjective complaints of traumatically brain injured patients reliable? Brain Inj 1998;12:505–12.
27. Jackson JC, Gordon SM, Ely EW, et al. Research issues in the evaluation of cognitive impairment in intensive care unit survivors. Intensive Care Med 2004; 30(11):2009–16.
28. Jackson JC, Hart RP, Gordon SM, et al. Six-month neuropsychological outcome of medical intensive care unit patients. Crit Care Med 2003;31(4):1226–34.
29. Hopkins RO, Weaver LK, Pope D, et al. Neuropsychological sequelae and impaired health status in survivors of severe acute respiratory distress syndrome. Am J Respir Crit Care Med 1999;160(1):50–6.
30. Rothenhäusler HB, Ehrentraut S, Stoll C, et al. The relationship between cognitive performance and employment and health status in long-term survivors of the acute respiratory distress syndrome: results of an exploratory study. Gen Hosp Psychiatry 2001;23(2):90–6.
31. Schillerstrom JE, Horton MS, Schillerstorm TL, et al. Prevalence, course, and risk factors for executive impairment in patients hospitalized on a general medical service. Psychosomatics 2007;46:411–7.
32. Schillerstrom JE, Horton MS, Royall DR. The impact of medical illness on executive function. Psychosomatics 2005;46(6):508–16.
33. Hopkins RO, Weaver LK, Collingridge D, et al. Two-year cognitive, emotional, and quality-of-life outcomes in acute respiratory distress syndrome. Am J Respir Crit Care Med 2005;171(4):340–7.
34. Suchyta MR, Hopkins RO, White J, et al. The incidence of cognitive dysfunction after ARDS. Am J Respir Crit Care Med 2004;169:A18.
35. Lyketsos CG, Toone L, Tschanz J, et al. Population-based study of medical comorbidity in early dementia and "cognitive impairment no dementia": association with functional and cognitive impairment - the Cache County Study. Am J Geriatr Psychiatry 2005;13:656–64.
36. Teunissen CE, van Boxtel MP, Bosma H, et al. Inflammation markers in relation to cognition in a healthy aging population. J Neuroimmunol 2003;134(1-2):142–50.
37. Yaffe K, Lindquist K, Penninx BW, et al. Inflammatory markers and cognition in well-functioning African-American and white elders. Neurology 2003;61(1):76–80.
38. Hopkins RO, Suchyta MR, Jephson A, et al. Hyperglycemia and neurocognitive outcome in ARDS survivors. Proc Am Thorac Soc 2005;2:A36.

39. Hopkins RO, Weaver LK, Chan KJ, et al. Quality of life, emotional, and cognitive function following acute respiratory distress syndrome. J Int Neuropsychol Soc 2004;10(7):1005–17.

40. Starr JM, Whalley LJ. Drug induced dementia. Drug Saf 1994;11:310–7.

41. Starr JM, Whalley LJ, Deary IJ. The effects of antihypertensive treatment on cognitive function: results from HOPE study. J Am Geriatr Soc 2002;44:411–5.

42. Pomara N, Willoughby L, Wesnes K, et al. Apolipoprotein E epsilon4 allele and lorazepam effects on memory in high-functioning older adults. Arch Gen Psychiatry 2005;62(2):209–16.

43. Kapfhammer HP, Rothenhäusler HB, Krauseneck T, et al. Posttraumatic stress disorder and health-related quality of life in long-term survivors of acute respiratory distress syndrome. Am J Psychiatry 2004;161(1):45–52.

44. Weinert CR, Gross CR, Kangas JR, et al. Health-related quality of life after acute lung injury. Am J Respir Crit Care Med 1997;156:1120–8.

45. Angus D, Musthafa AA, Clermonte G, et al. Quality-adjusted survival in the first year after the acute respiratory distress syndrome. Am J Respir Crit Care Med 2001;163:1389–94.

46. Cheung AM, Tansey CM, Tomlinson G, et al. Two-year outcomes, health care use, and costs of survivors of acute respiratory distress syndrome. Am J Respir Crit Care Med 2006;174(5):538–44.

47. Dowdy DW, Dinglas D, Mendez-Tellez P, et al. Intensive care unit hypoglycemia predicts depression during early recovery from acute lung injury. Crit Care Med 2009;36:2726–33.

48. Katon W, Sullivan MD. Depression and chronic medical illness. J Clin Psychiatry 1990;51:3–11.

49. Silverstone PH. Prevalence of psychiatric disorders in medical illness. J Nerv Ment Dis 1996;184:43–51.

50. Silverstone PH, LeMay T, Elliott J, et al. The prevalence of major depressive disorder and low self esteem in medical inpatients. Can J Psychiatry 1996;41:67–74.

51. Skodol AE. Anxiety in the medically ill: nosology and principles of differential diagnosis. Semin Clin Neuropsychiatry 1999;4:64–71.

52. Nelson BJ, Weinert CR, Bury CL, et al. Intensive care unit drug use and subsequent quality of life in acute lung injury patients. Crit Care Med 2000;28(11):3626–30.

53. Dowdy DW, Bienvenu OJ, Dinglas VD, et al. Are intensive care factors associated with depressive symptoms 6 months after acute lung injury? Crit Care Med 2009;37(5):1702–7.

54. Kress JP, Gehlbach B, Lacy M, et al. The long-term psychological effects of daily sedative interruption on critically ill patients. Am J Respir Crit Care Med 2003;168(12):1457–61.

55. Strain JJ, Liebowithz MR, Klein DF. Anxiety and panic attacks in the medically ill. Psychiatr Clin North Am 1981;4:333–50.

56. Pollack MH, Kradin R, Otto MW. Prevalence of panic in patients referred for pulmonary function testing at a major medical center. Am J Psychiatry 2009;153:110–3.

57. Katz IR. On the inseparability of mental and physical health in aged persons: lesions from depression and medical comorbidity. Am J Geriatr Psychiatry 1996;4:1–16.

58. Jackson JC, Hart RP, Gordon SM, et al. Post-traumatic stress disorder and post-traumatic stress symptoms following critical illness in medical intensive care unit patients: assessing the magnitude of the problem. Crit Care 2007;11(1):R27.

59. Foreman M, Milisen K. Improving recognition of delirium in the elderly. Prim Psychiatry 2004;11:46–50.
60. Sbordone R, Liter J. Mild traumatic brain injury does not produce posttraumatic stress disorder. Brain Inj 1995;9:405–12.
61. Malt L. The long term psychiatric consequences of accidental injury. Br J Psychiatry 1988;153:810–8.
62. Ursano R, Fullerton C, Epstein R. Acute and chronic posttraumatic stress disorder in motor vehicle victims. Am J Psychiatry 1999;156:589–95.
63. Bontke C, Rattok J, Boake C. Do patients with mild brain injury have posttraumatic stress disorder too? J Head Trauma Rehabil 1996;11:95–102.
64. Klein E, Caspi Y, Gil S. The relation between memory of the traumatic brain injury and PTSD: evidence from studies of traumatic brain injury. Can J Psychiatry 2003; 48:28–33.
65. Bryant RA. Posttraumatic stress disorder and traumatic brain injury: can they co-exist? Clin Psychol Rev 2001;21:931–48.
66. Brewin CR. A cognitive neuroscience account of posttraumatic stress disorder and its treatment. Behav Res Ther 2001;39:373–93.
67. Brewin CR, Dalgleish T, Joseph S. A dual representation theory of posttraumatic stress disorder. Psychol Rev 1996;103:670–86.
68. Schacter DL, Chiu CYP, Ochsner KN. Implicit memory: a selective review. Neuroscience 1993;16:159–82.
69. Sessler C. Top ten list in sepsis. Chest 2001;120:1390–3.
70. Jones C, Griffiths RD, Humprhis G. Disturbed memory and amnesia related to intensive care. Memory 2000;8:79–94.
71. Ely EW, Margolin R, Francis J, et al. Evaluation of delirium in critically ill patients: validation of the Confusion Assessment Method for the Intensive Care Unit (CAM-ICU). Crit Care Med 2001;29(7):1370–9.
72. Ely EW, Siegel MD, Inouye SK. Delirium in the intensive care unit: an under-recognized syndrome of organ dysfunction. Semin Respir Crit Care Med 2001;22(2):115–26.
73. Capuzzo M, Valpondi V, Cingolani E, et al. Post-traumatic stress disorder-related symptoms after intensive care. Minerva Anestesiol 2005;71(4):167–79.
74. Capuzzo M, Valpondi V, Cingolani E, et al. Application of the Italian version of the intensive care unit memory tool in the clinical setting. Crit Care 2004;8(1):R48–55.
75. Jones C, Griffiths RD, Humphris G, et al. Memory, delusions, and the development of acute posttraumatic stress disorder-related symptoms after intensive care. Crit Care Med 2001;29(3):573–80.
76. Jones C, Skirrow P, Griffiths RD, et al. Rehabilitation after critical illness: a randomized, controlled trial. Crit Care Med 2003;31(10):2456–61.
77. Heyland DK, Hopman W, Coo H, et al. Long-term health-related quality of life in survivors of sepsis. Short form 36: a valid and reliable measure of health-related quality of life. Crit Care Med 2000;28:3599–605.
78. Combes A, Costa MA, Trouillet JL, et al. Morbidity, mortality, and quality-of-life outcomes of patients requiring ≥14 days of mechanical ventilation. Crit Care Med 2003;31(5):1373–81.
79. Orme JF, Romney JS, Hopkins RO, et al. Pulmonary function and health-related quality of life in survivors of acute respiratory distress syndrome. Am J Respir Crit Care Med 2003;167:690–4.
80. Herridge MS, Cheung AM, Tansey CM, et al. One-year outcomes in survivors of the acute respiratory distress syndrome. N Engl J Med 2003;348(8):683–93.
81. Dowdy DW, Eid MP, Sedrakyan A, et al. Quality of life in adult survivors of critical illness: a systematic review of the literature. Intensive Care Med 2005;31(5):611–20.

82. Capes SE, Hunt D, Malmberg K, et al. Stress hyperglycemia and prognosis of stroke in nondiabetic and diabetic patients: a systematic overview. Stroke 2001;32(10):2426–32.

83. Sukantarat KT, Burgess PW, Williamson RC, et al. Prolonged cognitive dysfunction in survivors of critical illness. Anaesthesia 2005;60(9):847–53.

84. Toshima MT, Blumberg E, Ries AL. Does rehabiliation reduce depression in patients with chronic obstructive pulmonary disease? J Cardiopulm Rehabil 1992;12:261–9.

85. Robertson IH, Murre JM. Rehabilitation of brain damage: brain plasticity and principles of guided recovery. Psychol Bull 1999;125(5):544–75.

Index

Note: Page numbers of article titles are in **boldface** type.

Anesthesiology Clin 29 (2011) 765–773
doi:10.1016/S1932-2275(11)00098-X
1932-2275/11/$ – see front matter © 2011 Elsevier Inc. All rights reserved.

United States Postal Service
Statement of Ownership, Management, and Circulation
(All Periodicals Publications Except Requestor Publications)

1. Publication Title	2. Publication Number	3. Filing Date
Anesthesiology Clinics	0 0 0 - 2 7 7 7	9/16/11

4. Issue Frequency	5. Number of Issues Published Annually	6. Annual Subscription Price
Mar, Jun, Sep, Dec	4	$287.00

7. Complete Mailing Address of Known Office of Publication (Not printer) (Street, city, county, state, and ZIP+4®)

Elsevier Inc.
360 Park Avenue South
New York, NY 10010-1710

Contact Person
Amy S. Beacham
Telephone (Include area code)
215-239-3687

8. Complete Mailing Address of Headquarters or General Business Office of Publisher (Not printer)

Elsevier Inc., 360 Park Avenue South, New York, NY 10010-1710

9. Full Names and Complete Mailing Addresses of Publisher, Editor, and Managing Editor (Do not leave blank)

Publisher (Name and complete mailing address)

Kim Murphy, Elsevier, Inc., 1600 John F. Kennedy Blvd. Suite 1800, Philadelphia, PA 19103-2899

Editor (Name and complete mailing address)

Rachel Glover, Elsevier, Inc., 1600 John F. Kennedy Blvd. Suite 1800, Philadelphia, PA 19103-2899

Managing Editor (Name and complete mailing address)

Sarah Barth, Elsevier, Inc., 1600 John F. Kennedy Blvd. Suite 1800, Philadelphia, PA 19103-2899

10. Owner (Do not leave blank. If the publication is owned by a corporation, give the name and address of the corporation immediately followed by the names and addresses of all stockholders owning or holding 1 percent or more of the total amount of stock. If not owned by a corporation, give the names and addresses of the individual owners. If owned by a partnership or other unincorporated firm, give its name and address as well as those of each individual owner. If the publication is published by a nonprofit organization, give its name and address.)

Full Name	Complete Mailing Address
Wholly owned subsidiary of	4520 East-West Highway
Reed/Elsevier, US holdings	Bethesda, MD 20814

11. Known Bondholders, Mortgagees, and Other Security Holders Owning or Holding 1 Percent or More of Total Amount of Bonds, Mortgages, or Other Securities. If none, check box ☐ None

Full Name	Complete Mailing Address
N/A	

12. Tax Status (For completion by nonprofit organizations authorized to mail at nonprofit rates) (Check one)
The purpose, function, and nonprofit status of this organization and the exempt status for federal income tax purposes:
☐ Has Not Changed During Preceding 12 Months
☐ Has Changed During Preceding 12 Months (Publisher must submit explanation of change with this statement)

PS Form 3526, September 2007 (Page 1 of 3 (Instructions Page 3)) PSN 7530-01-000-9931 PRIVACY NOTICE: See our Privacy policy in www.usps.com

---

13. Publication Title	14. Issue Date for Circulation Data Below
Anesthesiology Clinics	September 2011

15. Extent and Nature of Circulation

		Average No. Copies Each Issue During Preceding 12 Months	No. Copies of Single Issue Published Nearest to Filing Date
a. Total Number of Copies (Net press run)		1370	940
b. Paid Circulation (By Mail and Outside the Mail)	(1) Mailed Outside-County Paid Subscriptions Stated on PS Form 3541. (Include paid distribution above nominal rate, advertiser's proof copies, and exchange copies)	463	403
	(2) Mailed In-County Paid Subscriptions Stated on PS Form 3541 (Include paid distribution above nominal rate, advertiser's proof copies, and exchange copies)		
	(3) Paid Distribution Outside the Mails Including Sales Through Dealers and Carriers, Street Vendors, Counter Sales, and Other Paid Distribution Outside USPS®	352	349
	(4) Paid Distribution by Other Classes Mailed Through the USPS (e.g. First-Class Mail®)		
c. Total Paid Distribution (Sum of 15b (1), (2), (3), and (4))		815	752
d. Free or Nominal Rate Distribution (By Mail and Outside the Mail)	(1) Free or Nominal Rate Outside-County Copies Included on PS Form 3541	90	81
	(2) Free or Nominal Rate In-County Copies Included on PS Form 3541		
	(3) Free or Nominal Rate Copies Mailed at Other Classes Through the USPS (e.g. First-Class Mail)		
	(4) Free or Nominal Rate Distribution Outside the Mail (Carriers or other means)		
e. Total Free or Nominal Rate Distribution (Sum of 15d (1), (2), (3) and (4))		90	81
f. Total Distribution (Sum of 15c and 15e)		905	833
g. Copies not Distributed (See instructions to publishers #4 (page #3))		465	107
h. Total (Sum of 15f and g)		1370	940
i. Percent Paid (15c divided by 15f times 100)		90.06%	90.28%

16. Publication of Statement of Ownership
☐ If the publication is a general publication, publication of this statement is required. Will be printed in the December 2011 issue of this publication.
☐ Publication not required.

17. Signature and Title of Editor, Publisher, Business Manager, or Owner

Amy S. Beacham – Senior Inventory Distribution Coordinator

Date September 16, 2011

I certify that all information furnished on this form is true and complete. I understand that anyone who furnishes false or misleading information on this form or who omits material or information requested on the form may be subject to criminal sanctions (including fines and imprisonment) and/or civil sanctions (including civil penalties).

PS Form 3526, September 2007 (Page 2 of 3)

Moving?

Make sure your subscription moves with you!

To notify us of your new address, find your **Clinics Account Number** (located on your mailing label above your name), and contact customer service at:

Email: journalscustomerservice-usa@elsevier.com

800-654-2452 (subscribers in the U.S. & Canada)
314-447-8871 (subscribers outside of the U.S. & Canada)

Fax number: 314-447-8029

Elsevier Health Sciences Division
Subscription Customer Service
3251 Riverport Lane
Maryland Heights, MO 63043

*To ensure uninterrupted delivery of your subscription, please notify us at least 4 weeks in advance of move.

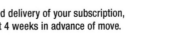

Printed and bound by CPI Group (UK) Ltd, Croydon, CR0 4YY

03/10/2024

01040460-0002